Gerontology Nursing Case Studies

Donna J. Bowles, MSN, EdD, RN, CNE, is a professor at the School of Nursing at Indiana University Southeast in New Albany, Indiana. Dr. Bowles coordinates and teaches the didactic courses in Alterations in Health I and II, with the corresponding Practicums, the Senior Capstone Practicum, and an NCLEX-RN© preparation class. Dr. Bowles has written three chapters for the textbook *Medical–Surgical Nursing, Second Edition,* edited by Daniels and Nicoll (2011) and "The Adult Client" chapter in Daniels's *Nursing Fundamentals: Caring and Clinical Decision Making,* second edition (2008). She was a coeditor with Mary Ann Hogan for *Nursing Fundamentals: Review and Rationales* (2002). She has published several peer-reviewed articles, including "Active Learning Strategies . . . Not for the Birds!" (*International Journal of Nursing Education Scholarship,* 2006), and "The Wizard of Oz: A Metaphor for Teaching Excellence" (*The Teaching Professor,* 2005), among others. Dr. Bowles is an active peer reviewer for several textbook publishers, the *International Journal of Nursing Education Scholarship, Nursing Spectrum,* and the *Journal of the Scholarship of Teaching and Learning.* She is the recipient of many teaching awards and fellowships and is a member of the following professional societies: STT, the Academy of Medical Surgical Nurses, Delta Epsilon Honor Society, the National League for Nursing, and the National Gerontology Nurses Association.

Gerontology Nursing Case Studies
100+ Narratives for Learning

Second Edition

Donna J. Bowles, MSN, EdD, RN, CNE

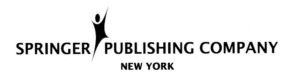

SPRINGER PUBLISHING COMPANY
NEW YORK

Springer Publishing Company, LLC
11 West 42nd Street
New York, NY 10036
www.springerpub.com

Acquisitions Editor: Elizabeth Nieginski
Composition: diacriTech

ISBN: 978-0-8261-9404-6
e-book ISBN: 978-0-8261-9405-3
Instructors' Material ISBN: 978-0-8261-9443-5

Instructors' Material: Qualified instructors may request supplements by e-mailing textbook@springerpub.com

15 16 17 18 / 5 4 3 2 1

The author and the publisher of this Work have made every effort to use sources believed to be reliable to provide information that is accurate and compatible with the standards generally accepted at the time of publication. Because medical science is continually advancing, our knowledge base continues to expand. Therefore, as new information becomes available, changes in procedures become necessary. We recommend that the reader always consult current research and specific institutional policies before performing any clinical procedure. The author and publisher shall not be liable for any special, consequential, or exemplary damages resulting, in whole or in part, from the readers' use of, or reliance on, the information contained in this book. The publisher has no responsibility for the persistence or accuracy of URLs for external or third-party Internet websites referred to in this publication and does not guarantee that any content on such websites is, or will remain, accurate or appropriate.

Library of Congress Cataloging-in-Publication Data
Bowles, Donna, author.
Gerontology nursing case studies : 100+ narratives for learning / Donna J. Bowles. — Second edition.
    p. ; cm.
Includes bibliographical references and index.
    ISBN 978-0-8261-9404-6 — ISBN 978-0-8261-9405-3 (e-book) — ISBN (invalid) 978-0-8261-9443-5
(Instructors manual)
    I. Title.
[DNLM: 1. Geriatric Nursing — methods — Case Reports. 2. Aged. 3. Aging — Case Reports. WY 152]
RC954
618.97'0231 — dc23

2015008185

Printed in the United States of America by Gasch Printing.

This one is for you, Mom . . .
JoAnn Elliott Nichols
(January 7, 1933 to March 8, 2014)

Contents

Foreword

The book *Gerontology Nursing Case Studies: 100+ Narratives for Learning, Second Edition,* by Donna J. Bowles, is a creative and informative compilation of everything that nursing students and new nurses need to know about care of the older adult. Kudos go to Donna Bowles for conceptualizing this and for the creative way in which she has used cases to capture the interest of students and motivate them to learn new information to help manage the cases in the chapters and the real-world patients they will encounter. It is written in an easy-to-read style. In fact, it is a book one could curl up with on a rainy day and enjoy! Each case's narrative section within the chapter provides numerous Internet references useful for the student to obtain additional information to answer the questions posed. The book is rather practical in the way in which it outlines content and topics. Rather than using a more traditional systems-based approach (head, chest, etc.) or disease-based approach (e.g., Alzheimer's disease, hypertension), material is organized in ways in which it would likely be used or experienced in the clinical setting. For example, the section on HIV is placed in the chapter that also includes management of cancer, chemotherapy, and hospice care. Likewise, anemia is placed in the chapter with cardiovascular disease because of the impact of anemia on cardiac function.

Overall, the new edition includes 21 chapters, although within each chapter there are three to eight case narrative sections that address different aspects of the topic. Chapter 1 starts with the critically important policies that every nurse should know when working with older adults. Such things as advance directives, health care decision making, use of restraints, issues about driving, and iatrogenesis are all reviewed. Essentially, this chapter presents the basics of providing legally competent and safe patient care. Chapter 2 focuses on the many losses that commonly occur with aging, such as the death of a spouse and the subsequent prolonged grief that can occur. The last case in this chapter on loss addresses death with dignity and provides the story, as told by a nurse, of a patient under the care of hospice who dies with the dignity that one would hope for for all patients. Chapter 3 covers the issues of neglect and abuse, both physical and financial, and provides guidance to new nurses caring for older adults as to how they can recognize abusive situations. Chapter 4 identifies and focuses on the most challenging psychosocial issues we encounter in geriatrics: depression and participation in risky behaviors, such as gaming and alcohol abuse. The next chapter, Chapter 5, is a terrific review of the individual and family dynamics affecting older adults, addressing such important issues as frailty, hoarding behavior, and health promotion for the elderly client. Chapter 6 addresses sexuality, presenting male and female issues in different narratives.

Chapters 7 through 14 review more traditional clinical problems and cover the sensory, dermatologic, musculoskeletal, neurologic, cardiovascular, pulmonary, endocrine, and genitourinary systems and the changes that occur with aging. Within each section, the most common problems we encounter are addressed with a case and management principles and resources. For example, the chapter on musculoskeletal disorders presents patient narratives that focus on degenerative joint disease, hip fractures, falls, immobility, osteoporosis, and foot problems.

Chapter 15 returns the reader to clinical issues and health and the topic of nutrition. This is not a simple regurgitation of nutritional guidelines. Rather, each case narrative poses the challenges related to achieving nutritional homeostasis in older adults due to mealtime issues, oral health, and gastrointestinal problems such as constipation or diverticulosis. Chapter 16 provides some general tips on chemotherapy, using the case of a woman with breast cancer, and then provides additional case narratives on colorectal cancer, as it is so prevalent in older adults. As noted earlier, this section also includes an overview of HIV and hospice. The five case narratives in Chapter 17, addressing cognitive impairment in the elderly, present realistic situations with regard to the common issues nurses encounter daily. Questions within the cases assist the reader to focus on evidence-based practice in order to assist those with the need for movement and wandering, who experience acute confusion and agitation or aggression. Dementia is compared and contrasted by cases that review early- and late-stage symptoms and approaches for nursing care.

Chapter 18 is a must-read for all health care providers as it gives an overview of cultural sensitivity in the first section and then an example of how to optimally manage a Hispanic patient. The information provided is practical and realistic and can be applied across settings.

Chapters 19 and 20 address common geriatric syndromes including pain and sleep disorders. The chapter on pain covers undertreatment of pain and how to recognize and manage this, pharmacological management of pain with opioids, a case narrative that reviews different types of pain (e.g., neuropathic) and use of adjuvant medications, and, lastly, a case narrative on noninvasive or behavioral interventions and prevention of pain. Chapter 20 addresses some prevalent sleep-related issues including restless legs syndrome and insomnia, as well as the much less commonly recognized hypersomnia experienced by some older adults.

This revised edition adds a wonderful new component with an entirely new Chapter 21, "Aging Issues Affecting the Family," and the incorporation throughout the text of 10 new case examples or focused topical areas on practical aspects of geriatrics, gerontology, and care of older adults. The new cases address such topics as health care disparities and the elderly, spirituality and aging, functional decline in the hospitalized aging, aging in place, health promotion for the elderly adult, challenges and solutions of leaving the homestead, long-distance caregiving, an overview of Medicare, catheter-associated urinary tract infections, and the cultural issues associated with generational aging as we face the aging of a large cohort of baby boomers. These cases are a wonderful source of information, with useful web pages and recommended resources, and provide practical information about how to best address these common aging issues and improve the lives of older adults.

In sum, this is a terrific text that provides nurses, and other health care providers, good basic information about clinical problems and challenges faced in providing care to older adults. It should be considered required reading in all undergraduate programs. While provided in a text format, the material is easy to read, thus, it will meet the needs of today's students who are used to accessing information quickly and easily on the Internet.

Barbara Resnick, PhD, CRNP, FAAN, FAANP
Professor
University of Maryland School of Nursing
Sonya Ziporkin Gershowitz Chair in Gerontology

Preface

The Process

Twenty contributors were recruited to assist with the first edition of this book. Combining the collective years of nursing practice of this group resulted in over several centuries' worth of expertise. The plethora of case study topics offered is highly unusual for a health care–associated text. In particular, psychosocial issues common in today's society such as gambling addiction, hoarding behavior, emergency preparedness, long-distance caregiving, and others, represent a holistic approach to geriatric nursing care. Many of the case studies reflect true events that have been transferred into a quality learning experience. The various roles and working environments inherent in the nursing profession are well represented, which came about rather serendipitously. These include encounters with the geriatric client in the home, hospital, long-term care, or rehabilitation facility, from a public health contact, a clinic, a hospice organization, as a neighbor, or through parish nursing. In addition, the health care provider may be a student, member of a nursing staff, advanced practitioner, or administrator.

The geriatric clients in the stories range in age from 65 to 91 years. Many are living predominantly healthy, productive lives with stable support systems. Considering the unfortunate ageism that exists in our country, this approach was purposeful in relation to countering myths and attitudes about getting older that undergraduate students may believe.

The Outcome

A comprehensive approach to addressing the physical, mental, and psychosocial needs and issues of the older adult are offered across the 100+ case studies in this text. Expected age-related changes, safety concerns, cultural awareness, and evidence-based practice pertaining to geriatric nursing are pervasive throughout the text. Ethical dilemmas are presented to encourage students to reflect on the "right thing to do" when planning or providing care. Each case provides 8 to 12 questions for the learner to address. Unlike electronic, "interactive" case studies available, students do not click response boxes of solely multiple-choice questions. Rather, they are often asked to use critical thinking skills; giving an opinion, conveying an experience, formulating a response, developing a plan, comparing and contrasting, and so on.

Gerontology Nursing Case Studies: 100+ Narratives for Learning, Second Edition has a multifaceted use for undergraduate students. The text can easily be integrated across the curriculum, or serve as an assessment piece in a stand-alone gerontology course. **A fully updated answer guide is available to professors who adopt the book from Springer Publishing Company by emailing textbook@springerpub .com.** The cases can be assigned as an out-of-class learning experience, stimulate a small group discussion, or be presented by the instructor to introduce or reinforce a specific lecture topic. The text design allows for heavy use of the Internet to explore answers and develop solutions to the various client situations.

These stories are highly varied with regard to the problem at hand, the role of the nurse, and unexpected events that occasionally surface. For example, a client with a postoperative pulmonary embolism placed on heparin therapy requires frequent lab work in order to receive safe care; a routine event for sure. However, she has a severe needle phobia. Or, a client who cannot afford medical services substitutes a beautiful hand-made quilt as payment. Should the nurse accept this gift?

This second edition has been revised fully, with updated links to relevant guides and resources. New case studies have been added, which cover topics such as aging in place, health care disparities, and the baby boomer culture. A new chapter on aging and the family delves into the roles of family caregivers, coping, and relationships.

It is with sincere intention that these stories were created to provide engagement of learning, encourage thoughtful discussion, and present students with a better understanding of the special needs of older people. Bridging the gap between theory and practice is a phrase many of us seasoned nurse educators have heard for years; this project was completed as a means to fill that gap. Enjoy.

Donna J. Bowles

Suggested Resources

Benner, P., Sutphen, M., Leonard, V., & Day, L. (2010). *Educating nurses: A call for radical transformation.* San Francisco, CA: Jossey-Bass.

Faculty Tool Kit. (2009). *The essentials of baccalaureate education for professional nursing practice.* American Association of Colleges of Nursing. Retrieved from www.aacn.nche .edu/education/bacessn.htm

1

Political, Ethical, and Legal Issues of Older Adults

Case 1.1 ■ Advance Directives

*M*elanie Hughes, RN, GNP, has two appointments this morning in regard to advance directives (ADs). She has been employed with a hospice facility for nearly a decade in the role of a nurse practitioner specializing in end-of-life care. The majority of her clients are elderly, and today she will meet with Tom Barker, an 80-year-old male diagnosed with colon cancer, and Margarita Ruiz, a 72-year-old with end-stage chronic obstructive pulmonary disease (COPD). Both individuals were recently hospitalized and were asked about the presence of an AD; neither has made formal arrangements although they both have opinions on the topic.

1. ***What federal law enacted in 1991 requires agencies and institutions receiving Medicare or Medicaid reimbursement to inform clients of their right to make health care decisions including completing an AD?***

Melanie generally begins a session with an unfamiliar client by assessing for any visual or hearing deficits and language barriers. She attempts to explore what quality of life means to the individual, along with how the client's illness and death will affect others insofar as emotional or financial impact. Melanie also asks the client what inspired him or her to seek assistance and assesses what is known about an AD. She provides written material and explains the details carefully. Reviewing terms and definitions is generally the first step in the process. Use the Hartford Institute for Geriatric Nursing website as a resource for the following two questions pertaining to an AD (Mitty, 2012) at http://consultgerirn.org/topics/advance_directives/want_to_know_more.

2. ***The authors of the evidence-based guideline point out less than 20% of Americans have an AD. What do you think may be contributing factors for this rate?***

3. ***What are the two types of ADs?***

Mr. Barker is the first appointment this morning. He has arrived with a document for his AD and explains to Melanie, "I may not have much time left on earth and want to make everything as easy for my daughter as possible." Mr. Barker was diagnosed with Stage IV colon cancer 8 months ago. He had surgery to remove a large section of malignancy; however, it was discovered metastases had spread to his peritoneum and spine. Hospice has been following him weekly for pain management; no palliative treatment such as chemotherapy or radiation was chosen by his request.

The client explains that his proxy will be his daughter and he needs assistance with several questions. He has determined, with his physician's awareness, if hospitalized, he does not want any form of resuscitation. When Melanie asks for him to clarify what treatments he chooses to forego, his response is, "I guess the cardiopulmonary resuscitation (CPR) part, what else is there?"

The National Cancer Institute Fact Sheet on Advance Directives (2013) may serve as a resource for the following questions. It is located at www.cancer.gov/cancertopics/factsheet/support/advance-directives.

4. As a nurse, what other medical directives would you review with a client?

Mr. Barker also asks Melanie about an AD being honored from one state to another. His daughter lives in a town only 10 miles away, but it is in a different state from his residency. He goes on to explain that if his health allows, he hopes to visit her for a few hours on the weekends for family meals and a change of scenery. Yet, he is concerned of the outcome, should he be hospitalized during a visit.

5. Is there reciprocity among states for an AD?

Finally, Mr. Barker tells Melanie that his daughter is also considering having an AD initiated. He states, "She's only 54 years old, what if medical technology advances and there are better options for her life when she's my age?"

6. Is an AD document permanent once it's signed?

Ms. Ruiz is accompanied by her long-term "boyfriend" when she visits the hospice facility. Her chronic lung condition requires continuous oxygen, multiple inhalers, and predominant bed rest. She had a physician visit in the same building this morning and asked to be seen in person although the offer for a home appointment was given. She stated over the phone that privacy was necessary and that was not possible in her house.

Ms. Ruiz presents Melanie with a document and asks for her opinion on the effectiveness of it. The document is known as "Five Wishes," originally disseminated from a grant by the Robert Wood Johnson Foundation in 1997. This document serves as a form of an AD, which does not require an attorney or notarization in order to be honored.

Ms. Ruiz goes on to explain that her immediate family, which consists of four adults and three teenagers all living in her home, has not accepted her condition as terminal. They were present when she had a hospice consult but refuse to believe she will likely decline physically to the point of death. Therefore, she has designated her boyfriend to keep a copy of her wishes and provide it when hospitalized. This event is purposely being kept "secret" from her family.

7. *Find a copy of the "Five Wishes" document and review it using the following link: www.agingwithdignity.org/five-wishes.php (Aging with Dignity, 2015). What are the actual five issues addressed?*

8. *From the information provided, can Ms. Ruiz name her boyfriend as a health care agent on this form?*

9. *Melanie has witnessed numerous family conflicts through the years as a hospice nurse pertaining to family thoughts on end-of-life care differing from the patient. Do you believe she should keep the "secret" of the "Five Wishes" document? Explain your rationale for this ethical dilemma.*

Ms. Ruiz was born in Mexico City and lived there until coming to the United States at the age of 40. She has a high level of acculturation, including reading, and speaking English fluently.

For an individual who may have cultural-based challenges with an AD, it is a nursing responsibility to be knowledgeable and sensitive toward the specific needs. The document in the following website, www.greaterniagarachamber.com/LinkClick.aspx?fileticket=F6VVHObJQWk%3D&tabid=203, offers numerous tips for effective communication with culturally diverse clients (Niagra Immigrant Connections Initiative, n.d.).

10. *Review the document and comment on a suggestion you found helpful, or new information that could be beneficial in your future practice.*

Suggested Resources

Aging With Dignity. (2015). *Five wishes*. Retrieved from http://www.agingwithdignity.org/five-wishes.php

Mitty, E. L. (2012). *Geriatric nursing standard of practice: Advance directives protocol*. Hartford Institute for Geriatric Nursing. Retrieved from http://consultgerirn.org/topics/advance_directives/want_to_know_more

National Cancer Institute. U.S. National Institutes of Health. (2013). *Advance directives*. Retrieved from http://www.cancer.gov/cancertopics/factsheet/support/advance-directives

Case 1.2 ■ Health Care Decision Making

Colby Hines sought employment in a large outpatient surgical center following 2 years of working on a medical–surgical floor after he became an RN. In this role, he rotates through all phases of the surgical experience; pre-, intra-, and postoperative patient care. Colby has been exposed to a variety of situations in his short career involving health care decision making and fully realizes the importance of this topic, in particular with older clients.

During his orientation period, two members of the Hospital Ethics Committee spoke to the new hires about the role and importance of this service. The speakers started their presentation reviewing the four core ethical principles, which set the foundation for the health care decision making process.

1. Respect for autonomy
2. Beneficence
3. Nonmaleficence
4. Distributive justice

> **1. Choose any two of the principles and create an example using a geriatric client to demonstrate understanding of the meaning of the terms.**

In addition, the Hospital Ethics Committee representatives emphasized repeatedly that individuals' right for self-determination includes not only the right to agree with a particular treatment but also the right to refuse. Colby witnessed a number of older people on the medical–surgical floor choose not to undergo a particular procedure, treatment, or modality that was presented by a physician.

One case involved a 90-year-old gentleman who was admitted for dehydration and weight loss. He became a widower 5 months prior, after being married for over seven decades; the couple had no children. His treatment plan called for insertion of a gastrostomy tube for feeding. It was explained to him that this could be a temporary measure, sustaining him nutritionally until he was able to take in sufficient calories again. The patient consistently refused consent each time he was asked. Colby reported that he believed it was disrespectful of this patient to be asked on four different occasions to give consent.

> **2. If this client asked you for your opinion on his decision, how might you respond?**

Colby is aware of the components involved with informed consent. There are several copies of the guidelines posted at the surgical center.

> **3. What requirements are to be included by the physician seeking consent for a treatment? Use the link, http://depts.washington .edu/bioethx/topics/consent.html (De Bord, 2014), to assist.**

> **4. Which of the following represents the RN's role with informed consent?**
>
> **a. Reviewing the anticipated postoperative discharge orders**
>
> **b. Providing literature on alternate treatments**
>
> **c. Developing a list of questions the client should ask the physician**
>
> **d. Witnessing the client's signature on the consent form**

Use the Hartford Institute for Geriatric Nursing website for evidence-based guidelines on health care decision making (Mitty & Post, 2012) found at http://consultgerirn.org/topics/treatment_decision_making/want_to_know_more to answer the remaining questions.

The determination of decision-making authority represents a significant event in the health care environment. Some patients purposefully choose to include others with this course of action and therefore use "assisted, supported, or delegated" autonomy with the decision-making process (Mitty & Post, 2012, p. 563). Assessment of an individual's capability for making decisions is often necessary.

5. Compare and contrast the terms "capacity" and "competence" in relation to decision making.

Colby distinctly remembers his time and contact with the elderly patient who refused a gastrostomy tube insertion. The gentleman had several co-morbid conditions, was very hard of hearing, and slept up to 15 hours of every 24-hour period. Yet, he possessed all elements of decisional capacity.

6. Identify the five essential elements.

During his 4 years of employment, Colby has worked multiple times with an advanced geriatric mental health nurse practitioner, Dr. Eads. Colby has great respect for Dr. Eads's clinical knowledge and communication skills after witnessing her interactions with families in the surgical center. In one case, an older client had a myocardial infarction preoperatively and died; another client experienced significant stroke activity postoperatively. In these events, Dr. Eads came to the clinical area with the hospital chaplain and provided emotional support during the crises.

In both cases, Dr. Eads assisted preoperatively in assessing the decision-making capacity for these two elderly patients. Colby attended these sessions and found them to be quite informative. Dr. Eads used an assessment tool, Screening Older Adults for Executive Dysfunction (Kennedy & Smyth, 2015), in both cases, which is located at www.nursingcenter.com/prodev/ce_article.asp?tid=828679.

7. What are the three instruments used to test for executive function representing best practice?

8. One of Colby's patients experienced a mild stage of dementia, the other was diagnosed with moderate mental retardation as a child. How does this affect their decision-making capacity?

In the past, Dr. Eads had shared a document with Colby from the *Best Practices in Older Adults: Dementia* (Mitty, 2012). Colby found the section on process guidelines particularly informative and uses the suggestions recommended in his practice frequently.

9. After review, what new information pertaining to decision making for clients with dementia was helpful to you?

Suggested Resources

De Bord, J. (2014). *Informed consent.* University of Washington School of Medicine, Ethics in Medicine. Retrieved from https://depts.washington.edu/bioethx/topics/consent.html

Kennedy, G. J., & Smyth, C. A. (2015). How to try this: Screening older adults for executive dysfunction. *American Journal of Nursing.* Retrieved from http://www.nursingcenter.com/prodev/ce_article.asp?tid=828679

Mitty, E. L. (2012). Geriatric nursing protocol: Advance directives. Hartford Institute for Geriatric Nursing and Alzheimer's Association. Retrieved from http://consultgerirn.org/uploads/File/trythis/try_this_d9.pdf

Mitty, E. L., & Post, L. F. (2011). Health care decision making. In B. Boltz, E. Capezuiti, T. T. Fulmer, & D. Zwicker (Eds.), *Evidence-based geriatric nursing protocols for best practice* (4th ed., pp. 562–578). New York, NY: Springer Publishing Company.

Mitty, E. L., & Post, L. F. (2012). *Nursing standard of practice protocol: Health care decision making.* Hartford Institute for Geriatric Nursing. Retrieved from http://consultgerirn.org/topics/treatment_decision_making/want_to_know_more

Case 1.3 ■ Physical Restraints

Joseph Deikel is a 78-year-old male admitted to a medical–surgical floor in an acute care facility. Three days before, he had visited his internist for nausea, vomiting, and a low-grade fever. At that time, he was provided with a prescription for promethazine (Phenergan) suppositories and returned home. Mr. Deikel has a strong aversion to any medications taken rectally and did not use the suppositories. The vomiting continued for another 48 hours and was followed by dry heaves. He barely was able to get out of bed at this point and had to hold onto furniture for support. His son found him lying on the bathroom floor, and he was transported to the local emergency department (ED).

Abnormal findings in the ED include Mr. Deikel's BP of 88/50, heart rate 114, temperature 100.1°F, oriented to person only, serum Na+ 128, blood urea nitrogen (BUN) 44, and creatinine 2.1. Intravenous fluids (IVF) of sodium chloride 0.9% were initiated at 140 mL/hr along with orders for multiple cultures.

On the medical–surgical unit, Mr. Deikel felt the need to urinate and attempted to get out of bed to go to the bathroom, and fell (no urinal had been provided). His son left, and he was put into a posey vest restraint. When given a dose of intravenous (IV) antibiotics shortly thereafter, he yelled out in pain as his entire arm with the IVFs had a tremendous burning sensation, so as a means of "self-preservation" he pulled the angiocath and tubing out. He now found himself with both wrists restrained.

Reviewing the events, it is apparent that Mr. Deikel, an elderly gentleman, was dehydrated by several days of fluid loss, as evidenced by abnormal vital signs and lab work, and thus became confused. The use of physical restraints described in this scenario was unfortunately not uncommon in years past. Hopefully, this will remain just that: a practice of the past. Use a document provided by the U.S. Food and Drug Administration (2014) at www.fda.gov/MedicalDevices/ProductsandMedicalProcedures/GeneralHospitalDevicesandSupplies/HospitalBeds/ucm123676.htm to assist with the following questions.

1. *When are full bedrails (aka, siderails) considered a form of physical restraint? What can be a negative outcome of having full bedrails up, surrounding a patient?*

2. *What psychological effects do you believe physical restraints can have on a patient?*

For Questions 3 to 7, use the Hartford Institute for Geriatric Nursing website at http://consultgerirn.org/topics/physical_restraints/want_to_know_more (Bradas, Sandhu, & Mion, 2012).

3. *What, if any, items listed under the definition of physical restraints were unfamiliar to you?*

4. *After reviewing the section "Morbidity and Mortality Risks Associated With Physical Restraints," choose any two items and discuss how physical restraints could lead to the specific problem.*

A thorough assessment of a client is the first step in planning an alternative to physical restraints of a patient in order to know whether physical or cognitive impairment exists, as well as risks for injury, such as falling. In addition, presence of medical devices in cognitively impaired patients can represent a risk factor, such as a urinary catheter, nasogastric tube, peripheral/central IV access device, and other invasive items. Finally, a diagnosis or presence of a psychiatric disorder such as drug withdrawal, posttraumatic stress disorder, panic attacks, and so forth should be known.

5. *Provide the name of the assessment tools and their primary purpose in the "Try This Series" listing.*

6. *If physical restraints must be used, which of the following must be implemented? Select all that apply.*

   a. *Choose the least restrictive device*

   b. *Ensure proper sizing and fit of restraint*

   c. *Reassess the patient's response at least every 4 hours*

   d. *Release the restraint at a minimum every 4 hours*

   e. *Renew orders every calendar day after evaluation by a licensed independent practitioner*

7. *After reviewing the information for alternate care strategies, which one(s) do you think might be the most challenging for a patient who is agitated and why?*

8. *The use of physical restraints often presents an ethical dilemma for nurses. Develop a statement to explain the conflict between beneficence (nursing) and autonomy (of the patient) in regard to restraints.*

Suggested Resources

Bradas, C. M., Sandhu, S. K., & Mion, L. C. (2012). *Use of physical restraints with elderly patients.* Hartford Institute for Geriatric Nursing. Retrieved from http://consultgerirn.org/topics/physical_restraints/want_to_know_more

Doerflinger, D. M. C. (2013). *Try this: Mental status assessment of older adults: The mini-cog.* Hartford Institute for Geriatric Nursing. Retrieved from http://consultgerirn.org/uploads/File/trythis/try_this_3.pdf

Hendrich, A. (2013). *Fall risk assessment for older adults: The Hendrich II Fall Risk Model.* Try this: Best practices in nursing care to older adults. Hartford Institute for Geriatric Nursing. Retrieved from http://consultgerirn.org/uploads/File/trythis/try_this_8.pdf

Horgas, A. L. (2012). *Assessing pain in older adults with dementia.* Try this: Best practices in nursing care to older adults. Hartford Institute for Geriatric Nursing. Retrieved from http://consultgerirn.org/uploads/File/trythis/try_this_d2.pdf

Horgas, A. L., Yoon, S. L., & Grall, M. (2102). *Pain assessment for older adults.* Try this: Best practices in nursing care to older adults. Hartford Institute for Geriatric Nursing. Retrieved from http://consultgerirn.org/topics/pain/want_to_know_more

U. S. Food and Drug Administration. (2014). *A guide to bed safety bed rails in hospitals, nursing homes and home health care: The facts.* Retrieved from http://www.fda.gov/MedicalDevices/ProductsandMedicalProcedures/GeneralHospitalDevicesandSupplies/HospitalBeds/ucm123676.htm

Waszynski, C. M. (2012). *The confusion assessment method (CAM).* Try this: Best practices in nursing care to older adults. Hartford Institute for Geriatric Nursing. Retrieved from http://consultgerirn.org/uploads/File/trythis/try_this_13.pdf

Case 1.4 ■ Patient's Bill of Rights (Long-Term Care)

*E*dward Newsom and his family are visiting a new skilled nursing facility to complete a preliminary assessment and ask questions before his admission on Monday. Mr. Newsom's daughter, son-in-law, and grandson are present at the assessment. Mr. Newsom is an 86-year-old, well-groomed man, who is 6 feet 3 inches and weighs 240 pounds. He is dressed seasonally appropriate in a navy cardigan, white long-sleeved shirt, khakis, and skid-proof loafers. He has a little pocket on his shirt in which he keeps a small notepad and a pencil to take notes. He pulls this notepad out as you start your assessment and leafs through previous notes that he has taken. You observe that Mr. Newsom is withdrawn and flustered in the process of answering questions about his medical history. Martha Smith, his daughter, pats her father on the leg and reassures him that they are there to help him answer questions.

Martha states that it was a hard decision to transfer her father from her family's care. They managed using an occasional sitter and a global positioning satellite (GPS) tracking device for the couple of times he had gotten lost when taking a "walk," while family members were at work and school. The family has had increasing concern about his safety and well-being, because all family members work full time and are unable to care for him 24/7. They have noticed that he has become more confused and gets agitated when he is unable to recall events.

Mr. Newsom served as a lieutenant colonel in the army and, in the past, loved to tell detailed stories about his military experience and leadership skills in running a battalion. Mr. Newsom has Stage IV (mild or early stage) Alzheimer's disease (Alzheimer's Association, 2014). His family appears stressed and anxious. He is expected to be admitted to the level I Alzheimer's care unit. Mr. Newsom states, "How do I know people are going to listen to me and not just assume I am an old, muttering fool?" Carol, the RN, states, "All nursing homes have to adhere to a patient's bill of rights, and would take seriously any concerns you might voice."

1. *The nurse knows that a patient's bill of rights was*

   a. *Established by county ordinances*

   b. *Always changing to allow flexibility and changes as the nursing home administration evaluates the residents' and staffing needs*

   c. *Set forth by the Omnibus Budget Reconciliation Act (OBRA) of 1987 that governs and protects resident rights in long-term care settings*

   d. *Created by the American Hospital Association*

Mr. Newsom asks, "What rights? I am here, aren't I? But I am trying to make the best of this situation, as I know my mind is getting cloudy."

2. *What are patient rights?*

3. *Go to http://ezinearticles.com/?Federal-Nursing-Home-Care-Reform-Act&id=1332677 (Devine, 2008) and review the Federal Nursing Home Reform Act from the OBRA of 1987. Outline these rights.*

Carol, the RN, explains to the family and Mr. Newsom that a patient's bill of rights must be posted in a clearly visible area of the unit. Every long-term care (LTC) facility must inform a resident or guardian of these rights. Martha takes an audible sigh of relief and states, "I want to make sure my father is getting the best care possible, what if we are not here or in town and he has a concern?" Carol explains all personnel must respect and honor these rights. The nurse explains that the National Long-Term Care Ombudsman (n.d.) program provides special oversight for resident care.

4. *The National Long-Term Care Ombudsman Resource Center has provided a video related to volunteering as an ombudsman. View the short program at www.youtube.com/watch?v=RdiqIifurOE and comment on what you learned about this role.*

5. *What is an ombudsman?*

6. *Use your Internet search engine (e.g., Google or Yahoo) and type the term "long-term care ombudsman" and your state name. List your area ombudsman contacts.*

Carol knows that all staff need to be knowledgeable about legal issues affecting older adults. She understands that laws vary from state to state and some states have adopted these rights plus additional ones, so it is essential to check state laws to obtain the full rights established.

7. ***What could occur if the ombudsman finds a violation or the facility fails to follow and grant rights?***

   a. Job loss

   b. Lawsuits and fines

   c. Imprisonment

   d. All of the above

Mr. Newsom's daughter pulls the nurse aside and asks, "As his condition worsens, I don't want to come and find him strapped to a wheelchair." The RN reassures Martha.

8. ***What are the laws from OBRA 1987 pertaining to restraint and use of physical and chemical restraints?***

Martha hugs the nurse and thanks her for taking the time to explain what patient rights are, and how her facility has concern for, and takes the time to explain these rights to, new residents and their families. Carol notices the family is visibly more at ease, and Mr. Newsom voices an interest in learning more on Monday about the activities for his care unit.

Suggested Resources

Alzheimer's Association. (2014). *Seven stages of Alzheimer's.* Retrieved from http://www.alz.org/alzheimers_disease_stages_of_alzheimers.asp

Devine, J. (2008). Federal Nursing Home Care Reform Act. Ezine articles. Retrieved from http://ezinearticles.com/?Federal-Nursing-Home-Care-Reform-Act&id=1332677

National Long-Term Care Ombudsman Resource Center. (n.d.). *Volunteer ombudsman* (Video file). Retrieved from http://www.youtube.com/watch?v=RdiqIifurOE

Tabloski, P. (2010). Principles of geriatrics. In P. Tabloski (Ed.), *Gerontological nursing* (2nd ed., pp. 75–77). Upper Saddle River, NJ: Pearson.

Case 1.5 ■ The Older Driver

Jane Kircher is an RN who volunteers two mornings a week as a parish nurse at her church. She has been contacted by several parishioners about a church member, Jack Billings, with regard to concerns of his driving capabilities. It is reported that Jack has been observed parked up to 6 feet from the curb in front of the church, backed into another member's car and didn't appear to realize it, and running a stop sign a few blocks away. The concerned members ask Jane for assistance in discussing these incidents with Jack, as they fear not only for his safety but others' as well. This topic is all too familiar to Jane as she has been worried about her own father's driving capabilities in recent years. A conversation she had with him was very similar to the short video found at www.usatoday.com/story/money/cars/2014/05/08/elderly-drivers-stop-keys/8852851.

Jane arranges a home visit with Jack and discovers the following information. He is 79 years old; lives alone in a small, well-kept home; and has been divorced for several decades. He has an estranged relationship with his only son who lives in another state. He states his health is "pretty darn good" and takes the following medications: Lopressor (metoprolol) 50 mg orally daily, Zocor (simvastatin) 40 mg orally at bedtime, and Prilosec (omeprazole) 20 mg orally daily. When asked about common side effects of these medications, Jack denies experiencing any. His height and weight are within proportionate norms; he walks with a steady gait and is oriented to person, place, time, and event. Jack states he drives daily, primarily to a local diner to have breakfast and talk with other older men over coffee. In addition, he goes to the grocery and church once a week, and the local Walmart twice a month.

For the first two questions, utilize the website www.maximhomecare.com/uploadedFiles/Resources/Checklist_content/MHC-Checklist-Elderly-Drivers.pdf.

1. At this point in Jack's interview, what other assessments might the nurse initiate within the confines of his home to evaluate driving risks?

Once Jane believes Jack feels comfortable with her, she initiates conversation regarding his driving, openly sharing that church members have witnessed problems. She reviews common events that can affect an older individual's ability to drive safely.

2. What might be several environmental factors to discuss with Jack?

Jane prepared for the visit by exploring websites on the Internet. She found the information distributed by the American Medical Association (AMA), titled "Older Driver Safety," particularly helpful.

3. What are six specific tests that the AMA recommends for Assessment of Driving-Related Skills (ADReS)?

4. Dealing with impaired older drivers can present ethical conflicts for the health care provider. What are several potential ethical issues you think might arise in Jack's situation?

Jack shares that he sees a local physician every 3 months for blood pressure checks. He has not had an eye exam in more than 5 years. Jane is aware of an ophthalmologist whose office is located in a nearby city, which requires using the interstate.

5. What transportation options might be suggested for Jack to explore?

In her role as parish nurse, Jane has frequently used the Eldercare Locator (n.d.), a public service of the U.S. Administration on Aging, to find services such as transportation.

> **6. Go to the following website, www.eldercare.gov/eldercare.net/ Public/Search_Results.aspx, and cite a source of transportation in your own community using Eldercare Locator services.**

A month later, Jack phones to relay that his eye exam showed bilateral cataracts. He will have surgery to remove these in the upcoming months.

> **7. How did the presence of cataracts adversely affect Jack's ability to drive?**

> **8. Use the simulator located at www.geteyesmart.org/eyesmart/ diseases/cataracts/vision-simulator.cfm to understand the progression of visual decline from cataracts. Describe this experience.**

Nearly a year has passed since Jane's initial visit with Jack, and she is aware of his upcoming 80th birthday through church records. She phones to wish him well. He tells Jane that he will be renewing his driver's license within a week and states, "I sure hope they don't hassle this old man."

> **9. If Jack were a resident of your state, what would the Bureau of Motor Vehicles require of him? Address the following: (a) how often a license is to be renewed based on age and (b) any special provisions. Compare your state to any other two of your choice. Use the following link for assistance: www.iihs.org/iihs/topics/ laws/olderdrivers.**

Suggested Resources

American Academy of Opthamology. (2014). Cataract vision simulator. Retrieved from http:// www.geteyesmart.org/eyesmart/diseases/cataracts/vision-simulator.cfm

Eldercare Locator. (n.d.). U.S. Administration on Aging. Department of Health and Human Services. Retrieved from http://www.eldercare.gov/eldercare.net/Public/Search_Results.aspx

Erb, R. (2014, May 8). Taking the car keys away from elder drivers. *USA Today*, Gannett Company. Retrieved from http://www.usatoday.com/story/money/cars/2014/05/08/ elderly-drivers-stop-keys/8852851/

Insurance Institute for Highway Safety Highway Loss Data Institute. (n.d.). *Older drivers. Highway safety research & communications.* Retrieved from http://www.iihs.org/iihs/ topics/laws/olderdrivers

Maxim Healthcare Services. (n.d.). Knowing when to put the breaks on older drivers. Retrieved from http://www.maximhomecare.com/uploadedFiles/Resources/Checklist_content/MHC-Checklist-Elderly-Drivers.pdf

Case 1.6 ■ Iatrogenesis and the Elderly

*B*etty Hamlin is attending a care conference at Rockville Manor, a long-term care (LTC) facility where her mother has resided for over 5 years. The facility director, clinical nurse manager, staff physician, and social worker asked Betty to join them for decision making in relation to sending her mother out to the local hospital for pneumonia treatment and monitoring. Betty is against this idea for a number of reasons.

Her mother is an 84-year-old woman who, prior to admittance, had a left hemisphere stroke resulting in right hemiplegia and dysphagia. Betty is the only child and has a home located across the road from the facility. She never learned to drive and walks to the grocery, bank, doctor, and church in the small town where she and her mother, Phyllis Hamlin, reside. If her mother transfers to the hospital, it would prevent Betty from being with her daily, which she greatly fears. The following is a description of three events that occurred at the local hospital, resulting in Betty losing all trust for the health care provision her mother will receive.

Phyllis Hamlin experienced fever, chills, and generalized fatigue a couple of years ago. She was transported to the ED with her records, along with a report from the staff physician at the LTC facility. It was determined she had a urinary tract infection and the decision was made to administer 72 hours of IV antibiotics. Following cultures, the ED physician ordered Levaquin (levofloxacin) 500 mg daily with the intention she would return to the LTC facility and take an oral dose for an additional 4 days. Betty got a ride to the hospital on the day her mother was to be discharged from the ED. She put her mother on the bedpan and noted blood in her urine, which was not present prior to admission. She also noted blood oozing from the IV site under the dressing. When she inquired about these findings, they were dismissed.

She contacted the staff physician at Rockville Manor to ask his opinion, and he suggested her INR (international normalized ratio) be checked prior to discharge. Phyllis had been using Coumadin (warfarin) 2 mg daily per gastrostomy tube (G-tube) for years following her stroke, which was continued in the hospital. When the results came back, Betty was told the discharge to the LTC facility was cancelled; her mother's bleeding time was "a bit high." In actuality, the INR was 9.4: over three times increased for patients on anticoagulant therapy.

Phyllis stayed another 3 days receiving many transfusions of plasma that required multiple IV sticks and transfer to a telemetry unit for cardiac monitoring. It was explained to Betty that the plasma would "dilute" the amount of circulating Coumadin (warfarin). She could not receive an explanation for what happened; her worry was that a much higher than usual dose of the anticoagulant had been given. The plasma transfusions triggered another problem; her mother's blood pressure stayed consistently high due to hypervolemia, and at one point on the monitor, Betty noted it was 198/120 mmHg; her fear was that another stroke would occur. In addition, she began having labored breathing and required oxygen therapy.

After her mother's return to the LTC facility, the staff physician explained to Betty that the reason for the dangerous increase in bleeding times was due to the combination of her particular antibiotic (a fluoroquinolone) and the Coumadin (warfarin).

Betty had the reference clerk at the local library look up information about this interaction and received volumes of information about the hazards.

> ### 1. Explore the Internet to determine what the potential risks for combining these two medications entails.

Approximately 1 year later, Phyllis returned to the hospital for elective surgery and an overnight stay for monitoring. She had cataract removal, along with three highly decayed teeth extracted. She tolerated the procedures well with no obvious complications. However, several days after returning to Rockville Manor, Phyllis had a thin, greenish drainage from the operative eye. In addition, the administrator of the LTC facility was informed by the hospital that a swab taken on the day of discharge for methicillin-resistant *staphylococcus aureus* (MRSA) was positive. The hospital infection-control nurse emphasized it was community acquired and Phyllis "brought it in with her," yet couldn't offer an explanation why the admission culture was negative.

Finally, the staff at the LTC facility noted Phyllis had a low heart rate, which continued to drop over a 24-hour period to the mid-40s. She was admitted to the local hospital for a cardiac evaluation and placed on a telemetry unit. It was determined she had a third-degree atrial-ventricular (AV) block and required a pacemaker implantation. Betty was there for the procedure and stayed until the next morning. She observed an evening shift nurse give her mother the nine routine morning medications withheld earlier due to her procedure. A cup containing them all (some liquid and some crushed) was brought to the room, and all the meds were inserted into her G-tube at once, and then it was plugged. Betty asked the nurse to flush the tube with water as she had witnessed at the LTC facility for years; the nurse complied with less than a tablespoon of water. Betty was worried this technique had been the norm for the several days prior when she couldn't be at the hospital. The next morning, a different nurse did the same thing before Phyllis was transferred back to the LTC facility.

As Betty feared, the G-tube that was inserted shortly after her mother's stroke was completely clogged after returning to the nursing home. The staff tried a variety of ways to get the tube opened; all were unsuccessful. Phyllis had to undergo another surgical procedure to replace her only source of feeding and medication administration.

> ### 2. Briefly describe the correct method for giving multiple medications through a G-tube.

The events Phyllis experienced are representative of the concept of iatrogenesis. The term comes from the Greek language; "iatros" means doctor or healer and "gennan" means "as a result" (Torrey, 2014). Questions 3 to 7 of this case require the use of the Hartford Institute for Geriatric Nursing website, http://consultgerirn.org/topics/iatrogenesis/want_to_know_more (Francis, 2012).

> ### 3. What is the definition provided for iatrogenesis? Do you believe any, or all, of the events described in this case fall under this definition?

> ### 4. The most common iatrogenic events result from which of the following? Select all that apply.

> #### a. Falling accidentally

> #### b. Hospital-acquired pressure ulcer

    c. Adverse reaction to a medication

    d. Inadequate staffing

    e. Prejudicial attitude of providers

5. **Adverse drug events (ADEs) are the most common form of iatrogenesis. In relation to the elderly population, what primarily contributes to drug–drug interactions in this age group?**

Phyllis Hamlin received a "therapeutic" treatment for her drug–drug ADE, supposedly, yet it caused additional health risks.

6. **Under the section titled "Adverse Effects of Diagnostic, Therapeutic, and Prophylactic Procedures," find a rationale for what transpired.**

7. **A hospitalized patient, who is immobilized due to a fractured hip develops a fecal impaction. How is this form of iatrogenesis labeled?**

A study presented by James (2013) suggests over 440,000 deaths due to medication errors in hospitalized patients occur each year; this would represent the third leading cause of death in the United States. A tremendous amount of focus has been put on evidence-based strategies toward medication reconciliation.

8. **What is the definition of medication reconciliation? Describe the three-step process used to accomplish this safety goal.**

The "Brown Bag Method" for reporting medications is briefly described at http://live.psu .edu/story/7079 (Penn State News, 2010).

    A major policy change for health care coverage and reimbursement occurred in late 2008 when Medicare chose to stop paying U.S. hospitals for eight preventable medical errors/events, all of which are addressed at the Hartford Institute for Geriatric Nursing website.

9. **Provide a list of these, and cite your source.**

The Quality and Safety Education for Nursing (QSEN) task force developed a number of competencies for schools of nursing across the nation. Review the section regarding safety at http://qsen.org/competencies/pre-licensure-ksas/#safety.

10. **What are three examples from your nursing program you believe assist in meeting the competency of being a safe provider?**

Betty told a friend, "I have to go to the hospital with my mother for surveillance [of all health care provided], not just support [emotional reassurance]."

11. **What is your reaction to this statement? Do you think patients truly need a family member or significant other with them when hospitalized to observe the care provided?**

Suggested Resources

Francis, D. F. (2012). *Iatrogenesis*. Hartford Institute for Geriatric Nursing. Retrieved from http://consultgerirn.org/topics/iatrogenesis/want_to_know_more

James, J. T. (2013). A new, evidence-based estimate of patient harms associated with hospital care. *Journal of Patient Safety, 9*(3), 122–128.

Penn State News. (2010). *Brown bag gives more complete picture of meds taken by older adults*. Retrieved from http://news.psu.edu/story/215617/2004/06/03/brown-bag-gives-more-complete-picture-meds-taken-older-adults

Quality and Safety Education for Nurses. (2006). *Pre-licensure competences*. Institute of Medicine. Retrieved from http://qsen.org/competencies/pre-licensure-ksas/#safety

Rosenthal, M. B. (2007). Nonpayment for performance? Medicare's new reimbursement rule. *New England Journal of Medicine, 357*, 1573–1575. Retrieved from http://content.nejm.org/cgi/content/full/357/16/1573; http://www.nejm.org/doi/full/10.1056/NEJMp078184

Torrey, T. (2014). Iatrogenic—What is the definition of iatrogenic? *About.com: Patient empowerment*. Retrieved from http://patients.about.com/od/glossary/g/iatrogenic.htm

2

Loss and End-of-Life Issues

Case 2.1 ■ Death of a Spouse

*H*arry and Alice were married when they were both 38 years old, and they celebrated their 50th wedding anniversary several months before Alice's death. For more than 20 years, they had lived in a condominium in a retirement community; then, in the years before Alice's death, they moved into an independent living apartment, which was part of a continual care community. Harry had dementia and was hard of hearing, but he was able to perform basic activities of daily living (ADL). Both gave up driving. Alice died at home from metastasized breast cancer. Both Harry and Alice enrolled in hospice, and as Alice's ability to care for herself declined, the care coordinator at the independent living facility arranged for her to have around-the-clock care; thus, Harry and Alice were able to stay together until Alice died.

During the hospice enrollment interview, which took place months before Alice's death, the nurse assessed Harry's mental status. She pointed to Alice and asked Harry who she was. Harry said, "That's my Alice." When the nurse asked, "And who is Alice to you?" Harry replied, "She is the world to me." This was one of their children's favorite moments, for it showed that even though both Harry and Alice were in decline, their relationship was still valuable to both.

Within a few days following Alice's death, Harry was moved along with his clothes, TV, bed, desk, and other personal belongings into an Alzheimer's unit, which was a part of the continuing care facility. Harry's sons gave away the personal belongings that Harry would not need, and that had no sentimental value to the family. Because of Harry's dementia, the sons took care of these tasks without consulting Harry, but this became a source of frustration for Harry in the months that followed.

Harry's family expected that he would die soon after Alice. At the time of Alice's death, he slept most of the day and seemed to care little about outside activities. He frequently said to family and friends, "You know my sad news about Alice" and "I miss Alice." Then, in the months after Harry moved into the Alzheimer's unit, he became more and more involved in the unit's activities. Members from his church took him to services on Sunday and to activities the church organized for individuals with Alzheimer's. Harry lived for 9 months in the Alzheimer's unit following Alice's death.

He was cared for by the hospice staff and died quickly thereafter from an acute illness. He had been visited by all his children in the months prior to his death.

1. *What physical symptoms are associated with grief? Cite your source.*

2. *What emotional symptoms are associated with grief? Cite your source.*

3. *Why might the recently bereaved be more at risk for death than individuals with living spouses? Use the link www.bbc.co.uk/news/health-16467182 to assist in finding information.*

4. *Give examples of how the stress and anxiety of grief might affect a number of body systems. Refer to the following website: www.nytimes.com/health/guides/symptoms/stress-and-anxiety/possible-complications.html.*

5. *Search the literature for an assessment tool that may be useful in looking at bereavement. Cite your source.*

6. *What are some benefits of an institutionalized older adult participating in social support programs?*

Use the information on grieving by Poinier and Zisook (2011) at www.mercy.net/healthinfo/aa122313 to give three examples for each of the remaining questions.

7. *What is different about older adults who are grieving?*

8. *Why does an older adult who is grieving need help?*

9. *What can be done to help an older person who is grieving?*

Suggested Resources

Poinier, A. C., & Zisook, S. (2011). *Helping older adults with grief.* Healthwise.org. Retrieved from http://www.mercy.net/healthinfo/aa122313

Roberts, M. (2012, January 10). *Bereavement raises heart attack risk, says study.* BBC News Health. Retrieved from http://www.bbc.co.uk/news/health-16467182

Simon, H. (2013). Stress and anxiety possible complications. American Accreditation Healthcare Commission. *New York Times Health Guide.* Retrieved from http://www.nytimes.com/health/guides/symptoms/stress-and-anxiety/possible-complications.html

Case 2.2 ▪ Prolonged Grief

*C*arlos Neves is a 77-year-old gentleman who is waiting anxiously to see a grief counselor affiliated with the local hospice agency. He is here at the insistence of his two adult daughters, whose opinion he values greatly. Carlos was born and lived in Peru for 55 years. He got married at the age of 19 to Anna, after she became pregnant with his child. The couple had another daughter several years later and ended the marriage shortly thereafter. Both of Carlos's parents died by the time he was 50 years old. He decided to pursue a lifelong goal and, with inheritance money, came to the United States to open a gambling casino in Miami, Florida.

Carlos worked night and day through the next decade building his casino business. He was a very wealthy man, overall had excellent health, and kept in contact with his daughters regularly. He developed a friendship with a lady named Nancy at the coffee shop he frequented nearly every morning. They shared many personal stories, laughed constantly and, over time, Carlos asked her to dinner. Within a year from that date, the couple was married.

Nancy and Carlos were best friends, went everywhere together, and both felt it was the happiest time in their lives. Their good fortune continued for years. While on a cruise for a 10th anniversary celebration, Nancy experienced shortness of breath, coughing, and hoarseness. She passed it off as a respiratory virus, initially. By the time she had a medical workup, it was determined she had adenocarcinoma of the lung with metastases to the spine. With hospice care, she lived for 6 months from the time of diagnosis.

For over a year, Carlos's daughters have encouraged him to see a physician, counselor, priest, or psychologist to assist with his profound, prolonged grief. He repeatedly refused this assistance, stating that a stranger who never knew Nancy would not be able to understand his loss. Finally, in response to his daughters' begging, Carlos agreed to meet with the primary nurse from hospice who managed Nancy's end-of-life care. This decision coincides with Carlos's Hispanic culture.

1. ***Using an article in MinorityNurse.com (Bougere, 2008), explain the probable rationale for Carlos agreeing to see his wife's hospice nurse for assistance. Go to www.minoritynurse.com/article/ culture-grief-and-bereavement-applications-clinical-practice.***

Use the article by Smith and Segal (2014), www.helpguide.org/mental/grief_loss.htm, to answer the next three questions

2. ***Review the following statements and determine whether each represents a fact or myth with regard to grief. State your rationale.***

   a. ***The pain will go away faster if you ignore it.***

   b. ***It's important to "be strong" in the face of loss.***

> *c. If you don't cry, it means you aren't sorry about the loss.*
> *d. Grief should last about a year.*

3. What are the five stages of grief?

Grief is a natural response to loss in one's life. After the death of a loved one, the reaction can be intense. However, even subtle losses, not necessarily of a person, can result in a grief.

4. What are examples of other life losses that can result in a grieving period?

Since Nancy's death a year and a half ago, Carlos has experienced a number of physical and mental health alterations. He was hospitalized twice; the first time for dehydration and generalized fatigue, which left him barely able to walk. Second, he was admitted for chest pain and had a thorough workup, which showed no underlying cardiac dysfunction. He takes a low-dose thiazide diuretic since the age of 60 for prehypertension; a beta-blocker and angiotensin-converting enzyme (ACE) inhibitor have been added to keep his systolic pressure under 140 mmHg. His weight has fluctuated from 180 to 140 pounds. He has great difficulty falling asleep and, as a result, he drinks four or more servings of alcohol each evening, whereas this had been his usual intake per *month*.

Carlos has difficulty concentrating. What was once a brilliant mind for business transactions and confident decision making has vanished. He can spend an hour choosing what shirt to wear or contemplating whether to pay a bill one day or the other. He has been asked regularly whether he believes he is depressed and responds angrily, "Who wouldn't be?" Suicide ideation has been firmly denied. There is minimal change to his voice or affect, which is a drastic alteration to his former gregarious personality. He will not participate in any American or Latino holiday or special event stating, "It wouldn't be right without my wife being able to enjoy the day with me." What concerns his daughters most, however, is his continued "obsession" with Nancy on a daily basis. Carlos has kept all of her clothes and holds and smells them regularly for the scent of her favorite cologne. He buys items for the house he has no need or use for, but believes Nancy would have enjoyed. All references to his wife are in present tense, for example, "She likes this television show."

5. Compare and contrast the following terms: grief, mourning, and bereavement.

The information provided at www.hospicenet.org/html/grief_guide.html can be helpful in answering the next three questions.

6. What phase(s) of grief does the client appear to be experiencing?

7. Does Carlos fit the article's description for experiencing complicated grief? Explain your opinion.

8. What tasks are involved when an individual undergoes grief therapy?

9. What healthy coping measures have you personally used when experiencing a loss in life?

After initially refusing therapy, Carlos agreed to one-on-one grief counseling. The psychotherapist that was recommended through hospice also lost a spouse years ago. Thus far, Carlos agreed to abstain from alcohol and to have two well-balanced meals daily. In addition, he joined a walking group, which meets three times a week at the local mall. His daughters continue their encouragement and hope their father returns to a productive, balanced life.

Suggested Resources

Bougere, M. H. (2008). *Culture, grief and bereavement: Applications for clinical practice.* Minority Nurse.com. Retrieved from http://www.minoritynurse.com/culture-grief-and-bereavement-applications-clinical-practice

National Cancer Institute. (n.d.). *PDQ's bereavement, mourning, and grief.* Retrieved from http://www.hospicenet.org/html/grief_guide.html

Smith, M., & Segal, J. (2014). *Coping with grief and loss.* Retrieved from http://www.helpguide.org/mental/grief_loss.htm

Case 2.3 ■ Death With Dignity

A few weeks after Don's mother died, he met with a nurse and a care coordinator who worked in the independent living facility where his parents lived during their last years. He told them both, "When nursing instructors like me dream of death with dignity, we dream of a death like Alice's."

Alice Kautz was 89 years old when she died 10 months before her husband, Harry, died. (Harry's life after Alice is described in Case 2.1 "Death of a Spouse.") Alice was fiercely independent all her life. She and Harry decided to leave the condominium where they had lived for over 20 years and move into an independent living facility after Alice found Harry "down" and had to call 911 twice in a month. A few weeks after Alice and Harry celebrated 50 years of marriage, Alice was diagnosed with breast cancer. Because she had some difficulty with problem solving, Alice knew about the tumor in her breast for months before she finally decided to seek treatment. When Alice had a mastectomy performed, the oncologist discovered that the breast cancer had metastasized to her liver. Alice lived for several months after the discovery of the metastases. Because she had several months to prepare prior to her death, Alice was able to make the arrangements she desired, which helped her die with dignity.

Alice and Harry were both enrolled in hospice, and they had weekly visits by an RN during the early summer months prior to Alice's death. They made changes to their wills and powers of attorney during that summer and made sure that all of their affairs were in order. They had saved money and lived frugally, and so they were financially secure. Their oldest son became their power of attorney and paid all of their bills during the last months of Alice's life.

Harry had dementia, and even though he was independent in his basic ADL, he was not able to problem solve or live independently. As Alice's endurance declined, the staff at the independent living facility made arrangements for personal care assistants (PCAs) to provide around-the-clock care for both Alice and Harry. The PCAs ensured that both Harry and Alice ate every meal, their laundry was done, and their personal needs were met. The care provided by the PCAs allowed Alice and Harry to live together until Alice died.

Alice and Harry's three children traveled from Colorado, New York, and Italy, to Arizona in order to visit Alice in the months before her death and to say good-bye. Alice was cognitively intact until her last days, and she had very little pain from the cancer. Alice's daughter was with her during the last 2 weeks before her death, and she returned to Italy the day before Alice died. Her family likes to think that Alice waited until her daughter arrived safely at home before dying. Her daughter made arrangements for all of Alice's children to talk to Alice one last time during the week before her death. Alice was regularly visited by members of the hospice team and her long-time minister and friend. Everyone involved in her care said that she "was at peace with dying" for several months prior to her death.

On the night Alice died, the PCA called the care coordinator, who came up to her room. The care coordinator later told me that she will always treasure the way Harry said good-bye to Alice after she had died, taking off her wedding ring to keep.

1. *An individual possessing mental capacity has the right to make his or her decisions regarding health care and end-of-life preferences. How would Alice's health care professionals have determined her decision-making capacity?*

2. *What are two types of advance directives available for individuals determined not to have the decision-making capacity?*

3. *The PCAs honored Alice's dignity by making provisions for her physical comfort during her final days. What are some other ways in which health care personnel could have enhanced her dignity during this time?*

Explore the website www.completingalife.msu.edu/audioon/intro.html to find information on important issues to address when assisting individuals to plan for their final hours of life. To answer Questions 4 to 7, go to the following specific sections of the website: last hours, goals, loss of control, health care, and family decisions.

4. *Using resources on the website, what are some additional arrangements and decisions that health care professionals could have assisted Alice and her family to identify and discuss regarding her desires for completing her life?*

Hospice is a philosophy of palliative care that uses a team of professionals to support the physical, emotional, and spiritual needs of an individual during end-of-life care.

5. *What professionals are involved in a typical hospice team and how do they ensure the dignity of their client(s)?*

6. *Alice's children all had the opportunity to visit with her and talk with her on the phone to say good-bye before her death. What are some other means of communication that can be used by an individual who wishes a final contact with those who may be unable to visit or talk on the phone?*

7. *Refer to "Planning for the Last Hours and After." What are some questions that an individual should consider if he or she wishes to plan for the last hours of life?*

Alice had only minimal cognitive impairment and was not demented. However, those with dementia also need nurses who will help them die with dignity. A new type of advance directive was created several years ago to allow for life planning while living with Alzheimer's disease and dementia. This document was the first of its kind focused on these specific challenges. With a purpose similar to a living will, the Alzheimer's and dementia directive aims to have a person's intentions known when the person isn't in a place to speak for himself or herself.

8. *Use the link www.deathwithdignity.org/2013/04/16/alzheimers-disease-and-dementia-mental-health-advance-directive to distinguish the difference of a traditional advance directive compared to the Alzheimer's directive.*

9. *Visit the following website to identify some assessment tools that might be used by the clinician to assess the functional status of Harry and Alice and determine the level of assistance they might require from the hospice team: http://consultgerirn.org/topics/palliative_care/want_to_know_more#item_2 (Gatto&Zwicker, 2006).*

Suggested Resources

Dastidar, J. G., & Odden, A. (2011). How do I determine if my patient has decision-making capacity? *The Hospitalist.* Retrieved from http://www.the-hospitalist.org/details/article/1309387/How_Do_I_Determine_if_My_Patient_has_Decision-Making_Capacity.html

Gatto, M. A., & Zwicker, D. (2006). *Want to know more: Palliative care.* Hartford Institute for Geriatric Nursing. Retrieved from http://consultgerirn.org/topics/palliative_care/want_to_know_more#item_2

Lorenz, J. M. (2014). *End-of-life issues.* Advance Healthcare Network. Retrieved from http://nursing.advanceweb.com/Continuing-Education/CE-Articles/End-of-Life-Issues.aspx

Michigan State University. (2001). *Completing a life.* Retrieved from http://www.completingalife.msu.edu/audioon/intro.htmll

Young, A. (2013). *Alzheimer's disease and dementia mental health advance directive.* Death With Dignity National Center. Retrieved from http://www.deathwithdignity.org/2013/04/16/alzheimers-disease-and-dementia-mental-health-advance-directive

3

Mistreatment of Older Adults

Case 3.1 ■ Physical Abuse

*A*n older woman comes to the clinic for a regular follow-up visit after left hip arthroplasty. The nurse, Christine, gleans the following information from the chart before meeting Mrs. Sable and making her initial assessment. Winnie Sable is an 84-year-old woman who lives with her husband, Alfred, age 89 years. The Sables have been married for 54 years and have no children. They reside in their own two-level home in a small suburban neighborhood where most of the neighbors keep to themselves. Winnie used to enjoy participating in church activities, but after "falling down the stairs" and breaking her hip 6 months ago, she does not venture out like she used to. Alfred has recently been diagnosed with mild cognitive problems (particularly progressive memory loss) suggestive of early Alzheimer's disease. Winnie depends on Alfred to drive them for groceries and to doctor appointments.

1. At this point, are there any risk factors for physical abuse for either Mr. or Mrs. Sable that the nurse should be alert to?

Christine obtains Mrs. Sable's height and weight. She is 5 feet 2 inches tall and weighs 91 pounds, reflecting a loss of 7 pounds in the past month. Mrs. Sable's vital signs are within normal limits, except her heart rate is 90 beats per minute. She seems quiet, withdrawn, does not make eye contact with the nurse, and seems hesitant when asked to put on a gown before the doctor comes to see her.

2. What signs, if any, suggest that the nurse should ask some follow-up questions regarding safety in the home for Mrs. Sable?

Mr. Sable is present in the room when Mrs. Sable is asked to put on a gown so the doctor can examine her. Christine asks Mr. Sable whether he would like to wait in the waiting room or step out for a minute. Mr. Sable answers the nurse angrily and refuses to leave the room, saying that his wife doesn't need to put on a gown to see the doctor. Seeing Mrs. Sable's obvious discomfort with having her husband in the examining room, Christine speaks calmly and quietly to Mr. Sable and offers him a cup of coffee. He reluctantly agrees to wait in the waiting room. Christine returns to

Mrs. Sable, who has donned a gown. The nurse notices bruises of various colors on her back and forearms.

3. At this point, what questions should the nurse be asking?

Christine asks how Mrs. Sable became bruised. Mrs. Sable lowers her eyes and whispers that she falls a lot. Christine makes a more thorough assessment and documentation of the bruising and gently probes for additional information. She uses the Elder Assessment Instrument (EAI; Fulmer, 2012) available through the "Try This Series" from the John A. Hartford Foundation to specifically record her findings.

4. What additional questions should Christine ask?

Mrs. Sable begins to cry and confesses that her husband hits and pushes her. She says it is not his fault, that since his memory began to fail, she has seen a change in his personality. He becomes angry and abusive over small things and hits her in the back and on the arms with his fists. Christine provides comfort to Mrs. Sable, documents her findings, and tells her that the doctor will be in soon.

5. What is the next course of action that Christine should take? Visit www.consultgerirn.com and look under the evidence-based geriatric topic of elder mistreatment and abuse. Explore the assessment tools and review the article.

Christine consults with the physician before he examines Mrs. Sable. She expresses her concern about the physical abuse and finishes documenting her findings using the EAI. While the doctor examines Mrs. Sable, Mr. Sable tells Christine that he isn't waiting anymore and wants to go home. He begins to yell and curse at the office staff.

6. What is the appropriate action for the staff to take?

While the office staff tries to calm Mr. Sable, the physician finishes his exam and tells Christine that he must make a report to Adult Protective Services (APS). He asks Christine to make a referral to social services immediately, and he does not want Mrs. Sable returning home with her husband. Mrs. Sable is willing to receive any help they will give her.

7. Since APS laws vary by state, find the guidelines for your particular state and apply them to this situation. What must the physician do to report physical abuse? Can he or she do so anonymously? Is reporting mandatory for him or her and/or Christine?

A social worker who is part of the interdisciplinary team at the clinic, where Mrs. Sable is a patient, visits the office and speaks with the doctor and Christine. She reviews the chart and then speaks with Mrs. Sable, who agrees that she does not feel safe to return home with her husband and is afraid for her life. Mrs. Sable continues to say that she feels that it is not her husband's fault, and she does not want him to get in trouble. She thinks he is just getting "senile" and cannot help his abusive behavior toward her.

The social worker initiates a plan to take care of Mrs. Sable's immediate needs and to make referrals and initiate help for her husband as well.

8. ***What do you think Mr. Sable's reaction will be to the fact that his wife is not going home with him? Do patients usually arrive at the decision to tell about abuse early in the process, or later after the abuse has become more serious? What types of assistance is this family going to need?***

Suggested Resources

Fulmer, T. (2012). *How to try this: Screening for mistreatment of older adults.* Hartford Institute for Geriatric Nursing. Retrieved from http://consultgerirn.org/uploads/File/trythis/try_this_15.pdf

Fulmer, T., & Caceres, B. A. (2012). *Elder mistreatment and abuse.* Hartford Institute for Geriatric Nursing. Retrieved from http://consultgerirn.org/topics/elder_mistreatment_and_abuse/want_to_know_more

Case 3.2 ■ Physical Neglect

*M*r. Edward McKay is an 82-year-old African American man who lives in a two-bedroom house with his daughter and son-in-law. Mr. McKay has a history of having had two cerebrovascular accidents (CVAs) that have left him partially paralyzed and unable to speak. He is bedridden with contractures of both lower extremities, incontinent, and dysphasic. His social history includes being married, having the one daughter whom he lives with, and two siblings who are in skilled nursing facilities. He does not have anyone who visits him on a regular basis. Mr. McKay is a retired plumber and his only income is his monthly Social Security benefit check.

Mr. McKay was referred to the local home health agency approximately 3 months ago by his medical doctor. His daughter states that they are unable to get him to a doctor's office for routine check-ups, so he is seen by a physician who makes home visits every 6 months. The doctor did not obtain any labs or weights the last time he visited the patient. The skilled nurse assigned to the case is visiting Mr. McKay for the third time today. The nurse obtained blood from the patient at the last visit and has the results with her today. The nurse notes that the patient's albumin level is 2.8 and his prealbumin level is 18. The nurse is still unable to obtain a height and weight on the patient because he is bed-bound, but the daughter does tell the nurse that her father is 6 feet 3 inches and that the last time he was weighed (which was over a year ago), he weighed 160 pounds. The nurse observes several things during this visit, and in previous visits, that she finds concerning. These issues include the following: (a) according to the daughter, she does not care for her father; she leaves the care to her husband, even though she does not work and is at home with the patient during the day; (b) the son-in-law feeds, cleans, and gives the patient his medicine, so when he is not there, the daughter does not do things for the patient, and she waits for her husband to get home; (c) the daughter is unable to answer any of the nurse's questions related to the patient's status; (d) the patient is developing a pressure ulcer on his sacrum; (e) every time the nurse has visited the home, the patient has had stool on him and his bed sheets appeared dirty; (f) there is cold food on the over-bed table and a glass of water is on the dresser (the patient is unable to feed himself and is dysphasic); and (g) when the daughter comes in the room, she is rough and harsh with the patient and he appears to be frightened of her. The nurse teaches the daughter about the dangers of aspiration and ways to prevent it, including carefully monitoring/assisting the patient when he is eating, not giving thin liquids such as water, not using straws, and so on. The daughter states, "Okay, I already know all that but since you think it is so important I will tell my husband who takes care of him." The nurse tries to set up a time when she can visit when the husband will be home, but the daughter states, "He works a lot. I can't tell you when he'll be here."

1. *What areas of the patient's assessment should the nurse concentrate on to evaluate his risk for physical neglect? Use the document by Robinson, Saison, and Segal (www.helpguide .org/mental/elder_abuse_physical_emotional_sexual_neglect.htm; 2014) to answer the following questions related to elder neglect.*

2. *Based on the information of where elder abuse most often occurs, who are the most common perpetrators?*

3. *What are Mr. McKay's risk factors for being the victim of physical neglect?*

4. *What are the general warning signs of physical neglect?*

5. *What are two psychosocial nursing diagnoses that Mr. McKay might be experiencing?*

6. *How should the nurse prioritize the physiological issues that Mr. McKay is experiencing?*

7. *What suggestions could be offered to a caregiver to avoid the strain that may lead to physical neglect?*

8. *What interventions/actions should the visiting nurse take to ensure this patient's safety and well-being?*

9. *An online article by Falk, Baigis, and Kopac (2012) provides an excellent overview on mistreatment of the elderly including information about the Elderly Justice Act. Briefly describe what this act offers to the older population. Go to http://nursingworld .org/MainMenuCategories/ANAMarketplace/ANAPeriodicals/ OJIN/TableofContents/Vol-17-2012/No3-Sept-2012/Articles- Previous-Topics/Elder-Mistreatment-and-Elder-Justice-Act.html.*

Suggested Resources

Falk, N. L., Baigis, J., & Kopac, C. (2012). Elder mistreatment and the elder justice act. *The Online Journal of Issues in Nursing, 17*(3). Retrieved from http://nursingworld .org/MainMenuCategories/ANAMarketplace/ANAPeriodicals/OJIN/TableofContents/ Vol-17-2012/No3-Sept-2012/Articles-Previous-Topics/Elder-Mistreatment-and-Elder-Justice-Act.html

Robinson, L., Saisan, J., & Segal, J. (2014). *Elder abuse and neglect.* Helpguide.org. Retrieved from http://www.minoritynurse.com/article/culture-grief-and-bereavement-applications-clinical-practice

Case 3.3 ■ Consumer Fraud and the Elderly

*F*ollowing a move from Los Angeles to the Gulf Coast several months ago, Nick Bergman is mentally and physically ready to start a major project in his career as an RN. Nick is 55 years old and has worked full time for over three decades. In his 20s, his clinical focus was critical care nursing, and at age 32, he returned to graduate school to achieve his nurse practitioner degree focusing on gerontology. He worked for a community health agency until his mid-40s and joined an internal medicine group where he practiced until his recent move.

Nick's life partner accepted a prestigious position with a Fortune 500 company and offered to financially support the couple if Nick was willing to go across the country with him. This change in lifestyle would allow Nick to concentrate solely on developing a nonprofit organization for senior citizens without the responsibility of earning an income. The focus of his altruistic endeavor is to heighten awareness of fraud by educating the public and advising older people to avoid being taken advantage of financially.

What motivated Nick to take on such a challenging project after years of providing direct health care services is multifaceted. When his own parents were in their 60s, they experienced consumer fraud, which he believes contributed to his father's stroke. Numerous similar situations were told to him by clients or their family members over the years. It seems as though he comes across these stories on the nightly news, the Internet, or in the newspaper at least weekly. He has spent years contemplating this project and has told those close to him it's as if a "spiritual calling" is leading him.

1. What is the definition of fraud?

2. What type of activities fall under the category of consumer fraud?

The following are examples of consumer fraud stories Nick has heard over the years as an RN.

Mary was an 85-year-old client Nick visited regularly as a home health nurse. She lived alone in a small home in need of multiple repairs. She could barely exist on her monthly income from Social Security yet was a pleasant, trusting woman. She was widowed, and her husband left her $400,000 from stock holdings. Mary planned to leave all of this to her church and rarely mentioned it to anyone. Diabetes, along with its various complications, resulted in weekly visits for a long period of time, and a friendship between Mary and Nick developed.

Mary was contacted by phone about a sweepstakes she won. The young lady explained that all subscribers to a magazine were eligible and Mary's name had been picked among thousands. She told the young lady that her husband had been the actual subscriber and died 4 years ago so it must be a mistake. The caller insisted Mary was the winner and suggested maybe her late husband was "trying to help her" in a mysterious form. After nearly a half hour, Mary was convinced the sweepstakes was legitimate and became as excited as the young lady on the phone had been from the onset of their conversation.

It was explained to Mary that she had to pay income taxes on the large sum immediately. Knowing she didn't have that amount, Mary remembered the bank account and told the caller she would need time to make a withdrawal. In an extremely helpful tone, the young lady offered to make the withdrawal over the phone for Mary so that she could get her windfall quicker. After account numbers were provided, the savings account was emptied without a trace of the perpetrator.

> **3. Use the website provided by the Federal Bureau of Investigation (FBI) located at www.fbi.gov/majcases/fraud/fraudschemes .htm After viewing "Tips to Avoid Telemarketing Fraud," what suggestions could have prevented consumer fraud from occurring in Mary's specific situation?**

James was an elderly patient Nick met when working in a busy internal medical practice. Due to chronic obstructive pulmonary disease, James seldom left his home. He had regular contact with his three children, their spouses, and his eight grandchildren via the phone and Internet. For Christmas one year, he bought gift cards from a variety of department stores, home improvement stores, and several popular restaurants for all 14 family members. James had ordered these on the Internet from the specific place of business. Every one of his "kids" made a point of letting him know what they purchased with their card or the great time they experienced eating out.

A few months later, James received an e-mail from a company advertising discounted gift cards for senior citizens. When he opened and read the message, he was shocked; every card he purchased for the holidays was listed. Typically, a $50 certificate only cost $30, and some were half off. The company emphasized how convenient and cost saving this service was for senior citizens. James had to list more personal information than usual when he made a purchase, such as his date of birth, Social Security number, and so forth. But, for the money he would be saving, he provided all the information requested. After ordering $350 worth of cards, they never arrived and the website vanished several weeks later.

LooksTooGoodtoBeTrue.com is a website sponsored by several government agencies and provides information to educate consumers about Internet fraud schemes. But, go to www.lookstoogoodtobetrue.com/pop/tip1.aspx.

> **4. After reviewing the online shopping tips, comment about a time in which you may have applied these recommendations, or other tips for safety not listed.**

Nick has witnessed that, more than any other kind of consumer fraud affecting the elderly, home improvement scams affect them the most. His own parents were affected to the tune of $75,000. Nick's father suffered from degenerative disc disease, which prevented him from taking on a dream project outside of their home. Through the years, he performed most of the repairs and remodeling himself, but he was unable to add a large deck and enclosed porch to the back of their home because of back pain and immobility. Nick's parents hired a contractor based on a referral from a home improvement store in their town. They paid $50,000 upfront for high-quality, maintenance-free materials, and most of the labor. The only service received was the removal of concrete steps leading to the back door and many shrubs and plants dug up in the area where the addition was to be built. The contractor never showed after 1 day of work, nor could he be reached by phone. The home improvement store manager apologized profusely, yet accepted no responsibility.

The additional $25,000 needed for the addition was put on a home equity loan; the contractor convinced Nick's father that it was the "best deal going," with payments less than $100 per month. What wasn't discussed was the interest rate of 18%; more than triple of what could be secured through a reputable lending agency.

Nick discovered a web source with very valuable information on this topic, provided by the National Committee for the Prevention of Elder Abuse (2008), at http://www.preventelderabuse.org/elderabuse/fin_abuse.html.

5. ***Check this site and share several deceptive sales tactics used with elderly homeowners.***

6. ***Older individuals are a common target for consumer fraud. Taking into consideration life changes associated with aging, identify a minimum of five reasons why this age group is at risk.***

7. ***After hearing the stories of consumer fraud from many geriatric clients he served through the years, Nick is still amazed at the number of incidents that go unreported. What may be the reason(s) for this?***

8. ***What consumer protection agencies are available in most states to assist with fraud?***

Nick continues to maintain contact with former classmates and many nursing coworkers from previous positions through his Facebook account. They are aware of his passion to develop the consumer fraud foundation, but he often receives a similar question, "What is it like to no longer be working as a nurse?" Nick replies that he is using the knowledge, skills, and values from the nursing profession toward his mission, daily.

9. ***What behaviors and actions do you believe Nick is referring to with regard to maintaining his nursing role?***

Suggested Resources

Federal Bureau of Investigation. (n.d.). *Common fraud schemes*. Retrieved from http://www.fbi .gov/majcases/fraud/fraudschemes.htm

National Committee for the Prevention of Elder Abuse. (2008). *Financial abuse*. Retrieved from http://www.preventelderabuse.org/elderabuse/fin_abuse.html

Case 3.4 ▪ Financial Mistreatment

*T*eresa Jones is a 70-year-old widowed woman residing alone in her own home in an affluent subdivision in a large midwestern town. Lisa is her friend and works as a nurse at the local assisted living center. Ms. Jones has three children and 10 grandchildren. Her oldest daughter, Marjorie, lives nearby and helps her mother with things around the house. Marjorie's teenage son, Joe, recently has moved in with his grandmother, because he does not get along with his mother. Although Ms. Jones is happy for the companionship and feels that Joe is "good" to her, she notices that some of her checks are missing, and she cannot find a few pieces of her gold jewelry. The jewelry is valued at over $11,000 and includes her precious wedding ring. These items were missing during the first 3 weeks after Joe moved in with her.

1. What risk factors for financial mistreatment are present in Ms. Jones's situation?

The bank calls to tell Ms. Jones that her checking account is overdrawn. They called as a courtesy because this has never happened before, and a check was cashed for a large sum; over $3,000. Ms. Jones goes to the bank and finds that someone has forged her signature on one of her checks. She suspects that Joe may have done it, but she says nothing to the bank officials about this. Ms. Jones rectifies the situation and returns home, then calls Lisa to ask her advice.

2. Is there additional information you would want to know about this situation? If so, what?

Ms. Jones confides that she thinks Joe stole some checks from her and now is cashing them. She tells Lisa that she talked to Joe and he denied everything, saying he was insulted that his grandmother would think he would ever do such a thing. Ms. Jones does not know what to do, but she is adamant that she will not allow anyone to steal her hard-earned money, even if it is a grandson.

3. Go to www.consultgerirn.org. Review the types of elder mistreatment found in the table of definitions from Fulmer

and Caceres's (2012) evidence-based practice guideline on elder mistreatment and abuse. What type of mistreatment or abuse is present in this situation?

Lisa tells Ms. Jones that this type of situation is not uncommon, citing 2014 statistics from the National Adult Protective Services Association (2014). "Estimates say that about 1 in 20 older adults indicate some form of perceived financial mistreatment occurring in the recent past. This is a form of mistreatment and it is not acceptable," says Lisa. Ms. Jones also confesses that her jewelry is missing. The two of them decide on an action plan that includes Ms. Jones first talking to her daughter Marjorie, Joe's mother.

Review the information from the agency previously mentioned at www.napsa-now.org/policy-advocacy/world-elder-abuse-awareness-day.

4. What facts are most surprising to you in relation to common ways family members and trusted others exploit vulnerable adults?

When Ms. Jones talks to Marjorie about her suspicions that Joe is stealing from her, Marjorie confesses to her mother that she kicked Joe out of her own house because he has a drug problem and had stolen money from her as well. Marjorie says she is sorry that she didn't tell her mother this before, but she was trying to protect her son and hoped he would change. Ms. Jones and Marjorie both agree that this theft must be reported to the police and they will go in person to talk to someone together the next day.

5. In reporting this to the police, what questions will Ms. Jones and Marjorie be asked?

6. By taking this action, are there any dangers that these women should be aware of?

Ms. Jones calls Lisa the next day to tell her that she and her daughter reported what they knew about the missing checks, stolen money and jewelry, Joe's possible forgery of one of Ms. Jones's checks, and Joe's drug problem. The police agree to investigate. Joe is now missing and nobody can locate him. He does not return any phone calls. Ms. Jones and Marjorie begin to be afraid that he will break into their homes to steal more money as he gets desperate to support his drug habit. They both have the locks changed on their doors and agree that Joe's behavior cannot be tolerated. Joe will no longer be welcome in their homes.

7. Are there any other actions that Ms. Jones could take to ensure that she is not a victim of any future financial mistreatment from her grandson or other family members?

The police find Joe and question him. There is enough evidence to arrest Joe for various other thefts and check forgery from Ms. Jones's neighborhood. Ms. Jones's jewelry had been sold from the local pawn shop and was not recovered. Joe is taken to juvenile detention.

8. How can older adults protect themselves from becoming victims of financial abuse or mistreatment?

Suggested Resources

Fulmer, T., & Caceres, B. A. (2012). *Elder mistreatment and abuse.* Hartford Institute for Geriatric Nursing. Retrieved from http://consultgerirn.org/topics/elder_mistreatment_and_abuse/want_to_know_more

National Adult Protective Services Association. (2014). *Elder financial exploitation.* Retrieved from http://www.napsa-now.org/policy-advocacy/world-elder-abuse-awareness-day

Case 3.5 ■ Health Care Disparities and the Elderly

*T*wo women live in an elderly housing complex and have many things in common about their lives. Both are 78 years old, and gave birth to one son and one daughter when in their 20s. Both were married for close to 20 years. Shared medical diagnoses include osteoporosis, hypertension, coronary heart disease, atrial fibrillation, and obesity. One woman, Eloise, receives $721 per month from Supplemental Security Income; her husband had sporadic employment as a general "handyman," was paid in cash for his services and had no savings. She was a waitress at a small diner and worked for tips only. Meanwhile, the other woman, Martha, never worked outside the home, her husband had 20 years with the railroad system before his death and she receives $1,450 per month from his pension.

The monthly rent each lady pays is $600, which includes utilities. Eloise chose to live at this site for safety, the proximity to public transportation, and from her children's encouragement because they reside a long distance away. She has no interaction with the hundreds of persons living in the complex with her. Martha sold the family homestead for a $500,000 profit and draws an extra $1,000 per month of interest from investing the money. She chose the housing complex as several of her long-term friends live there, so a convenient social circle exists, and she can use the parking garage for her car.

Last month each lady had another similar event occur; both experienced ischemic strokes. Martha was given a stroke warning card which she kept on her refrigerator and knew to contact 911 immediately when her speech became progressively slurred while on the phone. In addition, a recent screening for carotid artery stenosis revealed significant blockage and she received patient education from her primary care provider about this risk factor as likelihood of stroke. She took her Coumadin (warfarin) 5 mg tablet daily and never missed an appointment for international normalized ratio (INR) blood levels to evaluate clotting times. In addition to her Medicare standard coverage, she had purchased Part D so all her medications combined cost less than $40 per month.

Eloise uses a free clinic sponsored by the local health department that is staffed by volunteer physicians and nurses. It takes an hour to get there using the city bus and the round trip cost is over $10. She often waits up to 2 hours to be seen and, even then, feels rushed through the appointment. In the past, she was given forms to fill out for a reduced cost prescription program; the problem was she was illiterate and too proud to ask for assistance with the process. Therefore, Eloise has been cutting her 5 mg Coumadin tablets in half as $40 for this one drug each month is prohibitive.

Martha was inside a private hospital's emergency department and receiving tPA (tissue plasminogen activator) within 40 minutes of leaving her apartment. She recovered fully from her stroke with outpatient rehabilitation for mild hemiparesis in one arm.

On the day of Eloise's stroke, she became dizzy in her apartment and attempted to go from the kitchen table to her bedroom to lie down. However, her walking was so unstable, she more or less crawled to the room. She was quite scared and used prayer as a coping mechanism. She knew the older man next door went out each afternoon and returned at dusk. She decided to watch the daylight diminish from her bedroom window and would somehow make her way to his door to ask for assistance. Unfortunately, this never happened and Eloise died from complications within an hour.

There was one other difference between Martha and Eloise, and in this case, quite a significant one . . . the women's race; Martha was White while Eloise was Black.

Healthy People 2020 define a *health disparity* as "a particular type of health difference that is closely linked with social, economic, and/or environmental disadvantage. Health disparities adversely affect groups of people who have systematically experienced greater obstacles to health based on their racial or ethnic group; religion; socioeconomic status; gender; age; mental health; cognitive, sensory, or physical disability; sexual orientation or gender identity; geographic location; or other characteristics historically linked to discrimination or exclusion" (HealthyPeople.gov. Retrieved from www.healthypeople.gov/2020/about/foundation-health-measures/ Disparities).

1. *Compare and contrast the Healthy People goals in regard to disparities for the years 2000, 2010, and 2020.*

2. *List the disparities that Eloise experienced in contrast to Martha.*

3. *Report on the differences of African Americans and stroke compared to Whites using the following website from the National Stroke Association as a guideline: www.stroke.org/site/ PageServer?pagename=aamer*

4. *Using the statistics provided by the Administration on Aging (2013) website, www.aoa.gov/Aging_Statistics/Profile/2013/10 .aspx, compare the poverty rates for older Whites to African Americans, Asians, and Hispanics. Also, what group has the highest poverty rates in America?*

In the article *Social Justice, Health Disparities, and Culture in the Care of the Elderly* (Dilworth-Anderson, Pierre, & Hilliard, 2012), the authors focus on culturally correlated factors that perpetuate inequity using Alzheimer's disease as an example. Questions 5 to 8 will address these important social justice and disparity issues.

5. *In relation to "differences in perception about causes of the disease," what cultural belief do some Latinos believe about dementia?*

6. *The authors share information about African Americans' disparities in screening to validate the existence of Alzheimer's. What might be the underlying cause for this?*

7. *What are the two remaining disparities presented?*

8. *Watch* **The Faces of Disparity** *video, a 15-minute documentary that integrates personal stories of health care consumers with the perspectives of leading experts in health care and public health at www.ctmhp.org/press/faces-of-disparity-video. Comment on what comprises the CLAS Standards; a proposal for change.*

Suggested Resources

Administration on Community Living. (2013). *Administration on Aging (AoA). Poverty.* Washington, DC: U.S. Department of Health and Human Services.

Dilworth-Anderson, P., Pierre, G., & Hilliard, S. T. (2012). Social justice health disparities, and culture in the care of the elderly. *Journal of Law, Medicine & Ethics*, 26–32. Retrieved from http://oied.ncsu.edu/selc/wp-content/uploads/2013/03/Ditworth-Anderson-Social-Justice-Health-Disparity-and-Culture-in-the-Care-of-the-Elderly.pdf

National Conference of Health Legislators. (2014). *Health disparities overview.* Retrieved from http://www.ncsl.org/research/health/health-disparities-overview.aspx

4

Depression, Addiction, and Suicide

Case 4.1 ■ Alcoholism

An inner-city emergency department (ED) receives a report about an incoming 72-year-old man found disoriented, smelling of alcohol, and with a suspected hip fracture. Upon arrival to the ED, the patient, John Riley, has a blood alcohol level (BAL) of 0.17. He is 6 feet 1 inch tall and weighs 180 pounds. The ED doctor completes an x-ray of John's hip and does not find a fracture; however, the doctor notes old bruising on his arms and legs. His liver function tests of alanine aminotransferase (ALT) and aspartate aminotransferase (AST) are elevated (ALT = 53 IU/L and AST = 40 IU/L) so an additional gamma-glutamyltransferase (GGT) is ordered, indicating an elevated level at 72 IU/L.

1. ***What are the characteristic signs and symptoms of impaired liver function?***

The psych liaison nurse, Rob Pearson, RN, is paged to complete a psych evaluation on John to find out more about his alcohol consumption. John reports he only had two glasses of wine today.

2. ***Rob knows that John is minimizing his alcohol use and refers to http://hubpages.com/hub/How-to-calculate-BAC to estimate his actual consumption from the BAL Table for Men. Rob finds John has really consumed how many drinks?***

3. ***What does Rob realize about the importance of accurate alcohol screening?***

4. ***Rob understands that his questions should focus on which of the following?***

   a. ***Making John admit to his "real" alcohol consumption***

   b. ***Increasing John's feelings of guilt over his drinking, which will help him learn to stop***

   c. ***John's perceptions of his drinking behaviors and the consequences of his drinking***

   d. ***Teaching John the alcohol content in one drink***

Rob finds that John is drinking daily by administering the CAGE questionnaire (Ewing, 1984). He asks:

Have you ever felt you should **C**ut down on your drinking?

Have people **A**nnoyed you by criticizing your drinking?

Have you ever felt bad or **G**uilty about your drinking?

Have you ever had an **E**ye-opener drink first thing in the morning to steady your nerves or get rid of a hangover?

John states that he feels like he should cut down on his drinking and his daughter is constantly "on his case" about how much he drinks. He states, "If only I had the resources and ability to stop." John feels that he began drinking after his wife died 2 years ago. John relates when he tries to stop drinking, his hands start to shake, and he drinks a glass of wine to steady his nerves. He reports drinking 7 to 8 glasses of wine, on average, daily. The maximum amount John reports consuming is 1 gallon of wine.

5. What is one alcoholic drink defined as?

6. What are the potential risks with habitual and/or excessive alcohol use?

7. What additional signs and symptoms of alcohol-related abuse or dependence might be evident in the initial assessment?

Rob completes the Short Michigan Alcoholism Screening Test–Geriatric Version (SMAST-G) on John (www.positiveaging.org/provider/pdfs/alcohol_smast_g.pdf; Blow, 1991). John scores 9 out of 10, indicating alcohol is a problem. Rob also knows John has been drinking daily since his wife's death.

The American Psychological Association (APA) published the 5th edition of the *Diagnostic and Statistical Manual of Mental Disorders (DSM-5)* in May 2013. A major change from the earlier edition was that alcohol use disorders were broken down into two categories: *alcohol abuse* and *alcohol dependence*. According to the APA, the distinction between abuse and dependence was based on the concept of abuse as a mild or early phase, and dependence as the more severe manifestation. The most recent manual has a single diagnosis of alcohol abuse disorder which, according to the APA, will better match the symptoms that patients experience (Buddy, 2013).

8. Use the following web link to determine what criteria of the 11 identified must be met for John to be classified as having an alcohol abuse disorder: http://alcoholism.about.com/od/professionals/a/Dsm-5-Substance-Abuse-Disorders-Draws-Controversy.htm.

John states he will simply stop drinking on his own at home.

9. Rob strongly encourages John to transfer to the hospital's mental health floor and explains to John that receiving additional medical attention is imperative, because, if he attempts to stop drinking at home, he is at the highest risk for the following:

a. Withdrawal

b. Continuing to drink

c. Becoming nutritionally impaired

d. Increasing his isolation, putting him at risk for depression

John agrees to enter the detox program and signs in voluntarily for a transfer to the unit.

Suggested Resources

Blow, F. C. (1991). *Short Michigan Alcohol Screening Test–Geriatric Version (SMAST-G)*. Ann Arbor, MI: University of Michigan Alcohol Research Center.

Buddy, T. (2013). *DSM-5 substance abuse disorders draws controversy*. About.com Alcoholism. Retrieved from http://alcoholism.about.com/od/professionals/a/Dsm-5-Substance-Abuse-Disorders-Draws-Controversy.htm

Ewing, J. A. (1984). Detecting alcoholism: The CAGE questionnaire. *Journal of the American Medical Association, 252*, 1905–1907.

Case 4.2 ■ Prescription Pain Medication Misuse

*B*eatrice Christopher is an 80-year-old widowed Caucasian woman who has a history of benzodiazepine dependence. She has seen every prescriber in her small town to "prescription shop" and has received multiple prescriptions for her anxiety and pain. Beatrice has mild to moderate osteoarthritis (OA) and reports a score of 3 to 5 on a visual analogue scale for pain. Her Mini-Mental State Examination (MMSE), or Folstein test, indicates she has a score of 24, or no cognitive impairment. She is oriented to person, place, and time. She lives in her three-bedroom ranch style home with her grown son who has a history of mental illness.

1. What are the risks with multi-prescriber medication-seeking behaviors?

2. What steps can be taken to reduce the incidence of multiple prescriptions for the same controlled substance?

3. What questions should be asked to determine whether a patient's pain medications are being misused?

Beatrice makes an appointment with a new primary care provider. In her initial appointment, she describes to her doctor her history of OA and "severe" arthritic pain.

Her primary care physician prescribes propoxyphene napsylate (Darvon-N 50) and acetaminophen 325 mg one to two tablets every 4 to 6 hours. Her MMSE drops from 24 to between 10 and 12 (moderate cognitive impairment). Over the next 4 weeks, Beatrice falls three times and luckily is not severely injured. When attending church, her fellow church friends notice she has multiple bruises to her arms and face and is easily confused. Beatrice chuckles and states she has taken some falls. Her church pastor notices her struggles and hears from other parishioners the concerns they have for her health. Her pastor speaks with Beatrice and recommends a community program that helps the elderly with their health care needs.

Community Link is a volunteer program where nurses, clinical pharmacists, social workers, and other allied health professionals volunteer their time to improve the quality of life and health outcomes for the elderly in their community. After Beatrice's initial evaluation, Madelyn, one of the program's RNs, refers Beatrice to the clinical pharmacist to review her medications. Madelyn highlights her concerns about polypharmacy, medication misuse, and adverse events with the current regimen.

After Beatrice signs a consent form to release information, her primary care physician is contacted with regard to the clinical pharmacist's (Jim, RPh) recommendations to taper off and stop her propoxyphene. The physician states he has concern that she will simply ask for codeine or an oxycodone hydrochloride (OxyCotin) in the absence of some type of opioid pain medication.

> **4.** *Abruptly stopping benzodiazepines or opioids puts Beatrice at highest risk for which of the following? Select all that apply.*
>
> **a.** *Breakthrough pain*
>
> **b.** *Shopping for another doctor*
>
> **c.** *Finding another controlled substance as a substitute*
>
> **d.** *Symptoms of withdrawal*
>
> **5.** *What are the signs and symptoms of opioid withdrawal?*
>
> **6.** *When stopping opioids, how long until withdrawal symptoms are evident?*

After evaluating Beatrice's renal and liver function, Jim, recommends placing Beatrice on regular Tylenol (acetaminophen) 500 mg every 4 hours around the clock, 6 a.m., 10 a.m., 2 p.m., 6 p.m., and 10 p.m. The clinical pharmacist recommends she have a sixth dose, should she wake in the middle of the night with pain. The goal is to titrate the propoxyphene dose down to be discontinued, however, still allowing for pain coverage. She is transitioned to Darvon without acetaminophen, because starting her new medication regimen in addition to the existing acetaminophen would exceed the daily dose recommended of acetaminophen.

> **7.** *The clinical pharmacist also understands that the use of benzodiazepines and opioids puts Beatrice at significant risk for the following:*
>
> **a.** *Falls*
>
> **b.** *Constipation*

c. *Accidental overdose*

d. *All of the above*

The physician agrees to transition her benzodiazepines from Valium (diazepam) to Ativan (lorazepam) and then switch to Serax (oxazepam). This step-down program of shorter half-life benzos will attempt to convert her over to the shortest acting sedative possible to reduce the risk of falls. Beatrice admits that she has a history of depression, pain, and "horrible" anxiety, but agrees to this treatment plan. Beatrice's new treatment will be taking Buspar (buspirone) 30 mg daily for her anxiety, continue the acetaminophen, and, over the next 2 weeks, completely taper her off of the oxazepam.

Her primary care physician has doubts as to whether Beatrice will be able to adhere to this treatment plan, as her son reports she has a history of stealing his benzodiazepines and oxycodone. The case management records on Beatrice also note that she has reported her son steals her medications and, in the past, she has come up short at the end of the month.

8. *What recommendations could the nurse give to increase the probability that Beatrice will adhere to her new care plan?*

Suggested Resource

Townsend, M. (2007). Substance-related disorders. In M. Townsend (Ed.), *Essentials of psychiatric mental health nursing: Concepts of care in evidence-based practice* (4th ed., pp. 278–280). Philadelphia, PA: F.A. Davis.

Case 4.3 ■ Depression

James Edwards, an 88-year-old retired factory worker, resides in an independent living apartment in a continuing care retirement community (CCRC). He is relatively healthy, still able to care for his personal needs, and is able to drive. His four children, who all live within a 30-mile radius of the CCRC, have arranged for monthly cleaning of his apartment. They see him almost every weekend and once or twice during the week to go with him to appointments or to socialize. Mr. Edwards has a history of bladder cancer and has an ileal conduit for urinary diversion for which he provides his own care. He also has type 2 diabetes and is fully capable of injecting his own insulin, along with taking responsibility for self-care of this disease. All things considered, he has been relatively healthy in recent years, caring for his wife of 66 years who suffered from dementia and died 2 years ago. Since the death of his wife, Mr. Edwards has grown increasingly isolated. He used to play golf regularly and help other residents of the CCRC with transportation and other small projects for which they sought his help.

In recent months, however, Mr. Edwards has reported to his children that he no longer finds pleasure in golf or helping others, and prefers instead to sit in his apartment watching television, playing games on his computer, or even just sitting alone without engaging in any activities. The family has grown increasingly concerned about their father and has decided to investigate his symptoms, despite the fact that their father insists he is just fine.

Mr. Edwards's internist recommends a home visit from a nurse practitioner specializing in geriatric mental health. After taking a medical history from the client, the nurse practitioner explains he would like to use a questionnaire known as the Geriatric Depression Scale (GDS) to illicit further data.

1. *Using the website http://consultgerirn.org/uploads/File/trythis/ try_this_4.pdf, describe the purpose, reliability, and method of using the GDS (Greenberg, 2012). Would you consider implementing this scale in working with the elderly (explain your reason)?*

To answer Questions 2 and 3, refer to the American Psychological Association's (2014) website www.apa.org/helpcenter/aging-depression.aspx.

2. *What are some of the physical effects of depression on older people?*

3. *What are some actions a nurse might suggest to the family as they grapple with their father's symptoms?*

To answer Questions 4 to 6, please refer to the Centers for Disease Control and Prevention (2012) website at www.cdc.gov/aging/mentalhealth/depression.htm.

4. *Describe four of the many symptoms of depression.*

5. *The family asks the nurse, "How common is depression in older adults?" Which of the following is the best response?*

   a. *Depression is rare in older adults; it almost never occurs (< 1%).*

   b. *Depression is extremely common in older adults (> 50%); in fact, it is a normal part of aging.*

   c. *Depression estimates range from less than 1% (among community-dwelling older adults) to 13.5% (among those receiving home-based health care).*

   d. *Depression among older adults is only seen in those persons living in skilled care nursing facilities (about 25% of these older adults are depressed).*

6. *The family asks how depression might be different in their father than in a younger adult. What could the nurse tell them about depression in older adults?*

7. *The family wants to explore online information about depression among older adults. What are three reputable websites to which you might refer this family?*

Refer to the Geriatric Mental Health Foundation's (n.d.) website to answer Questions 8 and 9 at www.gmhfonline.org/gmhf/consumer/late_life_depression_trtmn.html.

8. *Mr. Edwards's family asks the nurse, "Is depression in older adults treatable?" What could the nurse accurately tell the family?*

9. *After Mr. Edwards saw the geriatric health care practitioner, he received an antidepressant medication as a treatment for his depression. The family asks the nurse, "How long will it take for our father to start to feel better from his symptoms of depression?" What is an accurate response to this question?*

10. *Mr. Edwards's daughter inquires about alternative and complementary measures to assist with his depression. What herbal and supplemental agents have been studied? What mind–body techniques have been used? Cite the source for your findings.*

Suggested Resources

American Psychological Association. (2014). *Aging and depression.* Retrieved from http://www .apa.org/helpcenter/aging-depression.aspx

Centers for Disease Control and Prevention. (2012). *Depression is not a normal part of growing older.* Retrieved from http://www.cdc.gov/aging/mentalhealth/depression.htm

Geriatric Mental Health Foundation. (n.d.). *Treatment options for late-life depression.* Retrieved from http://www.gmhfonline.org/gmhf/consumer/late_life_depression_trtmn.html

Greenberg, S. A. (2012). *Try this—Issue 4 the geriatric depression scale (GDS).* Hartford Institute for Geriatric Nursing. Retrieved from http://consultgerirn.org/uploads/File/trythis/try_this_4.pdf

Mayo Clinic Staff. (2014). *Depression (major depression) alternative medicine.* Retrieved from http://www.mayoclinic.com/health/depression/DS00175/DSECTION=alternative-medicine

Case 4.4 ■ Gambling Disorder

Jenny Parker is in her second year as a public health nurse in a small midwest river town. Prior to this position, she worked on a medical–surgical floor in a large teaching hospital for several years and then joined the home health services of that organization where she stayed for a decade. Jenny finds working with the community a challenging, yet rewarding, area of practice. She is the only RN within her public health department. She spent most of the first year of employment conducting a needs assessment and becoming familiar with the community.

What transpired the second year has definitely affected the social and economic climate of the community; a casino boat opened in a nearby town. A political vote was held, and the casino was highly supported by the majority. New jobs, a new tax base for the county, and a new source of entertainment became available. In addition, grant monies for education, health care, and social services were promised by the casino owners.

Despite all the excitement and favorable views, Jenny has been informed of problems, which have surfaced in recent months. The town mayor contacted her to be a member of a task force to explore the effects of gambling on the elderly population.

1. What other types of individuals from the community might be invited to serve as members on the task force with Jenny?

Jenny has read various e-mails sent to the mayor's office complaining about the casino and asking, actually demanding, that the top town officials take action. Letters from family members of elderly individuals address numerous concerns, such as those with Martha O'Riley. She is an 84-year-old widow who has been visiting the casino regularly for months. Her daughter states, "Everything was fine until the slot machines took over her life." Martha lives alone in the rural section of town and does not drive. She is an insulin-dependent diabetic and has hypertension and coronary artery disease. Her only hobby is working crossword puzzles. Otherwise, watching television, light housekeeping, and preparing simple meals describe her life since losing her spouse 4 years ago. Her daughter calls daily and stops by every weekend.

Martha saw an ad on television for "Senior Day" at the casino. There was valet parking, a buffet meal, door prizes every hour, and $20 worth of free tokens to play the slot machines. All the old people in the ad looked like they were having so much fun.

She knew her neighbor down the road had secured a part-time position at the casino, so she arranged a ride to the casino with the neighbor.

2. Martha's lifestyle situation is common to many older people. What do you think has attracted her to gambling?

Martha's daughter was not terribly concerned with her mother's early visits to the casino. The neighbor who provided transportation worked a couple of 4-hour shifts per week at the casino, and Martha initially went only once a week. However, when the neighbor changed to full-time status, Martha began leaving home to visit the casino at 7 a.m. and returning after 4 p.m.

3. Based on Martha's active medical problems, what concerns might her daughter have for her physical well-being while she is away from home for most of the day?

In addition to physical health concerns, Martha's daughter is concerned her mother might be developing a gambling disorder. One of Jenny's co-members on the task force is a psychologist. He shares these warning signs with the group:

1. Lying
2. Chasing losses
3. Always betting more
4. Being obsessed with gambling
5. Gambling out of need

6. Gambling to forget

7. Stealing or committing fraud to gamble

8. Gambling because it is the most important thing in the world (Gambling: Help and Referral, n.d)

Jenny shares a screening tool for assessing problem gambling she discovered in a recent nursing journal article.

> **4. Using the Internet, find at least two screening tools and cite the names, a brief description, and the reference source for each.**

> **5. Jenny asks the psychologist for information regarding risk factors for problem gambling. What would the psychologist likely share with the committee in regard to risk factors?**

Another member of the task force represents the state's Gaming Association. He shares that every state in the nation, with the exception of Hawaii and Utah, has some form of legalized gambling. Twenty-eight percent of people aged 65 and older visited a casino in the past 12 months according to the American Gaming Association (2014).

Martha O'Riley's daughter's other primary concern for her mother is financially focused. She states her mother is debt-free and she needs to remain so. She receives $1,400 per month from Social Security and has several hundred thousand dollars in stock investments her late husband left her. Martha has refused to tell her daughter any information about her spending at the casino. She has repeated several times, "I am an adult, fully competent, and it's my business only."

> **6. What are your thoughts on Martha's response? Is her daughter's concern justified?**

Another member of the task force is a 76-year-old female who was invited to join based on her past gambling experiences. Ethyl Moore played poker on the Internet after retiring from a lifelong career as a school teacher. She states that what started as a way to pass time for an hour or so a day became a compulsion, which took over her entire being. Over a 6-year span, Ethyl neglected her physical needs, became socially isolated, and took a second mortgage on her home to support the gaming. An intervention by her family and close friends was arranged, and she has not gambled in any form for nearly a decade. Ethyl is a member of Gamblers Anonymous (GA) and continues to attend meetings at least monthly.

> **7. Prepare a brief review of this support group. Include the date of origin, framework, and how GA is designed to assist those with a gaming addiction.**

After the initial meeting of the community task force, Jenny drafts a strategic plan for the group to discuss and further develop. Her overall goal is to "prevent gambling of any form to becoming a public health issue."

> **8. What are examples of devastating outcomes in the lives of gambling-addicted elderly people that Jenny is attempting to address?**

Suggested Resources

American Gaming Association. (2014). *2013 state of the states. The AGA survey of casino entertainment.* Retrieved from http://www.americangaming.org/sites/default/files/aga_sos2013_rev042014.pdf

Gamblers Anonymous. (n.d.). Retrieved from http://www.gamblersanonymous.org/ga/about.html

Gambling: Help and Referral. (n.d.). *10 signs of problem gambling.* Retrieved from http://www.jeu-aidereference.qc.ca/www/signs_problem_gambling_en.asp?cmpt=2

Mayo Clinic. (2014, February). *Compulsive gambling: Risk factors.* Retrieved from http://www.mayoclinic.org/diseases-conditions/compulsive-gambling/basics/risk-factors/con-20023242

Case 4.5 ▪ Risk for Suicide

*I*n a small college town, Susan Cooper, the nurse coordinator for the medical home initiative in a local primary care provider's office, assesses a new client. The nurse introduces herself and goes over the intake form with Helen Wright to plan for her care management. Ms. Wright was referred by the local ED because of repeated visits and complaints of "no one caring" for her or her well-being. The ED staff voiced concern for Ms. Wright, because she is estranged from her family, lives by herself, and has a long history of bipolar disorder. Ms. Wright's recent visits to the ED center on vague somatic complaints, and she often leaves before being seen by the doctor, stating that they are wasting her time and what is the point?

> 1. *What is a key benefit of medical home models for care coordination? Use the following link for assistance: www.commonwealthfund.org/publications/from-the-president/2009/can-patient-centered-medical-homes-transform-health-care-delivery (Davis, Abrams, & Haran, 2009).*
>
> 2. *Because of the referral information, what should the nurse assess in Ms. Wright's initial appointment?*

Nurse Susan reviews Ms. Wright's chart and finds she is a 72-year-old widow, who has lived in the same house for the past 40 years. Her husband died 7 years ago. Ms. Wright states her health has been poor, especially since she was recently diagnosed with diabetes. The ED report indicates her type 2 diabetes is well managed, along with her hypertension. Her clinical notes indicate that she often displays attention-seeking behaviors with vague physical symptoms. She reports taking Ambien (zolpidem) 10 mg, as needed at bedtime, due to an inability sleep; Remeron (mirtazapine) 15 mg at bedtime; Prozac (fluoxetine hydrochloride) 20 mg daily, admitting she sometimes forgets to take the morning dose, so sometimes she takes it in the afternoon or evening; Lithium 600 mg three times a day; Xanax (alprazolam) 0.50 mg as needed for anxiety; Glucophage (metformin) 500 mg twice a day with meals; and

Calan (verapamil) 240 mg daily. Her hemoglobin A1C is 6.5, her morning fasting blood sugar was 112, her lithium level is 1.0, and her blood pressure is 118/74. Ms. Wright states she often finds that life is not worth living and wishes she would die. Ms. Wright states her children are ungrateful and refuse to visit her. Notes on her chart indicate that family members have been present at ED visits in the past, but Ms. Wright is verbally abusive and her mood is labile at times.

3. ***What are common symptoms that the nurse should screen for with depression in Ms. Wright?***

4. ***What additional information would the nurse assess to determine suicide risk?***

5. ***What protective factors could help reduce suicide risk?***

Ms. Wright has a flattened affect and makes poor eye contact; she is oriented to person, place, and time. She reports difficulty sleeping at times and anxiety when she is unable to fall asleep. The nurse notes Ms. Wright is well-groomed and has a body mass index (BMI) of 23 with a petite 5-foot 2-inch frame. Ms. Wright has no limitations with her range of motion and states that she goes to the grocery store weekly. She states she used to attend church, but no longer attends because "those old cronies are just busy bodies."

6. ***What areas should the nurse probe in more detail to assess suicide risk with Ms. Wright?***

7. ***How should the nurse approach asking whether Ms. Wright is having suicidal thoughts?***

Nurse Susan asks, "How do you feel about living by yourself?" Ms. Wright crosses her arms and says, "Well I am fine, what a silly question . . . my family says I am not easy to live with, because some days I am up, but most days I am down. They get tired of listening, so now I am just tired of living." Ms. Wright reports to Susan that she feels passive about suicide and denies having a plan. She states she had attempted suicide about 20 years ago by overdosing on her medications; however, she denies a current suicide plan, stating she knows that would be wrong.

8. ***What type of safety plan should the nurse establish with Ms. Wright?***

Ms. Wright agrees to enter into a verbal contract and see the social worker at the practice to establish a mental health care plan, along with managing her diabetes and high blood pressure with the primary care doctor. Nurse Susan gives her a hotline number that is available 24/7, should Ms. Wright feel alone and want someone to talk with: National Suicide Prevention Lifeline at www.suicidepreventionlifeline.org; 1-800-273-TALK (8255).

The nurse takes this opportunity to review Ms. Wright's medications and develop a medication therapy management (MTM) plan to improve her care outcomes (Cooper & Burfield, 2007). The nurse reminds Ms. Wright to take her lithium after meals with plenty of water to reduce stomach upset, and to have her lithium level checked monthly.

9. Ms. Wright's medication regimen put her at the highest risk for which of the following? Select all that apply.

  a. Neurotoxicity

  b. Falls

  c. Constipation

  d. Bradycardia

Nurse Susan recommends a medication review by the clinical pharmacist and with the care planning team at their clinic. Susan explains that she has concern about the combination of her medications and the risk of medication interactions and her risk of falling. The nurse explains that her Prozac should only be taken first thing in the morning, as this medication can cause excitability, making it difficult to go to sleep if taken too close to bedtime. Ms. Wright verbalizes an understanding of her medications and agrees to return for further coordination of services. Ms. Wright states she feels much better having someone to talk to and knowing she can come to this one location and access all her care.

Suggested Resources

Centers for Disease Control and Prevention. (2012). *Web-based inquiry statistics query and reporting system (WISQARS)*. National Center for Injury Prevention and Control CDC Web site. Retrieved from http://www.cdc.gov/injury/wisqars/index.html

Cooper, J. W., & Burfield, A. H. (2007). Medication therapy management (MTM) strategies for geriatric patient interventions: Medicare part D implementation. *Annals of Long-Term Care: Clinical and Aging, 15*(7), 33–38.

Davis, K., Abrams, M. K., & Haran, C. (2009). *Can patient-centered medical homes transform health care delivery?* The Commonwealth Fund. Retrieved from http://www.commonwealthfund.org/publications/from-the-president/2009/can-patient-centered-medical-homes-transform-health-care-delivery

5

Assessment and Management of Individual Issues

Case 5.1 ■ Spirituality and Aging

*C*arly, a student in her first semester of nursing school, is currently taking a fundamentals course. The topic covered today was spirituality and nursing. She really enjoyed the instructor's presentation and it has her thinking about a number of things and wanting to know even more about this topic. Carly was raised in a Lutheran church; she still attends, although on a sporadic basis because she works as a pharmacy tech on weekends to help pay tuition.

Use the following resource in assisting with the first three questions: www .merckmanuals.com/home/older_peoples_health_issues/social_issues_affecting_ older_people/religion_and_spirituality_in_older_people.html.

1. The class started with comparing and contrasting the difference between an individual being religious or spiritual. What information can you find about this?

Carly's grandmothers are both in their mid-60s. She has thought a lot about the difference in their daily lives. Her father's mother is definitely religious; she is a member of a Baptist church and attends services every Wednesday evening and Sunday morning. In addition, she volunteers with both the cleaning of the inside and maintaining the flowers outside of the church building. Carly loves this grandmother immensely, but she has noticed in the past few years there are more "rules" she lives by than what she believes are necessary. For example, she will not associate with any person who drinks alcohol, she will only listen to church hymns and no other type of music, and doesn't seem to approve of Carly and her sister's choice of clothing.

On the other hand, her maternal grandmother has not attended a place of worship for decades. Grandma Nelson is the kindest person Carly has ever known. She helps at a homeless shelter, has loads of friends from "all walks of life," and has a wonderful sense of humor. Meditation is a regular event as well as a love for all things associated with nature. Grandma Nelson lives in a very small home, sparsely furnished, and jokes about being a "low-maintenance woman." Carly decides she is truly a spiritual person.

2. What statistics does the Merck Manual article share about the role of religion for older people in the United States?

Carly's nursing instructor used the following statement during her presentation in class. "People who are religious tend to have better physical and mental health than nonreligious people. However, experts cannot determine whether religion contributes to health or whether psychologically or physically healthier people are attracted to religious groups. If religion is helpful, the reason—whether it is the religious beliefs themselves or other factors—is not clear" (Kaplan & Berkman, 2013).

3. Provide an example of how religion can positively impact mental health, health promotion, and social experiences.

Carly is quickly learning about the need to assess patients prior to planning and implementing care. Her instructor reviewed the FICA Spiritual History Tool (Borneman, 2011) in class. She found this to be very user friendly and does not feel she will have any hesitation using it during her career.

4. Describe what the tool entails. It can be found from the Hartford Institute for Geriatric Nursing located at http://consultgerirn. org/uploads/File/trythis/try_this_sp5.pdf.

5. What other assessment measures are available for spiritual purposes?

Carly's class was encouraged to look at spirituality of older people insofar as ethnicity. Use the website http://cas.umkc.edu/casww/sa/Spirituality.htm for the remaining questions.

6. Match the following spiritual characteristics with the appropriate group listed here.

_____ **Strategies used in resolving adverse experiences include accepting reality, turning things over to a higher power, identifying life lessons, recognizing purpose and destiny, and achieving growth.**

_____ **Women, especially, use their religious and cultural traditions to adjust to their new country, sustain their families, and build more secure communities.**

_____ **The group vests many of their beliefs and spiritual powers in nature, the land, and animals.**

_____ **Programs to promote intergenerational healing among the four distinct generations in families are developing in communities.**

a. **African American women**

b. **Japanese Americans**

c. **Native Americans**

d. **Mexican Americans**

7. What six events do Ebersole and Hess (1998) classify as "Threats to Spirituality"?

8. Describe actions nurses can use to provide individuals with spiritual care.

Suggested Resources

Borneman, T. (2011). *Assessment of spirituality in older adults: FICA spiritual history tool.* The Hartford Institute for Geriatric Nursing. Retrieved from http://consultgerirn.org/uploads/File/trythis/try_this_sp5.pdf

Ebersole, P., & Hess, P. (1998). *Toward healthy aging: Human needs and nursing response* (5th ed.). St. Louis, MO: Mosby.

Kaplan, D. B., & Berkman, B. J. (2013). *Religion and spirituality in older people.* Merck Manuals. Retrieved from http://www.merckmanuals.com/home/older_peoples_health_issues/social_issues_affecting_older_people/religion_and_spirituality_in_older_people.html

Case 5.2 ■ Frailty

*A*shton Hayes is a 25-year-old senior nursing student beginning a capstone course, which requires 150 clock hours over the semester. She has chosen a facility that offers skilled and assistive living, along with an Alzheimer's/memory care unit. Ashton volunteered here during her high school freshman and sophomore summers. Assisting the activities director was an enjoyable experience because it was an Eden Alternative facility, which Ashton found impressive. She helped the residents plant and care for outside flower gardens, gave the unit's dogs baths, prepared homemade ice cream, and had cookouts on the patio. But the most memorable part was the interaction with the senior citizens, hearing their stories and observing how low stressed their lives appeared.

During Ashton's junior year of high school, her maternal grandmother moved in with her family. At the time of arrival, her "Grammy" was 70 years old and needed short-term help after knee replacement surgery. Unfortunately, an ischemic stroke that followed resulted in much more around-the-clock care over the years. Ashton's mother worked full time to support the family, so Ashton tended to her siblings and Grammy's needs. This meant delaying college for 3 years.

Selecting a capstone experience was not a tough decision for Ashton. Although she enjoyed most of her coursework and clinical rotations in nursing school, geriatrics was her favorite area and hopeful future career focus. She will be working with Carla Sanchez, clinical services director, who will be her designated preceptor at the facility. The pair met and planned a tentative schedule for the upcoming rotation. Goals and objectives were developed by Ashton, which Carla approved and then added specific activities to assist with learning.

This week, Ashton will study, observe, and apply material related to the topic of frailty. When attending doctor visits with her grandmother several years back, she often heard Grammy referred to as "frail" from health care providers. She tells Carla, "I don't really know the difference between frailty, disability, and a term my nursing instructors use regularly: co-morbidity." Carla explains the terms are actually inter-related and that frailty is considered a syndrome.

Assessment of frailty is the next topic for exploration. Carla and Ashton look at the nursing literature for evidence-based tools. The facility uses an adaptation of Fried et al.'s *Phenotype for Frailty* (2001). Criteria to measure with this tool include shrinking, exhaustion, strength, slowness, and low physical activity. Carla requests that Ashton utilize the tool with Mrs. Gibson, a 91-year-old resident at the facility.

Through physical assessment and reading her history, Carla finds Mrs. Gibson's spouse of nearly seven decades died within the past year. Since that time, she had a gastrostomy tube insertion for nutrition following a 14-pound weight loss, in addition to becoming fatigued with any physical activity, and requiring a wheel-chair for mobility (previously ambulated without assistance). Mrs. Gibson has with-drawn verbally to the point that it was not possible to assess cognitive function. Ashton determines Mrs. Gibson meets the criteria for primary frailty; she then con-trasts her own grandmother's situation and recognizes secondary frailty was the challenge in her case.

Use the Hartford Geriatric Institute for Nursing website for the following questions. *Frailty and Its Implication for Care* (Benefield & Higbee, 2007) is located at http://consultgerirn.org/topics/frailty_and_its_implications_for_care_new/want_to_know_more.

1. **Compare and contrast the definitions for frailty, disability, and co-morbidity.**

2. **Explain why frailty is considered a syndrome.**

3. **View the frailty assessment tool and determine Mrs. Gibson's actual score.**

4. **Differentiate primary versus secondary frailty.**

Ashton completes a number of assigned readings regarding research on frailty. She discovers there are four broad categories scientists attribute as risk factors. These include physiologic events, presence of certain medical illnesses, sociode-mographic/psychological data, and disability. Once again, she thinks back to her grandmother's risk factors and certain ones that may have been avoidable, or at least controlled better.

Use the article *Risk Factors for Frailty in the Older Adult* (Espinoza & Fried, 2007) at www.geroupr.com/Risk_Factors_for_Frailty_in_the_Older_Adult.doc to answer the following questions.

5. **What criteria comprise the six physiologic-based risk factors for frailty?**

6. **Discuss the sociodemographic and psychological risk factors presented in the article.**

7. **Which of the risk factors reviewed for frailty would not be modifiable?**

8. *What may be a preventive approach to avoiding frailty with aging? Watch an interview with Dr. Linda Fried via PBS at www .pbs.org/lifepart2/exclusives/dr-linda-fried-frailty-and-how-fight-it.*

In discussing the interventions for treating the frail elderly, Ashton is aware that the overall goal is to minimize further weight loss, decline of muscle mass and strength, and reduce fall risk factors to help maintain a state of homeostasis. She has a strong interest in complementary and alternative medicine and uses many approaches herself for stress management while in nursing school. In relation to weight loss and frailty, Ashton reads an article that provides an overview of suggested methods for the management and treatment of fraility (Morley, 2002) found at www.thedoctorwillseeyounow .com/content/aging/art2070.html.

9. *Using the acronym FRAILITY, what measures are suggested?*

10. *Using the same Internet source, discuss how tai chi may be an appropriate intervention.*

Ashton concentrates on outcomes that institutions will demonstrate to meet the various goals. She notes that on the Hartford Institute for Geriatric Nursing website, one outcome is "environments that reflect universal design sensitive to older adult needs" (Benefield & Higbee, 2007). She is unfamiliar with the term "universal design" and plans on learning more about this concept when she returns to clinical next week.

11. *What are specific examples used in facilities/agencies that implement universal design?*

Suggested Resources

Benefield, L. E., & Higbee, R. L. (2007). *Frailty and its implication for care.* Hartford Institute for Geriatric Nursing. Retrieved from http://consultgerirn.org/topics/ frailty_and_its_implications_for_care_new/want_to_know_more

Espinoza, S. E., & Fried, L. P. (2007). *Risk factors for frailty in the older adult.* Johns Hopkins Medicine. Retrieved from www.geroupr.com/Risk_Factors_for_Frailty_in_the_Older_Adult.doc

Fried, L. P., Tangen, C. M., Walston, J., Newman, A. B., Hirsch, C., Gottdiener, J., et al. (2001). Frailty in older adults: Evidence for a phenotype. *Journals of gerontology. Series A, Biological sciences and medical sciences.*

Morely, J. (2002). *Fraility: Management and treatment.* Retrieved from http://www .thedoctorwillseeyounow.com/content/aging/art2070.html

Case 5.3 ■ Functional Decline in the Hospitalized Elderly

June Evans is a 72-year-old retired school teacher who traveled from the East to West Coast several weeks ago to assist her daughter in a very important mission. Through artificial insemination, June's daughter gave birth to twin boys as a single mother; the babies are now home and weigh 6 pounds each. June promised to stay a month to allow her daughter to form a routine and find a full-time nanny prior to returning to work as an accountant.

All went well the first week; the infants primarily slept, and the ladies traded off nighttime feedings. However, during the second week, June tripped over an infant carrier in the darkness and experienced an intertrochanteric fractured hip as a result. She was admitted to the local hospital for a total hip arthroplasty procedure.

Initially, the physical pain was not nearly as uncomfortable as the emotional pain associated with this accident. June felt immense guilt leaving her daughter to tend to the babies alone. Whether it was driven by being overwhelmed, worry, or perhaps just personality, June's daughter spoke harshly to her mother while waiting for an ambulance. "How could you do this to me? What am I suppose to do now? You are so clumsy" were but a few of the accusations made. June did not hear from her daughter prior to having surgery the next afternoon.

The first 72 hours in the hospital were miserable. June felt completely powerless insofar as having no input into her care or participating with the simplest decisions. She refused to eat anything but fruit on her meal tray because the food had no seasoning. In addition, there was no access to the cola drink that served as her main form of fluid intake; the water pitcher was not within reach at her bedside. The narcotic she received made her nauseous; therefore, she chose not to take it. The two physical therapists assigned to her case were very friendly but she felt they were too "rough" with her so she began refusing to get out of bed. No one came in to help her change position. She had a different RN every shift and felt they were much more interested in her bowels than anything else.

The discharge planning nurse was an exception; she would visit June twice a day. Her cell phone constantly buzzed, yet the nurse ignored it and focused on June exclusively. She contacted June's daughter repeatedly for input on a rehab facility in the area but did not receive a return call. The discharge planner felt sympathy for June's situation, but "had a job to do" and explained to June that she would be transferred to another site for extensive rehabilitation.

June actually liked the environment better at the new health care facility. It was quieter and she was left alone to sleep or watch television for extended periods of time. On day four June was told she had developed pneumonia and would require intravenous antibiotic therapy. On day six, June became disoriented to place and time, likely triggered by a urinary tract infection.

June was transferred back to the hospital on day 10 of the rehab program. She was found to have a 12% postoperative weight loss, a Stage II pressure ulcer over the sacrum, and multiple electrolyte imbalances, with the admitting diagnosis of acute respiratory failure. Her daughter was contacted and made a do not resuscitate order for her mother as she needed ventilator assistance. June could not participate in this decision due to extensive cognitive decline. She died several days later. The discharge planner stayed with her during the last hour of life.

June's story represents an all-too-common occurrence within the acute care system for elderly clients; the complication of functional decline. Many acute care hospitals, and the nurses who work in them, are using best practices to avoid this event through delivering holistic-based assessments and interventions with a comprehensive approach to avoidance. The questions that follow will focus on these overall approaches.

1. *Let's first begin with learning more about the term deconditioning.*
   Provide a definition and indicate what is the most predictable
   body system affected. An article by Lewis and Shaw (2012) found
   at http://occupational-therapy.advanceweb.com/Features/Articles/
   Preventing-Deconditioning-in-Older-Adults.aspx may be helpful.

Use the evidence-based guidelines from Chapter 11 of *Patient Safety and Quality: An Evidence-Based Handbook for Nurses* (2008) for answering Questions 2 to 5 at www.ahrq.gov/professionals/clinicians-providers/resources/nursing/resources/nurseshdbk/KleinpellR_RFDHE.pdf.

2. *Table 1 in this handbook reviews the physiologic effects of bed rest*
   for a hospitalized elderly individual. Review these and comment
   on what material was new to your knowledge base.

3. *Deconditioning and functional decline from baseline was found*
   to occur by which day of hospitalization in elderly patients?

4. *Preadmission health and functional status of the elderly*
   can indicate risk of further functional decline associated
   with hospitalization. Although no details were provided about
   June's history, what are common indicators research supports
   to be predictive?

"Comprehensive geriatric assessment (CGA) is used to create a plan of care for hospitalized elders. A specific goal of the CGA is early identification of elder care needs in order to provide interventions to minimize high-risk events such as falls or the onset of delirium" (Kleinpell, Fletcher, & Jennings, 2008, p. 4).

5. *What are the components of a geriatric comprehensive assessment?*

A framework was developed by the American Academy of Nursing's Expert Panels on Acute and Critical Care, Aging and Quality Health Care on the theme Healthy Care Environments for Older Adults—Creating a Culture of Care. A schematic diagram is shown on the Hartford Institute for Geriatric Nursing at http://consultgerirn.org/uploads/File/trythis/try_this_31.pdf.

6. *List the eight elements representing goals for creating a healthy*
   care environment for elderly adults.

7. *Best practice literature for promoting nutrition in the*
   hospitalized elderly includes "rescinding restrictive (dietary)
   orders." What is your opinion about June's food and fluid
   preferences not being met? What suggestions can you offer?

8. *What occurred in the case study regarding social support for*
   June? Did you find her daughter's reaction to hospitalization
   uncommon?

Suggested Resources

Kleinpell, R. M., Fletcher, K., & Jennings, B. M. (2008). Reducing functional decline in hospitalized elderly. In R. G. Hughes (Ed.), *Patient safety and quality: An evidence-based handbook for nurses*. Agency for Healthcare Research and Quality. U.S. Dept. of Health and Human Services. Retrieved from http://www.ahrq.gov/professionals/clinicians-providers/resources/nursing/resources/nurseshdbk/KleinpellR_RFDHE.pdf

Lewis, C., & Shaw, K. (2012). *Preventing deconditioning in older adults*. Advance Healthcare Network. Retrieved from http://occupational-therapy.advanceweb.com/Features/Articles/Preventing-Deconditioning-in-Older-Adults.aspx

Case 5.4 ■ Aging in Place

*L*indsay and Matt Kisch are a couple in their early 30s who have been married for 5 years. They have been invited to have dinner with Matt's parents this evening and were told, "We have some news to share with you." Lindsay is concerned her in-laws are going to announce a move to Florida as they are both retiring in the near future. This is a concern because Lindsay has just confirmed a first pregnancy, and very much wants grandparents nearby to assist in raising their child. Her father lives on the West Coast, far away from their Ohio residency, and his health has declined significantly after her mother died several years ago.

Matt's parents, Joan and Bob Kisch, are in their mid-60s and have owned a home improvement store for more than three decades. A buyout offer came by surprise from a local contractor and they immediately agreed to sell the business. They have considered a variety of options for housing and a potential move out of Ohio. Both are in good health, Matt is an only child, and neither have any obligation to their own parents, as they are no longer living.

When the family got together that evening, Bob got the conversation started by telling the kids, "We have made a decision about where to live once the business is gone, and are very pleased with our choice." Matt and Lindsay sat in silence, expecting there would be a home on the real estate market before their baby was born.

Joan shared that she had been reading and "studying" an option they first learned about at a home improvement trade show. She went on to explain since about 2011, they were seeing and experiencing a huge trend toward appliances, fixtures, flooring, and a multitude of other new items for homeowners to increase safety, as well as make transitioning into older age more comfortable and flexible. She asked the couple, "We are going to age in place; have you heard of this concept?"

1. Find a definition on the Internet for "aging in place" (AIP).

Matt's dad went on to explain they loved their neighborhood of many years, did not want to navigate a new town with heavy traffic, change churches, and make new friends; since their home was paid off, they would be investing only a few thousand dollars for the necessary changes. He also said, "We cannot imagine being in Florida in the event you all ever give us a grandchild, or two." At that point, Matt and Lindsay shared their own good news and had many questions related to this new idea of AIP.

Dr. Patick Roden created a website and blog with a focus on AIP. Use the tabs at the top of the page found at http://aginginplace.com/mini-2/key-ingredients/ for Questions 2 to 5.

2. *Under AIP Key Ingredients, two of the benefits the author discusses are preserving brain function through "environmental press" and exposing adults to "environmental complexity." Explain what each of these concepts mean in relation to a positive outcome of AIP.*

3. *The areas of most challenge in adapting a home to meet an aging person's needs include the entry and exit points, going up and down stairs, and safety in the bathroom. Review the recommendations and comment on what information was new to you.*

4. *What are the seven principles of universal design?*

5. *Residents in Boston's Beacon Hill neighborhood planned the country's first "virtual" retirement community; briefly describe what this model for AIP entails.*

6. *Watch the video* Imagine the Future of Aging *found at www .youtube.com/watch?v=SBH9dkCZsXQ#t=448. Comment on several items that increased your awareness of technology currently available to allow older persons to remain in their home as they age.*

Use information found in the article *As Senior Population Grows, Aging in Place Gains Popularity: Communities Conducting Outreach* (McGill, 2013) found at http://thenationshealth.aphapublications.org/content/43/8/1.2.full for Questions 7 and 8.

7. *Describe the potential financial savings offered by elderly persons AIP.*

8. *The author states, "As universities work to expose more students to geriatrics, there are potential federal and state solutions to address future workforce shortages." What are some examples?*

Suggested Resource

McGill, N. (2013). As senior population grows, aging in place gains popularity: Communities conducting outreach. *The Nation's Health, 43*(8), 1–16. Retrieved from http://thenationshealth.aphapublications.org/content/43/8/1.2.full

Case 5.5 ◼ Hoarding Behavior

*M*ary Jane Jenkins, RN, is the clinical coordinator for a rehabilitation unit located within a community hospital. She has arranged for a patient care conference to discuss the future plans for a 73-year-old client named Shirley West. Those attending the meeting include the unit's discharge planner, social worker, two staff nurses, an occupational and physical therapist, and the orthopedic surgeon who operated on Shirley 2 weeks prior.

Shirley came to the hospital's emergency room (ER) with a fractured left greater trochanter via the local emergency medical service (EMS). It was reported a 911 call was generated from Shirley's home stating, "I fell and cannot walk due to terrible pain." When the EMS workers arrived at her home, Shirley was just outside her front door, laying on the porch with her purse in one hand and a portable phone in the other. She reported falling off a step stool in her kitchen approximately 2 hours earlier. When the technicians asked why she delayed calling for help and was currently outside the home, her response was, "I thought maybe it was just a bad sprain and didn't want to trouble you all to have to bring a stretcher inside."

In the ER, Shirley was triaged and found to have an elevated blood pressure and heart rate and all lab work was within normal limits. As far as her medical history, Shirley stated she was treated with antidepressants for fibromyalgia in her 50s, which "eventually went away," and she did not seek any regular health care until age 65 when "my Medicare finally kicked in." She sees a local family practitioner biannually for a 6-month prescription of Crestor (rosuvastatin calcium) and Lopressor (metoprolol). She was alert and oriented, cooperative, with minimal eye contact, and expressed appreciation for all service provided.

The health assessment interview of Shirley's social history was quite challenging for the ER staff. Shirley stated there was not a single individual to list as an emergency contact or next of kin. She had been divorced for 30 years and lived alone since that time. Shirley had long-term employment at the local library and retired 10 years ago. The triage nurse inquired about extended family, neighbors, a church affiliation, former coworkers, her ex-husband/his family, friends, or acquaintances, and Shirley was adamant no one was available to serve this role. Shirley described herself as a "simple woman who is quite content staying inside my home talking to no one." She stated she had no pets, walked to the grocery when necessary, and although she owned a car, "it quit working years ago and sits out back." Alcohol or illicit drug use was denied.

During the hospital admission, Shirley was in Buck's traction for 48 hours, followed by an intramedullary nailing of the left fractured hip. Her postop course on the orthopedic unit for three additional days was unremarkable; no complications of any kind were observed. Since being transferred to the rehabilitation unit, she has worked diligently with the physical therapists and can get in and out of bed, ambulate with a walker 100 feet, and go up and down three stair steps solo. The occupational therapist's evaluation is not quite as promising. Due to standard postop restrictions of avoiding prolonged sitting, bending over, and extended time standing, Shirley's ability to perform activities of daily living is deemed as requiring daily in-home support. Specifically, having assistance with bathing, cooking, dressing, and routine housekeeping is recommended.

The social worker reports offering the client either an assisted-care facility placement or daily home health aides for a month. Although polite, Shirley firmly declines either option. She states, "I want to go home alone and will be careful. Stop badgering me about someone coming to my house, it will not happen."

1. At this point, what are some alternative options for care or assistance you think may be helpful for Shirley's situation?

Mary Jane spends the next workday discussing this patient care dilemma with the hospital's attorney (exploring legal restraints to prevent discharging her home), the chair of the hospital's Ethics Committee (seeking input as to patient rights overriding safety), and other nurse managers. She decides to have one last conversation with Shirley alone to explore discharge options.

Shirley finally agrees to have the social worker and occupational therapist come into her home when she is discharged the following day to assess her capabilities and provide a safety assessment related to falls risk. However, she refused home health services with the statement, "I'm not a good housekeeper and this would upset me far greater than provide help."

What the two health care members witnessed the next morning at Shirley's residence was quite overwhelming. Shirley had been a long-term hoarder. There was barely a pathway through the house. Old cardboard boxes were stacked to the ceiling in the living room; every piece of furniture was piled high with newspapers, magazines, catalogs, and plastic bags. The kitchen counters, a dinette set, and stove top could not be seen due to empty food containers, used paper plates, and hundreds of canned goods. One bedroom door could only be opened partially due to all the items stored behind it. Shirley's bed had less than a fourth of it cleared to lie down. There were perhaps a 1,000 paperback books that filled half the room, stacked up to 6 feet high. Hundreds of skeins of unused yarn were everywhere. Stacks of clothes covered the dresser, nightstands, and floor.

Several dozen empty shampoo bottles, multiple packages of toilet tissue, the bathtub piled high with old clothing, and a multitude of threadbare towels were present in the bathroom. The hallways were full of shopping bags filled with receipts, old mail, and boxes of unused greeting cards, file folders, brochures, tax returns, and lists.

Although the home had a full basement, the health care workers chose not to enter this area. When the door was opened, the steps were covered with plastic trash bags filled to capacity. It was assumed the furnace and perhaps a washer and dryer were housed there. Looking out the back door, the yard was relatively clear. Entering the one-car garage was avoided as well.

Shirley stood inside the doorway as the social worker and therapist went silently through her home. Her walker was too wide to navigate the 2-foot clearance through the rooms. After a brief walk-through, the social worker put her arm around Shirley as she quietly wept. The occupational therapist went outside to call Mary Jane at the hospital. He relayed, "The secret has been discovered, we will be returning shortly, and bringing the patient with us. . . ."

2. *Hoarding is defined as the acquisition of, and inability to discard, worthless items even though they appear (to others) to have no value. Why do people hoard? Use the website http://understanding_ocd.tripod.com/hoarding1_why.html to identify a common misconception for each of the following reasons for hoarding: (a) sentimental value, (b) decision making, (c) organizing, (d) responsibility, (e) control/ perfection, (f) scared of forgetting/perfection, and (g) letting go.*

3. *How would you distinguish the difference between being a collector and a hoarder?*

Use the resources found at http://www.nfpa.org/safety-information/for-consumers/ hoarding-and-fire-safety for Questions 4 through 7. The brief video clips on the website are very useful in further understanding hoarding.

4. *Why do people become hoarders?*

5. *What mental health issue is considered an underlying cause of hoarding behavior?*

6. *What safety factors come into play with Shirley's home and her current medical condition?*

7. *Some individuals believe that when the hoarder is away, such as when Shirley is hospitalized, the perfect opportunity arises to complete a "surprise clean-up." Do you believe this is an effective method? Provide a rationale for your answer.*

8. *Shirley can be classified as a "closet hoarder" because driving by her home or looking around her yard showed no signs of the serious problem inside. Other forms of hoarding can pose a community health risk. What are some examples? Cite the Internet source used for your answer.*

Suggested Resources

National Fire Protection Association. (2014). *Hoarding and fire safety.* Retrieved from http://www.nfpa.org/safety-information/for-consumers/hoarding-and-fire-safety

Understanding Hoarding. (2003). *Why people hoard.* Retrieved from http://understanding_ocd. tripod.com/hoarding1_why.html

Case 5.6 ■ Health Promotion for the Elderly Client

Donna and David Ellis are 65 and 68 years old, respectively. They have been married for 2 years. Both were single for quite awhile, but never gave up on the idea of finding a partner. After reading so many ads, seeing commercials on TV, and being encouraged by family, the couple joined an Internet singles program. Within 3 months, they met and a year later were married.

Donna has just started receiving Medicare benefits and her Social Security payment. She read through the material and discovered a program known as "Welcome to Medicare" preventive visit and made an appointment.

> **1. What services will be offered? What is the cost for an individual who has Part B Medicare coverage?**

David has not participated in preventive health his entire life. He believes if you take good care of yourself, there is no need to see a health care provider and spend the time or money. Other than smoking in recent years, he has been conscientious in most all lifestyle choices. He has stayed physically active through being a mail carrier and playing on a men's softball team, eats three balanced meals with no snacking and has abstained from alcohol and recreational drugs. Donna has had issues with maintaining her ideal body weight since menopause, drinks wine almost daily, and takes an antihypertensive and statin drug. Yet, she has the philosophy, "an ounce of prevention is worth a pound of cure."

> **2. Watch the several-minute video, What Can Happen When Men Don't Go to the Doctor? found at www.youtube.com/ watch?v=JrJGnKgmpCE. Comment on the reason the patient featured shares to not seek preventive health care. Do you know anyone like this?**

Donna and David have a number of conversations about his lack of preventive health care. She emphasizes repeatedly how much she loves him and wants to live many years of marriage together. David finally concedes to her request and schedules an appointment for a full physical exam with labwork and screenings—only after Donna agrees to learn to play golf with him.

Use the website Health Screening for Men Over 65, found at www.nlm.nih.gov/ medlineplus/ency/article/007466.htm for the next three questions.

> **3. David smoked (as a means of stress relief) from the time he became a widower at age 55 until he turned 65; he smoked a half pack of cigarettes per day. Based on this information, should he undergo a lung screening examination?**

> **4. What other test is recommended for men ages 65 to 75 who have ever smoked?**

5. *Which of the following exams are recommended health screenings in relation to colon cancer screening? Select all that apply.*

   a. Barium enema annually

   b. A stool guaiac test done every year

   c. Flexible sigmoidoscopy every 5 to 10 years

   d. Colonoscopy every 10 years

Donna has not had a dual energy x-ray absorptiometry (DEXA) scan since her early 40s. This took place at a health fair and involved putting her heel on a metal plate. She has heard "whole body" scans are now the norm and fears the amount of radiation exposure, as well as becoming claustrophobic.

6. *Find a short video that would serve as a visual teaching aide of a DEXA scan to alleviate Donna's concerns. Cite the source.*

7. *Donna completed menopause at age 50. Since that time, she had one Pap smear at age 52 when a friend insisted she be checked due to some slight vaginal bleeding. Is there any need for her to continue this exam at age 65? Use www.nlm.nih.gov/ medlineplus/ency/article/007463.htm as a resource.*

8. *What immunizations should the couple consider receiving related to their ages?*

9. *The couple are screened for hearing loss. The process begins with them completing an assessment tool. Describe the Hearing Handicap Inventory for the Elderly Screening Version (HHIE-S), considered a best practice tool found at http://consultgerirn.org/ uploads/File/trythis/try_this_12.pdf (Demers, 2013).*

10. *Review the National Council on Aging's (2012) sponsored project, Evidence-Based Health Programs for Older Adults, at www.ncoa.org/improve-health/NCOA-Health-Promo-Issue-Brief.pdf. The Sustainability Framework calls for developing partnerships from a variety of community aspects. What are the five other strategies proposed to maintain sustainability?*

Suggested Resources

Demers, K. (2013). *Hearing screening in older adults.* Hartford Institute for Geriatric Nursing. Retrieved from http://consultgerirn.org/uploads/File/trythis/try_this_12.pdf

Greenberg, D. (2014). *Health screening—Men age 65 and older.* Medline Plus. Retrieved from http://www.nlm.nih.gov/medlineplus/ency/article/007466.htm

National Council on Aging. (2012). *Evidence-based health programs for older adults: Key factors and strategies contributing to program sustainability.* Retrieved from http://www.ncoa .org/improve-health/NCOA-Health-Promo-Issue-Brief.pdf

Case 5.7 ■ Overview of Medicare Services

*M*organ Houchins graduated from her nursing program last weekend and is looking forward to beginning her career. She has a "promised" position for hire at a local hospital based on passing her NCLEX-RN®, which is scheduled in 9 weeks. She was planning on an extensive study schedule for the exam, resuming her daily workouts at the gym, catching up with friends, and not much else for the upcoming months.

Her mother has another idea for Morgan. The ladies group at her church is in need of an educational presentation and she asks her daughter to provide a program. The church budget allows $500 annually for the group to have outside speakers and the money must be used in the upcoming month or it will go back to the general fund. Her mother knows Morgan could really use the extra income and has total faith her daughter could create a quality presentation; she did several while in nursing school.

Morgan is reluctant to take on this request for a variety of reasons. She first wants to know what topic the ladies group has in mind, telling her mother, "I am not an expert in anything." Her mother does not have an answer, stating, "How about I ask everyone what they are interested in most and will let them know you will provide basic information, rather than from a specialist's viewpoint?" Morgan states she is willing to go this far with the request.

Mrs. Houchins's ladies group is composed of about 30 regular members. Their ages range from mid-50s to mid-80s, with the mean age at 65 years old. She proposes the idea of Morgan being the speaker for an hour-long program next month to the group, and it is accepted with enthusiasm. When a topic for the presentation is discussed, two are ruled out as not meeting the needs for the majority of members; these are long-term care insurance and adjusting to widowhood. The third suggestion is met with full approval: an "Overview of Medicare Services."

Morgan initially tells her mother "no way" when she hears what the topic will be; however, the speaker's fee remains an enticement. Plus, she remembers from her last nursing course, Transitions Into Practice, the instructor encouraging students to begin building their resumes as soon as possible. Volunteering for employee-based committee work, participation in a professional nursing organization, attending continued education offerings, and providing community education were examples shared with her class.

So . . . Morgan concedes and begins developing her program. She wants to begin with a history of how Medicare was initiated in the United States. Her plan is then to organize the material by referring to the "Top Ten Things to Know About Medicare."

Use any of the following websites (or cite additional resources) to explore what information Morgan would likely find, discuss, and share with the church ladies group.

- www.medicareinteractive.org/page2.php?topic=counselor&page=script&script_id=1670
- www.ncbi.nlm.nih.gov/pmc/articles/PMC2790649
- www.medicare.gov/forms-help-and-resources

1. *What led to the creation of Medicare in the United States and when was this program first initiated?*

2. *The Medicare program is often confused with Medicaid; compare and contrast these services.*

3. *What groups are covered by Medicare?*

4. *How is Medigap utilized in relation to Medicare?*

5. *Describe what health care–related needs are covered by Part A.*

6. *Describe what health care–related needs are covered by Part B.*

7. *Create a listing of the health promotion services covered by Part B Medicare for older adults.*

8. *What is the Medicare Advantage Plan and who is eligible for this?*

9. *Explain the Part D component of Medicare.*

10. *What are the costs associated with the various Medicare programs?*

Morgan's presentation was evaluated as exceptional by the group. She passed her NCLEX, began her hospital residency as a new graduate RN, and committed to providing another program in the near future for the ladies group.

6

Sexuality

Case 6.1 ■ Erectile Dysfunction

Donald Vissing is a 68-year-old male who is en route to an appointment with the urology clinic at the Veterans Affairs Medical Center, his health care provider for several decades. Donald is thinking about how to approach a worrisome and personally embarrassing topic after his annual prostate screening is completed.

The client was married for more than 40 years when he became widowed 5 years ago. In the past year, he was approached at church by Susan, an attractive divorcee in her late 50s. Susan invited Donald to her home for dinner and the couple have had daily contact ever since. Both individuals live alone and have adult children and grandchildren with whom they visit regularly. Donald considers his general health to be "good." He was diagnosed with hypertension shortly before his wife died and uses Tenormin (atenolol) 50 mg daily. He had a mitral valve replacement due to prolapse at age 55, and is on lifelong prophylactic Coumadin (warfarin) 2 mg daily. Otherwise, his total cholesterol count has remained within normal range, which he attributes to exercise and proper diet. He is 69 inches tall and weighs 170 pounds.

Donald's relationship with Susan has been nothing but pleasurable. They have similar interests, personalities, and share many of the same acquaintances in their small community. His current concern focuses on physical intimacy. The couple regularly cuddles, and although they have taken naps together, sexual intercourse has not transpired. Donald has experienced erections with Susan, however, lasting no longer than a minute. He desires to move forward with their intimacy, yet believes it may not be possible.

The client chose to use the herb gingko after seeing a television commercial about the positive effects this supplement can have for older people. Believing it may help his erectile dysfunction, he took the recommended dose for more than a month with no results.

1. Based on Donald's prescribed medication, what adverse effect was he at risk for when using gingko?

Donald has his prostate screening by a male nurse practitioner, Kevin Mercer. He approaches the topic of impotence by saying to the nurse, "Did I tell you I have a lady friend I really like?" The two talk for several minutes on this topic, and as Donald gets up to leave he states, "I may want to ask you some questions about a personal problem related to my masculinity, sometime." Kevin asks whether Donald would like to talk over the phone or return for an additional visit. It is agreed the nurse practitioner will call him the next day.

Kevin begins the phone conversation by telling Donald a bit of his background in nursing. This includes 10 years as an RN with three of those as a practitioner specializing in men's health. He read over the client's chart prior to the conversation and asks whether they can discuss Donald's sexual history in general terms. Kevin was introduced to a screening tool during his graduate program for assessing sexuality in older adults, which guides his approach.

2. *Using the website consultgerirn.org from the Hartford Institute for Geriatric Nursing, what is the name and components of the evidence-based practice tool Kevin used (Wallace, 2012)?*

3. *What information would be shared with the client in relation to common age-related changes of the male reproductive system contributing to erectile dysfunction?*

Kevin reviews medications that can impair the ability to sustain an erection.

4. *Which of these drugs are known to possibly contribute to erectile dysfunction? Select all that apply.*

a. *Antiplatelet aggregates*

b. *Hypnotics*

c. *Tranquilizers*

d. *Antidepressants*

e. *Thyroid hormone replacement*

f. *Anticholinergics*

Kevin next shares information about the role contributing factors, such as lifestyle behaviors and illnesses, can have on erectile dysfunction.

5. *Which of these items would he include? Select all that apply.*

a. *Diabetes*

b. *Alcoholism*

c. *Angina*

d. *Smoking*

e. *Hypertension*

f. *Visual impairment*

In an effort to be supportive, Kevin commends Donald's overall physical condition, healthy lifestyle choices, and preventive care activities. The client asks, "Do most men approaching 70 years old have this problem?"

6. *What statistical information would be shared on the incidence of erectile dysfunction in older men?*

Treatment options for erectile dysfunction are reviewed by Kevin. He begins with discussing penile implants, which Donald immediately rejects.

7. *What are three other devices or methods of treatment (nonpharmacological) that should be included?*

Donald tells the nurse practitioner, "What I'd like to consider is trying a medication, something that will actually work since that herb sure didn't." Kevin suggests a prescription for Cialis (tadalafil), which the client is very interested in trying.

8. *What teaching with regard to use, and potential adverse effects, will Kevin share about this drug?*

The phone conversation concludes. Kevin is documenting the consultation and begins with the required nursing care plan computer entry. He chooses the nursing diagnosis, sexual dysfunction.

9. *What defining characteristics will be entered for Donald to support this diagnosis?*

A year goes by, and Donald returns to the urology clinic for his annual prostate screening. He shares with Kevin, "I need a refill for the 'miracle drug' you prescribed last year. By the way, Susan and I are getting married next month; life is great."

Suggested Resources

Arena, J. M., & Wallace, M. (2008). Issues regarding sexuality. In E. Capezuti, M. Mezey, T. Fulmer, & D. Zwicker (Eds.), *Evidence-based geriatric nursing protocols for best practice* (3rd ed., p. 632). New York, NY: Springer Publishing.

Mauk, K. L., & Hanson, P. (2010). Management of common illnesses, diseases, and health conditions. In K. L. Mauk (Ed.), *Gerontological nursing competencies for care* (2nd ed., pp. 418–419). Sudbury, MA: Jones and Bartlett.

Skidmore-Roth, L. (2014). *Mosby's 2014 nursing drug reference* (27th ed.). Atlanta, GA: Elsevier.

Wallace, M. (2012). *Nursing standard of practice protocol: Sexuality in older adults.* Hartford Institute for Geriatric Nursing. Retrieved from http://consultgerirn.org

Case 6.2 ■ Vaginal Dryness and Dyspareunia

*D*ottie Jones is a 76-year-old widow who moved into an independent living center 2 years ago. Bill Jones, her husband of 50 years, died several years earlier of long-standing heart disease and diabetes. Bill had been a lifelong smoker and also had chronic lung disease. Because of Bill's poor health, Dottie and Bill had not been able to have intercourse for many years prior to his death. Dottie is an independent and very active 76-year-old. She goes to the YWCA 5 days a week and participates in swimming and low-impact aerobics classes. She is not overweight, and her only health problems are type 2 diabetes and long-term hypertension, which appear to be genetic. Dottie controls her diabetes with diet and Glucotrol (glipizide) therapy. Her blood pressure is under control with a daily regimen of Lasix (furosemide), Lopressor (metoprolol), and Cardizem (diltiazem). Dottie has had vaginal dryness for several years, ever since she started taking this regimen of medications. Fortunately, she has never experienced a vaginal infection, or felt concern about the vaginal dryness, likely due to not having a sexual partner.

Since moving into the independent living center, Dottie has become very active in the social events, including playing bridge, attending concerts and lectures, as well as many other indoor and outdoor activities. Over the past year, she has gradually moved from a friendship to a romantic relationship with Chris Stevens, a 72-year-old resident. Chris is in good health and is able to achieve an erection through the use of his "little blue helper," Viagra. Over the past month, Chris and Dottie have had penile–vaginal intercourse three times. Even though Dottie has been able to climax with manual stimulation of her clitoris by Chris, intercourse has been painful each time. Dottie wants to know what she can do to overcome her dyspareunia during intercourse. Refer to the following three web sources to answer the questions that follow:

- "Issues Regarding Sexuality" provides evidence-based content found on the Hartford Institute for Geriatric Nursing website at http://consultgerirn.org/topics/sexuality_issues_in_aging/want_to_know_more (Wallace, 2012)
- Stoppler, M. C., & Needleman, M. D. (2013). *Vaginal dryness and vaginal atrophy*. MedicineNet.com Retrieved from www.medicinenet.com/vaginal_dryness_and_vaginal_atrophy/article.htm
- Harvard Health Publications. (2014). *When sex gives more pain than pleasure*. Retrieved from http://healthyliving.msn.com/health-wellness/women/sex/when-sex-gives-more-pain-than-pleasure-1?pageart=2

1. *Use the website to discuss the stages of the PLISSIT model to conduct a sexual assessment.*

2. *When should vaginal dryness be treated in a woman who is not sexually active?*

3. *What are some reliable over-the-counter artificial water-based lubricants?*

4. *What are some daily hygiene practices that might help Dottie decrease her symptoms of vaginal dryness?*

5. *What type of hormone replacement therapy products might be appropriate for Dottie to discuss with her health care practitioner to help with her vaginal dryness?*

6. *If Dottie and her practitioner decide to initiate estrogen therapy to help with her vaginal dryness, what is a general time frame within which Dottie should see results?*

7. *What are some methods that might assist Dottie to overcome her dyspareunia during intercourse?*

8. *What are some other recommendations for Dottie and her partner to consider for decreasing her dyspareunia? Select all that apply.*

   a. *Experiment with sexual positions/activities that minimize painful intercourse*

   b. *Communicate with her partner to let him know what feels good and what is painful*

   c. *Spend time doing other intimate activities that do not involve intercourse or orgasm*

   d. *Increase her dietary intake of omega-3 fatty acids and vitamin E*

Suggested Resources

Harvard Health Publications. (2014). *When sex gives more pain than pleasure.* Retrieved from http://healthyliving.msn.com/health-wellness/women/sex/when-sex-gives-more-pain-than-pleasure-1?pageart=2

Stoppler, M. C., & Needleman, M. D. (2013). *Vaginal dryness and vaginal atrophy.* MedicineNet. com. Retrieved from http://www.medicinenet.com/vaginal_dryness_and_vaginal_atrophy/article.htm

Wallace, M. (2012). *Issues regarding sexuality.* Hartford Institute for Geriatric Nursing. Retrieved from http://consultgerirn.org/topics/sexuality_issues_in_aging/want_to_know_mor

Case 6.3 ■ Sexual Problems Due to Physical Limitations

*L*ibby Smith and Warren Nystrom were high school sweethearts, but went separate ways after graduation. Each of them found a new partner and had a family. After many years of being married, Libby lost her husband to heart disease, and Warren lost his wife to cancer. They reunited after moving to the same independent living center and seeing each other regularly in the exercise program provided by the center. After a lifetime apart, they easily rekindled their romance, and after a 6-month courtship, they married.

Both Libby and Warren have significant health problems. Libby, who is 64, has had rheumatoid arthritis since her early 40s, which has progressed rapidly, and she now uses a scooter to get around. She is independent in her activities of daily living (ADL), but long ago gave up driving. Warren, who is 65, smoked all his life until 5 years ago when he quit after a myocardial infarction. He also has significant chronic obstructive pulmonary disease (COPD) and wears continuous oxygen. He has lost more than 100 pounds in the past several years due to a declining appetite. For several years, he slept in a recliner chair. Libby and Warren each gave up having sexual intercourse with their former spouses many years ago. For Warren, this was due to his breathing difficulties and frequent inability to get an erection; for Libby it is related to her limited hip movement, which causes her pain during sex.

After attending a healthy living seminar at the independent living center, Libby and Warren decided they were interested in increasing their ability to engage in sexual activities. However, they know they need a lot of information in order to do so. Warren has also noticed he has started getting spontaneous erections since losing weight. They have come into the nurse's office at the independent living center requesting information and advice.

Answer the first two questions by visiting the website provided by the American College of Rheumatology, www.rheumatology.org/Practice/Clinical/Patients/Diseases_And_Conditions/Sex_and_Arthritis/ (Leong, 2012).

> 1. *Libby asks the nurse, "How can I have sex without pain?" What are three recommendations from the section "Plan Ahead for Sex" to minimize the effects of pain and fatigue?*
>
> 2. *Libby expresses concern that medication she uses for rheumatoid arthritis may have an impact on her sexuality. What medications may affect her libido?*
>
> 3. *What other sexual activities can Libby and Warren try to satisfy themselves that don't require intercourse?*

Libby wants to know where she can get additional information on how to enjoy sex while living with arthritis.

> 4. *Find two additional websites that provide information on "sex with arthritis" and cite the sources.*

Warren also has concerns about being able to participate in sexual activities without becoming short of breath and fatigued. Refer to suggestions related to COPD and sexual intimacy at www.webmd.com/lung/copd/features/copd-sex (Kam, 2010) for the following questions.

> 5. *If a client with COPD can accomplish certain physical activities, participation in a sexual relationship may be possible. What are some examples?*
>
> 6. *What are suggestions for ridding the bedroom of irritants that may affect breathing?*
>
> 7. *What position for sexual activity may be most tolerated?*

As the baby boomer generation continues to age, more couples like Libby and Warren will be seeking advice from health care providers for participating in a physically intimate relationship. It is not uncommon for nursing students, or registered nurses, to feel uncomfortable discussing sexuality. Keeping in mind Maslow's Hierarchy of Needs, first published in the 1940s and revised several times, Libby and Warren's health conditions do not affect their desire, although a sexual relationship may be challenging physically.

> **8. What need from Maslow's theory is being sought? Describe your level of comfort at this point in the profession of nursing insofar as including sexuality as a component of patient care.**

Suggested Resources

Kam, K. (2010). *COPD and sex*. WebMD. Retrieved from http://www.webmd.com/lung/copd/features/copd-sex?page=3

Leong, A. L. (2012). *Sex and arthritis*. American College of Rheumatology. Retrieved from https://www.rheumatology.org/Practice/Clinical/Patients/Diseases_And_Conditions/Sex_and_Arthritis

Case 6.4 ■ Sexual Expression for Institutionalized Older Adults

Jill Talley is a 75-year-old widow living in an extended care facility. She had a stroke 2 years ago and has hemiplegia of her right arm and leg and expressive aphasia. She is clearly able to understand others, and she regularly directs her care. She occasionally needs assistance with hygiene and dressing, although she is independent most of the time. She is able to tolerate a regular diet and eats without assistance; she has no difficulty chewing or swallowing. The only medicines she is on are Lasix (furosemide) and aspirin 80 mg a day. Her blood pressure is well controlled. Jill has a daughter living about an hour away who visits two or three times a month.

Ross Walton is a 70-year-old widower living in the same extended care facility. He is completely independent in his ADL and walks without assistance. Ross is moderately impaired due to dementia. He knows where he is and who he is, but he cannot tell what day it is. Staff members need to be sure he has bathed and is wearing clean clothes. Ross likes to walk and sit outside, and he is extremely social. He frequently visits other residents and talks with them about their day. Ross also loves to be an escort for Carrie, a 10-year-old golden retriever owned by one of the staff. Ross takes Carrie from room to room, walks outside, and loves to sit with the dog for hours.

Jill also loves Carrie. The nurses at the extended care facility have noticed a recent trend in the "rounds" that Ross makes during his room-to-room stops with Carrie. Jill's room has become his last stop during the indoor visits with Carrie. Jill then accompanies Ross and Carrie on the short walk to the outside bench, where they have been seen sitting with Carrie and talking while holding hands.

"Sexuality is at the core of who we are and has an impact on our lives in so many ways. It does not stop once we hit the age of 60 or 70 or 90 or even 100 despite the myths and assumptions of society. Sexual desire does not necessarily dissipate with age, but the physical, cognitive, and psychosocial changes that can occur with aging may interfere with sexual outcomes. Issues of sexuality with older adults often become a taboo topic; whether it is the expression of desire or the inappropriate sexual acting out of the individual with disinhibition secondary to dementia" (Tavolaro-Ryley, 2013).

Watch the 3-minute video *Freedom of Sexual Expression* found at www.youtube .com/watch?v=qRPcdG8mCDY.

1. *Sexual expression has major benefits for an older person. What are these?*

2. *The statement, "A hundred staff members can have 100 different personal, moral, and religious approaches to sex, but there can only be one institutional approach." How do you believe this goal can be accomplished?*

3. *Why are written policies addressing sexual expression imperative for long-term care facilities?*

4. *One of the speakers in the video represented the Hebrew Home of Riverdale, which houses the Center for Older Adult Sexuality. What is special about this facility in relation to sexual expression?*

5. *Using the link www.hebrewhome.org/uploads/ckeditor/files/ sexualexpressionpolicy.pdf, what are the five rights for each resident in relation to sexual expression?*

6. *Find the state of your residence on the map provided by Bloomberg and note what the nursing home regulations are regarding conjugal visits. Use www.bloomberg.com/ infographics/2013-07-22/lets-talk-about-sex-in-nursing-homes .html.*

7. *What are some ways in which the older adult might demonstrate his or her sexuality?*

Suggested Resources

Dressel, R., & Ramirez, M. (2013). *Policies and procedures concerning sexual expression at the Hebrew Home at Riverdale.* Retrieved from http://www.hebrewhome.org/uploads/ ckeditor/files/sexualexpressionpolicy.pdf

Tavolaro-Ryley, L. (2013). *Sex and the retirement community: Sexuality and the older adult.* Advancing Care Excellence for Seniors. National League for Nurses. Retrieved from http:// www.nln.org/facultyprograms/facultyresources/aces/Sexuality/sexuality.pdf

YouTube. (n.d.) *Freedom of sexual expression* [Video file]. Retrieved from http://www.youtube .com/watch?v=qRPcdG8mCDY

7

The Aging Sensory System

Case 7.1 ■ Gustatory and Olfactory Disturbance

Dorothy Heln is a 72-year-old female living alone in her own home. She is visiting with her nurse practitioner, Sarah Stewart, for follow-up after a bout with food poisoning. She had been brought to the hospital emergency room by her daughter, Sheryl, after vomiting for 2 days. In reviewing Dorothy's food intake history, it was revealed that she ate some bad tuna salad 2 days prior to her emergency room evaluation. She is no longer affected by the food poisoning incident. Sheryl is very concerned about her mother's sense of smell and taste because her mother had reported that, "the tuna salad smelled just fine to me." Sheryl has also noticed that her mother, who had always had a great sense of style, is wearing more perfume than is acceptable and that when she was babysitting one of the grandchildren recently, she failed to detect a dirty diaper for several hours. Dorothy had also had some weight loss prior to the food poisoning incident.

1. List some risks that might result from impairment of smell and/or taste.

Sarah's visit with Dorothy reveals the following. Dorothy is 64 inches tall and weighs 120 pounds. She notes in her chart that Dorothy's previous weight was 125 pounds. She is not taking any medications. She is a nonsmoker. Dorothy complains that she "just doesn't feel much like eating anymore, food just doesn't taste that good." Evaluation of her oral and nasal cavities does not reveal any disorders. She has not had a recent history of viral infections and lists no known allergies. Her preliminary neurological exam is normal. She is oriented to time and place, and her daughter confirms that she is lucid and that they have not had concerns. She does not complain of any dental problems, does not wear dentures, and when asked confirms that she has received regular oral care.

2. Explain the importance, in this case, of evaluating the patient's medication history.

3. Why is evaluation of the oral and nasal cavities an appropriate evaluation for the patient's complaints?

4. What is the relevance of the neurologic exam?

5. Why is it important to note that the patient is not complaining of any dental problems?

Sarah arranges a follow-up visit to try to characterize the nature of the smell and taste loss. Exposure to one nostril at a time to basic smells, like vanilla bean, coffee, and a floral smell, indicate that Dorothy is not able to identify some common household items. Tests of sour (lemon), sweet (sugar), bitter (aspirin), and salty (salt) on the surface of her tongue reveal Dorothy does not have difficulty identifying the tastes. Sarah refers Dorothy to a neurologist for further evaluation, suggesting she obtain an MRI or CT scan. Results of the MRI are negative for the presence of masses or lesions on the cribriform plate.

Conclusions:

It would appear that Dorothy is suffering from olfactory impairment, which subsequently has affected her gustatory function. Unfortunately, smell and taste disorders are prevalent, whereas:

- Twenty-four and a half percent (15 million) of Americans 55 years old or older have a problem with their sense of smell
- Thirty percent of Americans between the ages of 70 and 80 have a problem with their sense of smell
- Nearly a third of people over 80 have a problem with their sense of smell (Aging .com, 2014)

Follow-Up:

6. What advice might you give this patient to enhance her quality of life?

7. What advice regarding safety might you give this patient?

8. Watch the 1-minute video available at www.youtube.com/ watch?v=WavjbJhiRAE to reinforce your learning. What would be the top three items you would personally miss having the ability to smell?

Suggested Resources

Aging.com. (2014). *Problems with the sense of smell in the elderly.* National Institute on Aging, National Institutes of Health. Retrieved from http://www.agingcare.com/ Articles/When-elderly-lose-sense-of-smell-133880.htm

American Academy of Otolaryngology—Head and Neck Surgery. (2014). *Smell and taste.* Retrieved from http://www.entnet.org/content/smell-taste

Fried, M. P. (2012). *Smell and taste disorders.* Merck Manuals: Online Medical Library—Ear, Nose, and Throat Disorders. Retrieved from http://www.merck.com/mmhe/sec19/ch221/ ch221j.html

National Institute on Aging. (n.d.). *Adult problems with smell.* Retrieved from http:// nihseniorhealth.gov/problemswithsmell/aboutproblemswithsmell/01.html

National Institute on Deafness and Other Communication Disorders (NIDCD). (2014). *Smell disorders.* Retrieved from http://www.nidcd.nih.gov/health/smelltaste/pages/smell.aspx

Case 7.2 ■ Hearing Loss

*M*r. John Callahan, age 71, is a new resident at the Golden Years Assisted Living Facility. He had been living alone for the past 18 months, following the death of his wife. He entered the facility at the insistence of his two daughters, who both live out of state. They reported to the admissions nurse that their father had always been the life of the party and had always enjoyed family gatherings and social events until the past few months. They have noticed him becoming withdrawn. For example, they reported that at Christmas, when the family gathered, he sat quietly in the corner instead of participating in conversation. When his daughter asked him whether he was feeling well, his reply was, "Yes, I like the snow." The daughters urged him to sell his house and move into the assisted living facility, because they felt he was lonely and depressed due to the loss of his wife.

Mr. Callahan's medical history includes hypertension, osteoarthritis, and a mild MI 5 years ago. Current medications include Lopressor (metoprolol) 50 mg daily, aspirin 81 mg daily, and Tylenol Arthritis (acetaminophen) 650 mg twice a day. He was also started on Zoloft (sertraline hydrochloride) 50 mg daily for depression about 6 weeks ago.

Molly Sanders, the RN director of the facility, has been observing Mr. Callahan in the day room. She suspects that Mr. Callahan may be suffering from hearing loss instead of (or in addition to) depression. She sits down near him in the day room and engages him in conversation. He reports that he has not made any friends at the facility and complains that "everyone mumbles." She notices that he focuses on her face as if he is trying to read her lips.

1. List the behaviors that may indicate that Mr. Callahan has a hearing loss.

The nurse decides to do some screening to detect any signs or symptoms of hearing loss. First she checks the ear canal for cerumen (ear wax) impaction, but finds none. As a geriatric nurse, she relies on professional resources such as the Hartford Institute for Geriatric Nursing to find evidence-based guidelines for caring for elders. Go to their website at http://consultgerirn.org/topics/sensory_changes/want_to_know_more.

To learn about hearing loss in the elderly, read the material by Cacchione (2005) and answer the following questions.

2. Name the three types of hearing loss common in the older adult.

3. A normal change of aging results in the secretion of drier cerumen, which easily becomes impacted in the ear. What type of hearing loss is caused by impacted cerumen?

4. Presbycusis results in difficulty hearing what type of sounds?

On the first page of the website listed earlier, click on Try This Issue 12—Hearing Screening in Older Adults—A Brief Hearing Loss Screener (Demers, 2013). The first page of the screening tool provides information to answer the following questions.

> *5. **What is the prevalence of hearing impairment in the older adult?***
>
> *6. **Name at least five risk factors for hearing impairment.***

Nurse Sanders uses this screening tool to assess Mr. Callahan. He scores five out of eight points, which indicates a need for further assessment.

To find other assessment techniques for hearing impairment, Ms. Sanders uses techniques such as in the video www.youtube.com/watch?v=FNy7dgOwu30.

After conducting the whispered-voice test, as well as the Rinne and Weber tuning-fork tests, she determines that Mr. Callahan has indications of bilateral, nonconductive hearing loss. She discusses her findings with Mr. Callahan, and with his permission, she schedules an appointment with an audiologist. After testing, he is fitted with bilateral hearing aids.

In the meantime, Ms. Sanders instructs the facility staff in interventions to improve communication with Mr. Callahan. Based on Cacchione's (2005) evidence-based findings, answer the following questions about techniques to facilitate effective communication with Mr. Callahan.

> *7. **When speaking with him, name at least three adaptive techniques staff should use.***
>
> *8. **Name at least three environmental modifications or devices that will enhance Mr. Callahan's ability to hear and participate in conversations.***

In the following weeks, Ms. Sanders observes improvements in Mr. Callahan's adjustment to the facility. He makes friends and sits with them in the dining room for meals. He participates in planned social activities such as bingo and goes on outings to the mall. He no longer appears withdrawn or depressed. When his family visits to celebrate his birthday, he interacts "like his old self," talking and laughing and enjoying being with them.

Suggested Resources

Cacchione, P. (2005). *Want to know more: Sensory changes*. Hartford Institute for Geriatric Nursing. Retrieved from http://consultgerirn.org/topics/sensory_changes/want_to_know_more

Demers, K. (2013). *Hearing screening in older adults: A brief hearing loss screener*. Hartford Institute for Geriatric Nursing. Retrieved from http://consultgerirn.org/uploads/File/trythis/try_this_12.pdf

MedicineNet.com. (2006). *Hearing loss and aging*. Retrieved from http://www.medicinenet.com/script/main/art.asp?articlekey=20432

YouTube. (2007, May 4). *Cranial nerve VIII—auditory acuity, Weber & Rinne Tests 20* [Video file]. Retrieved from http://www.youtube.com/watch?v=FNy7dgOwu30

Case 7.3 ■ Somatosensory Disturbance

*J*uleen Stokes, a 79-year-old retired, married elementary school teacher, has been relatively healthy her entire life. She has no known chronic conditions and takes only vitamins. Then, one day in the middle of her usual 1-mile walk around the neighborhood, she experienced severe chest and arm pain. She was found to have a 95% occluded left-anterior coronary artery and significant blockage in two other coronary arteries. In spite of her advanced age, she underwent emergent coronary bypass surgery. After coming off the ventilator and being discharged from the intensive care unit (ICU), it was clear that Mrs. Stokes's mental status had changed.

The day after transfer from the ICU, Mrs. Stokes began to pick at bugs in the air, reporting to her husband that she saw bugs climbing up the wall of her hospital room. She was quite distressed, becoming agitated as she described what she saw. Her vital signs were BP 126/84, pulse 88, respirations 18. Her blood counts and electrolyte panel were all within normal limits. Her medications included morphine 2 mg IV every 4 hours as needed for pain and aspirin 81 mg every day. She had three doses of morphine since her surgery for complaints of pain. Within 45 minutes of each dose, she reported relief of her acute pain. The doctors and nurses initially suspect it is the opiates that are causing her problem.

Use the following article, "Opiates and Elderly: Use and Side Effects" (Chau, Walker, Pai, & Cho, 2008), found at www.ncbi.nlm.nih.gov/pmc/articles/PMC2546472 to answer Questions 1 and 2.

1. What might be the cause of Mrs. Stokes's hallucinations?

2. The nurse reports to her health care practitioner that Mrs. Stokes is having visual hallucinations. Based on this article, what treatments might the nurse anticipate to be ordered for Mrs. Stokes?

It is suspected that Mrs. Stokes may be experiencing delirium. The opiates are stopped, and 2 days later, Ms. Stokes pain is well controlled with around-the-clock dosing of Toradol (ketorolac). She is now eating upright, walking with assistance, and her surgical sites are healing nicely, with no clinical manifestations of infection. She still has times when she reports seeing bugs on the wall.

Use the resource, "Visual Hallucinations: Differential Diagnosis and Treatment" available at www.ncbi.nlm.nih.gov/pmc/articles/PMC2660156 to answer Questions 3 through 6.

3. What other acute health problems might be the underlying causes of Mrs. Stokes's hallucinations?

4. *The physicians start Mrs. Stokes on Seroquel (quetiapine) to treat her hallucinations. What would you teach her and her family about this medication?*

5. *Seroquel (quetiapine) is also recommended for those with Parkinson's disease; what is the rationale?*

A CT scan and MRI are done to see whether Mrs. Stokes has suffered a stroke or other event. These tests show only "age-related changes." The physicians believe Mrs. Stokes may have suffered mild brain anoxia while she was having open-heart surgery and on the heart-lung bypass machine. Mr. Stokes insists on taking his wife home as he is adamant in his belief that it is being in the hospital that is causing her problems. Their daughter Lilly and 17-year-old granddaughter, Carol, come to stay with them and help out. While most of the time Mrs. Stokes is appropriate, her affect is quite "flat," and she still has occasions when she is having visual hallucinations, which are very upsetting to 17-year-old Carol.

6. *Use the section on the causes of visual hallucinations to develop an explanation of the hallucinations to 17-year-old Carol.*

Refer to the web article "Hallucinations & False Ideas" at www.fightdementia.org.au/services/hallucinations-false-ideas.aspx when answering the following questions.

7. *Carol says she understands, but wants to know what to say when her grandmother says she is seeing bugs. What may be a therapeutic response?*

Several days later, all are rested and seem to be doing well at home. The Stokes's daughter and granddaughter plan to return to their home as the hallucinations appear to have resolved.

8. *What are some examples of distracters that may be helpful when an individual is hallucinating?*

9. *What value could keeping a record, or diary, of when hallucinations occur serve?*

Suggested Resources

Chau, D. L., Walker, V., Pai, L., & Cho, L. M. (2008). Opiates and elderly: Use and side effects. *Clinical Interventions in Aging.* Retrieved from http://www.ncbi.nlm.nih.gov/pmc/articles/PMC2546472

Teeple, R. C., Caplan, J. P., & Stern, T. A. (2009). Visual hallucinations: Differential diagnosis and treatment. *The Primary Care Companion to the Journal of Clinical Psychiatry.* Retrieved from http://www.ncbi.nlm.nih.gov/pmc/articles/PMC2660156

Case 7.4 ■ Macular Degeneration

*B*ill Sanchez is a 66-year-old Hispanic American who moved from a comfortable life in a Chicago suburb to an Alabama coastal town 6 months ago to be near his only child. Much more than his address has changed in the past 18 months. Bill ended his career as a stockbroker at age 65 and planned for years to have the "dream retirement." His financial planning, physical health, and long-term marriage were in great shape.

Several weeks following his retirement, Bill's daughter, Maria, was diagnosed with multiple sclerosis. Her symptoms were initially mild; with hired household help and her husband's support, it appeared his daughter would continue to function reasonably well.

About a year later, his wife died suddenly following an abdominal hysterectomy. Bill was devastated and grieved deeply for months. His plans for traveling, hobbies, and social activities postretirement came to an abrupt halt.

He decided to move to new surroundings and be near his daughter in order to provide her with assistance and to see his grandchildren on a daily basis. Although Bill enjoyed the warm southern climate, he noticed an immediate change when on the beach; the bright light from the sun hitting the ocean caused considerable haziness in his sight.

In addition, other visual symptoms have occurred with increased frequency, which Bill attributed to fatigue or stress. When using his computer, he has noted blurriness while viewing a spreadsheet. His daughter commented on the difficulty he had maneuvering around when entering her dimly lit basement. Lastly, Bill has experienced a small blind spot in his central vision twice in the last week. He realized this when trying to write a check and again when reading a recipe on the back of a box. Bill makes an appointment with an ophthalmologist at his daughter's urging. To experience what Bill's visual changes have entailed, please view the simulation at http://www.geteyesmart.org/eyesmart/diseases/age-related-macular-degeneration/macular-degeneration-vision-simulator.cfm.

Following a thorough eye exam, the physician tells Bill that he likely is experiencing macular degeneration. Looking at the health history form Bill filled out earlier, he states, "You don't have the usual risk factors, other than age."

1. What are the most common risk factors for macular degeneration?

The physician explains what occurs with age-related macular degeneration (AMD). It is presented to Bill as a painless disease whereby the macula gradually breaks down due to the development of drusen: fatty, yellow, and metabolic waste products, which accumulate beneath the retina. The progress is slow and results in mild to moderate loss of sight, which usually leaves reading vision intact. Loss of central vision occurs with continued degeneration. He shows Bill a large diagram of the eye and then discusses the two types of macular degeneration, dry and wet.

2. What are the primary differences between wet and dry macular degeneration?

Bill is noticeably upset and asks the ophthalmologist whether AMD is common as he's never heard the medical term before.

3. What response would you expect from the health care provider in relation to prevalence?

Bill is provided with an Amsler grid. It is suggested he place it on the refrigerator to self-monitor any changes in vision on a daily basis.

4. What instructions should be provided to Bill in relation to using the Amsler grid? Watch a brief video demonstration at www.youtube.com/watch?v=ou1vzX17nY0.

Bill is also advised to increase his intake of antioxidants and zinc. His food preferences are culturally based in the Hispanic tradition.

5. What are examples he might add to his daily diet based on preferences?

Bill emphasizes to the ophthalmologist how very "unfair" he believes it is to be diagnosed with AMD. He states he has worked diligently to have a healthy lifestyle; he quit smoking a decade ago after a 40-pack-year history, has maintained an ideal body weight, drinks alcohol moderately, and exercises every morning. He asks what else he might have done to avoid the macular degeneration. The physician relays that he has been following evidence-based practice research, and it appears consumption of omega-3 fatty acids has a positive influence in prevention. He also reminds Bill to include his smoking history on health forms in the future.

Bill's daughter Maria attends the office visit with him and detects how upset her father is over the diagnosis. She picks up a brochure in the waiting room called "Low Vision Aides" to look over after they return home.

6. What type of items might be included for purchase in this brochure?

7. Discuss the treatment of anti-VEGF therapy and how it is administered.

In the weeks following the diagnosis of AMD, Bill realizes his coping skills are essentially depleted. He confides his sorrow, anger, and feelings of hopelessness to a neighbor who happens to be an RN. She suggests counseling for Bill, which he agrees to. Within several months, his outlook has improved considerably He decides to begin volunteer work to help others with macular degeneration.

8. What agencies are available for Bill's volunteerism in relation to support groups or foundations?

Suggested Resources

Bauer, J. (2014). *How food affects macular degeneration*. Retrieved from http://www.joybauer.com/vision/how-food-affects-macular-degeneration.aspx

Genentech. (n.d.). *Age-related macular degeneration fact sheet*. Retrieved from http://www.gene.com/patients/disease-education/amd-fact-sheet

Macular Degeneration Partnership. (2014). *Experience what AMD looks like*. Retrieved from http://www.amd.org/what-is-amd/experience-amd.html

Sheppard, J. D. (2012). *Macular degeneration*. emedicine health. Retrieved from http://www.emedicinehealth.com/macular_degeneration/page12_em.htm

YouTube. (2010). *Amsler grid eye test* [Video file]. Retrieved from http://www.youtube.com/watch?v=ou1vzX17nY0

Case 7.5 ■ Visual Alterations

*M*rs. Margaret Cooper is a 70-year-old African American female, who has come to Eastridge Family Health Center (EFHC) for an annual physical examination. Mrs. Cooper is a widow who lives alone in a small second-floor apartment and is a retail sales clerk. EFHC admission nurse John Barton conducts a health interview with Mrs. Cooper and notes that Mrs. Cooper is alert and oriented, dressed appropriately for the weather, and answers questions readily and completely.

Mrs. Cooper states that she is allergic to dust mites and mold, and takes Claritin-D (10 mg loratadine/240 mg pseudoephedrine sulfate) every day. She reports that she has osteoarthritis in both hips and knees and takes 650 mg of Tylenol (acetaminophen) every 6 hours. She also takes Restoril (temazepam) 15 mg at bedtime for sleep.

During the interview, Mrs. Cooper complains of being "unable to see cars coming up alongside when driving," but denies any eye pain. Mrs. Cooper reveals that she is experiencing "blind spots," which are darkening and increasing in size and number, and that she is losing visual acuity and is beginning to see "halos" around lights. Mrs. Cooper's daughter has accompanied her to the clinic visit and notes that Mrs. Cooper has had several small fender bender car accidents in the past year.

John performs standard admissions assessments on Mrs. Cooper and notes that she has an absence of the red reflex in the right eye and that her Snellen chart reading is 20/40 (left), 20/50 (right), and 20/50 (both eyes). He observes that she has difficulty rising from a chair, has trouble finding her way from the intake area to the exam room, and collides with the door frame.

1. What history or physical examination findings should be the greatest concern to the admissions nurse?

John continues to talk with Mrs. Cooper and discovers that she has fallen four times on the steps leading to her apartment and has been tripped by rugs and furniture in her home in the past 3 months. She states, "I have more trouble seeing the keys on the cash register, and I am afraid I might get fired."

> ***2. What other assessments might the nurse perform to evaluate safety risks for Mrs. Cooper? Go to the following website and evaluate the fall risk of Mrs. Cooper: http://consultgerirn.org/ uploads/File/trythis/try_this_8.pdf (Hendrich, 2013).***

Mrs. Cooper says, "I hope that some stronger reading glasses might help; I don't think Medicare covers eye care. I don't have the money for a prescription drug plan through Medicare."

> ***3. What resources might John identify to assist this patient? Go to the following websites and evaluate the resources that might be available to assist Mrs. Cooper: www.alcon.com/en/corporate-responsibility/patient-clinic-inst-assistance.asp and http://www .medicareinteractive.org/page2.php?topic=counselor&page=script& script_id=1593.***

After the clinic visit, Mrs. Cooper has been given a referral for a complete eye exam, including tonometry (a test of intraocular pressure). John arranges an appointment with a local ophthalmologist, who participates in a no-cost vision screening program for low-income patients. Mrs. Cooper calls after the appointment and reports that the tonometry tests revealed that she has open-angle glaucoma.

> ***4. What is the difference between closed-angle and open-angle glaucoma?***

> ***5. Why was Mrs. Cooper at high risk for glaucoma?***

The ophthalmologist writes prescriptions for the treatment of Mrs. Cooper's glaucoma. Mrs. Cooper brings them to EFHC and asks John to give her more information about the medications.

> ***6. What medications are used in treatment for glaucoma? List the medications, including classifications, drug interactions, and side effects.***

> ***7. What medications should be avoided by patients with open-angle glaucoma?***

> ***8. What instructions should John give to Mrs. Cooper?***

One month later, Mrs. Cooper visits the EFHC with her daughter and tells John that her vision has improved. Mrs. Cooper says, "I worry about my daughter having problems with her eyes."

> ***9. What could you teach Mrs. Cooper's 30-year-old daughter about protecting her vision?***

Suggested Resources

Alcon Cares, Inc.–U.S. Patient Assistance. (2014). *U.S. patient, clinic & institutional assistance.* Retrieved from http://www.alcon.com/en/corporate-responsibility/patient-clinic-inst-assistance.asp

Glaucoma Research Foundation. (n.d.). *Are you at risk for glaucoma?* Retrieved from http://www.glaucoma.org/learn/are_you_at_risk.php

Hendrich, A. (2013). *Fall risk assessment for older adults: The Hendrich II Fall Risk Model™.* The Hartford Institute for Geriatric Nursing. Retrieved from http://consultgerirn.org/uploads/File/trythis/try_this_8.pdf

Medicare Interactive. (n.d.) *When does Medicare cover eye care?* Retrieved from http://www.medicareinteractive.org/page2.php?topic=counselor&page=script&script_id=1593

National Eye Institute. (2014). *Facts about glaucoma.* Retrieved from http://www.nei.nih.gov/health/glaucoma/glaucoma_facts.asp

8

Integumentary Disorders and Infectious Diseases of the Elderly

Case 8.1 ■ Venous Insufficiency in a Homebound Elder

Robert Stein is an obese 78-year-old male, who is a retired truck driver and lives with his wife in a one-story suburban home. He was recently hospitalized for an infected wound of his left lower extremity. He received intravenous (IV) antibiotics while hospitalized, heparin therapy for deep vein thrombosis prevention, and his usual home medications. Following hospitalization, he was discharged to a long-term care facility for 4 additional weeks of IV antibiotic therapy, wound care, and subacute rehabilitation therapy for weakness, gait, and balance disturbance. He received 6 weeks of therapy and progressively improved in his ambulation distance, steadiness of gait, and balance. His infection cleared, the peripheral inserted central catheter (PICC) line was removed, and his left lower extremity wound closed. He has been discharged with an order for home health care nursing and physical therapy follow-up.

The home care nurse is seeing Mr. Stein today for evaluation. In further reviewing Mr. Stein's history, the nurse learns he has a past medical history of hypertension, obesity, congestive heart failure, hyperlipidemia, osteoarthritis of the knees, chronic venous insufficiency, and chronic recurrent venous leg ulcers. His home medications are Hyzaar (hydrochlorothiazide/losartan) 50/12.5 mg, one tablet orally daily; Mevacor (lovastatin) 40 mg, one tablet orally every night; aspirin 81 mg, one tablet daily; Tylenol (acetaminophen) 500 mg, two tablets orally every 12 hours as needed for arthritis pain.

Mr. Stein explains to the home care nurse that what led to his hospitalization was an injury he sustained to his leg. He reports that he and his wife were on their way out for breakfast when he caught his leg between his walker and a coffee table when ambulating through the living room. He reports this caused his leg to "open up . . . and really bleed." After his wife helped him clean the wound and the bleeding stopped, they applied a dressing and went out to breakfast. He states that the next morning he noticed the leg to be more painful, red, and swollen. A visit to the emergency department (ED) resulted in admission to the hospital with a diagnosis of left leg cellulitis.

Additionally, the nurse learns that Mr. Stein has been ambulatory with a walker, although he states, "I don't get out much . . . I mostly sit and watch television. My main exercise is walking to the mailbox . . . but I am too weak to do that now.

I am hoping to get stronger." He states he is independent with toileting, eating, and taking his medications; however, he receives assistance from his wife with bathing and dressing.

Social history reveals that he is married with three grown children and six grandchildren, two of the children live out of state, and one daughter lives within 30 minutes and visits weekly. Mr. Stein reports his height is 5 feet 9 inches and weight is 285 pounds. He denies food or drug allergies. The nurse completes the review of systems. Mr. Stein denies complaints except for an "aching and sometimes heavy feeling" in his legs and some tenderness over the site of the healed wound if his leg is touched. He reports that "walking around a little . . . or elevating my legs by sitting in the recliner" relieves the heaviness and aching.

Use the article located at http://emedicine.medscape.com/article/1085412-clinical# aw2aab6b3b3 (Weiss, 2012) to facilitate answering the first several questions.

1. *What are the risk factors this patient shows for chronic venous insufficiency?*

2. *What are some complications of chronic venous insufficiency?*

3. *Which complications has Mr. Stein experienced and which complications does he remain at risk for?*

4. *What symptoms of venous insufficiency does Mr. Stein report?*

The nurse performs a physical examination and finds the following: blood pressure 128/84, heart rate 75, and respirations 22. The calculated body mass index rounded is 42. General: obese elderly male in no acute distress. HEENT: upper and lower dentures, oral mucosa moist, no oral lesions. Respiratory: lungs clear to percussion and auscultation. Cardiovascular: regular rate and rhythm, apical heart rate: 78 beats per minute. Abdomen: obese, nontender, bowel sounds present. Extremities: upper extremities pulses +2 equal, lower extremities +1, pitting edema toes to knees, brown hyperpigmentation discoloration of the skin from mid-calf to ankle, absent hair of the lower extremities, light pink irregularly shaped area of the medial left lower extremity that is slightly tender to touch, distended, and torturous veins are visible from just above the knee posterior and medially extending to the lower calf bilaterally, feet are warm to touch. Pulses: popliteal not assessed due to body size and difficulty positioning to palpate properly, post-tibial and pedal pulses +2 bilaterally, feet show scaly dry skin with thick yellow toenails, sensation is intact.

5. *What assessment findings does Mr. Stein have that are consistent with venous insufficiency?*

6. *Are there any additional examination maneuvers the nurse could perform to assess for chronic venous insufficiency?*

The nurse asks Mr. Stein if he recalls having any tests to assess the circulation in his legs while he was hospitalized or in the rehabilitation facility. Mr. Stein states, "They did a Doppler test on both of my legs and told me I didn't have any blood clots or artery occlusions."

7. *What is a Doppler test? What role does this exam play in diagnosis and treatment decisions in chronic venous insufficiency? Cite your source.*

Mrs. Stein tells the nurse that her husband was given a prescription for "some kind of stockings" and asks the nurse if she should get them for her husband. She tells the nurse, "I really want to help him get better. Is there anything else we can do to help his condition and avoid the development of 'leg sores?'"

Use the website www.uptodate.com/contents/chronic-venous-disease-beyond-the-basics (Alguire & Mathes, 2013) to assist with answering the remaining questions.

8. *What type of compression stocking is used for chronic venous insufficiency?*

9. *What type of medications and herbal supplements are used?*

10. *What are three vein ablation procedures that can be implemented?*

Suggested Resources

Alguire, P. C., & Mathes, B. M. (2013). *Patient information: Chronic venous disease (beyond the basics)*. UpToDate. Retrieved from http://www.uptodate.com/contents/chronic-venous-disease-beyond-the-basics

Weiss, R. (2012). *Venous insufficiency*. Medscape. Retrieved from http://emedicine.medscape.com/article/1085412-clinical#aw2aab6b3b

Case 8.2 ■ Pressure Ulcer in an Acute Care Setting

*T*homas Montoya is a 70-year-old Hispanic male with a history of type 2 diabetes mellitus (DM). He has been admitted to the medical–surgical unit for stabilization of his blood sugar. Kristin Lee will be the primary care nurse for Mr. Montoya. She completes an admission history and physical exam for Mr. Montoya.

Mr. Montoya has lived in the United States for 40 years, and shares in a two-story house with his wife of 50 years. His son, daughter-in-law, and their three children also live in the home. Mr. Montoya had a below-the-knee amputation (BKA) of the right leg 2 years ago, after he developed gangrene in his right foot.

Mr. Montoya states that for 3 weeks, he has had frequent urination and blurry vision. In addition, he has lost 12 pounds in the past month. Since his surgery, he has been less physically active. He did see a dietitian, postoperatively, and does self-monitoring of blood glucose (SMBG) "once in a while." He takes Glucophage (metformin) 500 mg twice a day and Zestril (lisinopril) 20 mg daily. He drinks 8 ounces of beer with dinner each evening, and smokes one half of a pack of cigarettes per day.

Initial assessment shows that Mr. Montoya is 64 inches tall and weighs 205 pounds. Peripheral pulses are 2+ radial, left dorsalis pedis 1+. His left foot is cool, with capillary refill of 5 seconds. His blood pressure is 158/98, heart rate 84, and respirations 20.

Results of laboratory tests:

- Glucose (nonfasting): 240 mg/dL
- Creatinine: 1.6 mg/dL
- Blood urea nitrogen: 22 mg/dL
- Sodium: 141 mg/dL
- Potassium: 4.3 mg/dL

Lipid panel:

- Total cholesterol: 220 mg/dL (normal: < 200 mg/dL)
- HDL cholesterol: 36 mg/dL
- LDL cholesterol: 184 mg/dL
- Triglycerides: 177 mg/dL
- A1C: 8.1% (normal: 4%–6%)
- Urine micro albumin: 45 mg

1. *What history, laboratory results, and physical examination findings should be of the greatest concern to the admissions nurse?*

2. *What problems should Kristin consider in creating a plan of care for Mr. Montoya?*

3. *What risk factors does Mr. Montoya have for the development of pressure ulcers?*

4. *The Braden Scale for Predicting Pressure Sore Risk (Bergstrom, Braden, Laguzza, & Holman, 1987) is used to assess Mr. Montoya's risk for pressure ulcers; what six categories will be addressed? What will be his score? A resource is available at http://consultgerirn .org/uploads/File/trythis/try_this_5.pdf.*

Three days after admission, Kristin is performing an early morning assessment on Mr. Montoya. She notes a 1-cm blister on Mr. Montoya's left heel. Kristin promptly notifies Mr. Montoya's primary care provider (PCP) about the finding, who orders that the heel be elevated off the bed, and that Mr. Montoya be in the chair for an hour at least three times a day.

5. *What other nursing interventions might Kristin initiate to reduce Mr. Montoya's risk of skin breakdown?*

Despite the interventions, Mr. Montoya's left heel blister worsens to the extent that the nurses document it as a Stage II pressure ulcer, 2 cm in diameter.

6. *How does the National Pressure Ulcer Advisory Panel (2007) define a Stage II ulcer?*

7. *There are a multitude of dressings and skin products on the market; identify the categories of dressing treatments. The website www.fairview.org/healthlibrary/Article/84022 may be helpful.*

The PCP orders a hydrocolloid dressing be applied to the heel. The nurses continue to provide meticulous care, assessing the pressure ulcer every shift, and increasing the turning schedule to every hour while Mr. Montoya is in bed. Mr. Montoya is slowly able to regain 3 pounds, his blood sugars stabilize, and he becomes much more alert. His left heel ulcer improves, decreasing in size to 1 cm; there is no sign of infection. Mrs. Montoya will be caring for her husband's pressure ulcer at home. Home care nurses will monitor Mr. Montoya weekly.

8. *Find a type of hydrocolloid dressing on the market and prepare teaching instructions for proper use at home.*

Suggested Resources

Ayello, E. A. (2012). *Try this: Predicting pressure ulcer risk.* Hartford Institute for Geriatric Nursing. Retrieved from http://consultgerirn.org/uploads/File/trythis/try_this_5.pdf

Bergstrom, N., Braden, B. J., Laguzza, A., & Holman V. (1987). The Braden scale for predicting pressure sore risk. *Nursing Research, 36*(4), 205–210.

Cooper, K. L. (2013). Evidence-based prevention of pressure ulcers in the intensive care unit. *Critical Care Nurse, 33*(6), 57–67. Retrieved from http://ccn.aacnjournals.org/content/33/6/57.full

National Pressure Ulcer Advisory Committee. (2007). *Pressure ulcer stages revised by NPUAP.* Retrieved from http://www.npuap.org/pr2.htm

Case 8.3 ■ Burns and the Elderly

Grace Townsend is an 83-year-old female, who has lived in a New York City high-rise apartment since the structure was built in 1972. She was an early participant in the state's rent-controlled stabilization program and cannot imagine any other lifestyle. She has often been asked through the years why she would choose to pay monthly rent versus own a home or condo, and her standard answer has been, "Because I can."

Grace was married to her high school classmate for close to 30 years. The couple had no children, although they enjoyed their contact with nieces and nephews. Her husband drowned when they visited Atlantic City one summer; she never dated, nor had any interest in a romantic relationship after the tragedy. She focused her time and energy on her career. This entailed being the buyer for the women's hat department at Macy's department store. That is, until hats were no longer the expected fashion accessory; she then transferred to department manager for purses. Grace retired on her 70th birthday.

As the youngest of six, only one of Grace's siblings is still living. Her twin brother, John, experienced a hemorrhagic stroke several years ago and resides in a rehabilitation facility in upstate New York. His two children and grandchildren also reside in that area, and she has at least weekly contact with some of them.

On this particular blistery cold winter morning, Grace is phoned by her grandniece, Katie. She is still in bed at 9 a.m., as she stayed up late reading. She turns up the portable space heater in her bedroom, puts on her robe, and proceeds to have a conversation standing in front of the much needed warmth. Her niece is excited about sharing news of her engagement; she received a proposal and ring the prior evening.

Approximately 5 minutes into the conversation, Grace moves away from the space heater as the back of her legs are becoming far too warm. She sits on the side of the bed and then smells something burning and sees smoke. She jumps up and pulls the back of her robe around to the front of her body and sees actual flames. Screams of "I'm on fire" alternate with "Someone help me!" On the other end of the phone, her grandniece is yelling, "Stop, drop, and roll." Grace realizes in a split second the floor space in her room is minimal; she lies on her bed instead, rolling back and forth.

She repeats this action over and over and barely manages to stand up again. She attempts to take her silky robe and gown off; however, the lower part of the garments have melted onto the back of her legs. Grace becomes nauseated, is shaking violently, and feels she is going to pass out; she lies down on her bed once again.

Many hours later, Grace arouses to find herself lying prone on a stretcher in a very noisy ED. She realizes she is wearing an oxygen mask and it feels like she has nails driven into each lower forearm, which are attached to clear tubing pumping fluid into her. She can see a digital monitor above her, which shows a blood pressure of 189/99 and a heart rate of 100. Another number says 88%, but she is unclear what that represents. The pain to the back of her legs from the ankles to her gluteal folds is like nothing she has ever known; she thinks to herself that she has multiple hot irons going up and down her extremities.

Suddenly the grandniece she spoke to earlier on the phone is by her side. Katie is tearful and expresses gratitude her aunt is still alive. She shares that she stayed on her cell phone for close to an hour while waiting for emergency medical services (EMS) to arrive and provide treatment; she contacted help via a landline in her parents' home as soon as she heard the word "fire."

Katie tells Grace that the ED physician said she has second-degree burns, is being assessed closely for potential complications, and will be admitted when a bed is available in the critical care unit. Grace inquires about damage to her apartment and if the fire spread to other units (it did not). A nurse interrupts to put medicine in the IV tubing, which she explains is "a little morphine we are giving you at regular intervals." Grace doses back into a restless sleep.

> 1. *The elderly (as well as young children) suffer from a higher incidence of burn injury compared to all other age groups. What predisposing factors increase the vulnerability for burns in the aging population? Use the article as a source found at www.unchealthcare.org/site/Nursing/nursingmedialibrary/ articles/burn.pdf?searchterm=in&searchterm=in.*

2. *When EMS arrived at Grace's apartment, she was immediately assessed for the total body surface area (TBSA) burned using the Rule of Nines tool. What percent do you think was reported? A brief video may be helpful in understanding this tool; it is available at https://vimeo.com/62746412 (mysafela.org, 2013).*

3. *It was stated that Grace experienced second-degree burns. Most health care providers use the term "burn depth" when classifying the severity. Compare and contrast the three levels using the following table as a guideline. (Use a medical–surgical nursing textbook or the Internet for the next three questions and cite your source.)*

Depth of burn	Skin involved	Symptoms	Wound appearance

4. *Morbidity associated with burns in the elderly is influenced by age-related changes of integumentary functioning. Briefly explain how alterations in this system may be involved.*

5. *A vital need immediately following a burn is fluid and electrolyte resuscitation. What IV fluids were initially used for Grace in the ED? Provide the rationale why potassium (K+) excess and sodium (Na+) deficit occur during the emergent stage of burns.*

While Grace was in the ED, her grandniece made contact with Joseph Barnes, the designated power of attorney and health care proxy for her greataunt. Joseph is the son of Grace's lifelong friend. He was able to provide basic health care information about Grace; for example, she is allergic to penicillin, and takes medication for hypertension and osteoporosis. She had colon cancer resulting in a transverse colostomy sometime after her retirement, a knee replacement at the age of 75, and has never smoked or used recreational drugs; her alcohol consumption is rare. He has a copy of her advanced directives, which he agrees to fax to the hospital. In addition, he provides the name and number of the internist Grace has used for over a decade. This physician will follow her while she is hospitalized, along with the critical care intensivist.

Grace is fully alert and oriented the next morning and is placed on IV hydromorphone (Dilaudid) 0.2 mg every 6 minutes with an 8 mg lockout at 4 hours, per a patient-controlled analgesia (PCA) pain pump. A nurse checks the history at the end of his shift, and it shows there were 32 demands with 10 doses of the narcotic administered.

6. *What should the nurse do first about this finding?*

   a. *Contact the MD for either a larger dose of the opioid or shorter intervals between doses.*

   b. *Exchange this PCA pump for another; there is an obvious error in this reading.*

> c. *Assess Grace's understanding of how she uses the PCA pump for pain management.*
>
> d. *Consider giving Grace her "break-through" dose of Dilaudid (hydromorphone) IV push.*

It is apparent Grace's sense of humor is still intact despite the trauma she has experienced. The primary nurse assigned to her in the ED noted the presence of an ostomy and made the remark, "This is actually a blessing." Grace has since used this term repeatedly such as, "My blessing needs emptying," "I need more supplies ordered for my blessing," and so on.

7. *Why did the nurse refer to her colostomy as a "blessing"?*

Grace is transferred on day 4 of hospitalization to a transitional care unit (TCU).

A nurse unfamiliar to her announces she will change the dressings on Grace's legs after lunch.

She brings in many supplies and states a nursing student would like to observe, which Grace approves. Lying in a supine position and using deep breathing techniques in anticipation of the discomfort, Grace cannot see the nurse or student. The nurse drops a package of opened 4 × 4 gauze dressings on the floor, picks them up, and places them on the sterile field.

8. *As a student observing this event, discuss how you would handle this issue.*

Two potential complications are removed from the nursing care plan developed for Grace during the emergent phase following her accident. These include the potential for development of compartment syndrome and Curling's ulcer.

9. *Explain why Grace was at risk for these complications following her burn injury.*

Nutritional support is a primary focus of care for burn patients. Grace was eating 50% to 75% of a high-calorie regular diet by the third day of hospitalization. After an extensive dietary consult, the decision was made to use enteral feedings as a supplement. Grace had a small bore feeding tube inserted and received supplemental feedings from 7 p.m. to 7 a.m., until she was discharged to a rehabilitation facility on day 10 following her burn.

10. *What was the likely rationale for significantly increasing her caloric intake postburn? Select all that apply.*

> a. *Hypermetabolism occurs with burns*
>
> b. *Healing of the burn consumes large quantities of energy*
>
> c. *Increasing fat intake is essential for homeostasis*
>
> d. *Appetite may be diminished related to pain and/or anxiety*
>
> e. *Reserve fat deposits are catabolized*

Grace was transferred to a rehabilitation facility an hour outside of New York City, which allowed for various members of her extended family to visit daily. She recovered there for 2 weeks and returned to her apartment in early spring.

11. What areas of health care not addressed in Grace's story do you think received attention during the rehab phase?

Suggested Resources

Fenicle, J. D. (2010). Management of patients with burn injury. In S. C. Smeltzer, B. G. Bare, J. L. Hinkle, & K. H. Cheever (Eds.), *Brunner and Suddarth's textbook of medical–surgical nursing* (12th ed., p. 1720). Philadelphia, PA: Lippincott Williams & Wilkins.

Grant, E. J. (2013). Preventing burns in the elderly. *Home Healthcare Nurse, 31*(10), 561–573. Retrieved from https://www.unchealthcare.org/site/Nursing/nursingmedialibrary/articles/burn.pdf?searchterm=in&searchterm=in

My Safe: LA. (2013). *Rule of nines* [Video file]. Retrieved from http://vimeo.com/62746412

Case 8.4 ■ Dermatologic Drug Reaction

*H*elen Schneider is a retired, 72-year-old Chinese American woman who is hospitalized with community-acquired pneumonia. Her past medical history includes chronic obstructive pulmonary disease (COPD), hypertension, and osteoarthritis. She has had several bouts of community-acquired pneumonia over the past 2 years, which have been difficult to treat because Helen has multiple drug allergies. She reports allergy to sulfonamides, fluoroquinolones, and penicillin. You have just received an order to administer Ceftriaxone 1 gm IV every 24 hours and Azithromycin 500 mg IV every 24 hours. You wonder whether it is safe to follow this order since Helen is allergic to penicillin. You also wonder what the alternatives might be.

1. What questions should you ask Helen to elucidate the details of her previous drug reactions?

Her penicillin allergy came into being many decades ago when she was given ampicillin by mouth for a sore throat. She vaguely remembers developing a rash over her whole body but doesn't remember any details about how long she had been taking the medication when the reaction began. Helen tells you that she thinks she took Benadryl to make the rash subside. She has avoided all penicillins and cephalosporins since that time.

She experienced a reaction on the fourth day of a course of Bactrim for a urinary tract infection. Redness and itching on the palms of her hands appeared, in addition to itching in the back of her throat with wheezing. She took Benadryl and an Albuterol nebulizer to remedy the problem. It took about a week after stopping the drug before the palmar itching completely subsided. She has avoided sulfonamide antibiotics, diuretics, sulfite-containing preservatives, and any other drugs with sulfa since that time.

When she takes Levaquin, she gets abdominal pain and diarrhea. The symptoms subside after discontinuing the drug without treatment. She doesn't have this problem with ciprofloxacin. These allergies do not surprise her because she tells you that everyone in her family has multiple drug allergies.

2. *Which of the reactions previously listed is most likely to be IgE-mediated hypersensitivity? The following link may be helpful: http://emedicine.medscape.com/article/136217-overview.*

3. *What is a common cause of rash with administration of ampicillin?*

4. *Did any of Helen's reactions meet the diagnostic criteria for an anaphylactic reaction? Use the article by Mustafa (2014) found at http://emedicine.medscape.com/article/135065-overview.*

5. *How common are anaphylactic reactions after administration of penicillin?*

6. *How does Helen's age affect her risk for development of a penicillin allergy?*

7. *If Helen had a true allergy to sulfonamide antibiotics, what other drugs should she avoid?*

8. *If Helen had a true allergy to penicillin, what other drugs should she avoid?*

9. *Is there any way that you can be absolutely sure if Helen has a true allergy to sulfonamides and penicillins?*

Suggested Resources

Kerr, M. (2012). *Sulfa allergies vs. sulphite allergies.* Healthline. Retrieved from http://www.healthline.com/health/allergies/sulfa-sulfite#2

Mustafa, S. S. (2014). *Anaphylaxis: Practice essentials. Medscape.* Retrieved from http://emedicine.medscape.com/article/135065-overview

Solensky, R. (2013). *Patient information: Allergy to penicillin and related antibiotics (beyond the basics).* UpToDate. Retrieved from http://www.uptodate.com/contents/allergy-to-penicillin-and-related-antibiotics-beyond-the-basics

Warner, J. (2014). *When is an allergic reaction an emergency?* Everyday Health.com. Retrieved from http://www.everydayhealth.com/health-report/anaphylaxis-severe-allergy-guide/allergic-reaction-emergency.aspx

Case 8.5 ■ Postoperative Infection (*Clostridium difficile*)

*M*r. Barnett, 80 years old, was admitted to the hospital for a right hip nailing after falling from his front porch. Surgery took place the following morning. Mr. Barnett was unable to urinate for 8 hours postoperatively and required an indwelling catheter. When the physical therapy department had him up on a walker the next day, the catheter was removed with the goal being that Mr. Barnett could stand at the bedside to use a urinal. However, this still was not possible and his catheter had to be reinserted. His surgeon believed that the narcotics used with the PCA pump may have affected his ability to urinate. The morphine was discontinued and pain was controlled with Vicodin (acetaminophen/oxycodone) alternated with Toradol (ketoralac).

On the fourth postoperative day, Mr. Barnett displayed some mild confusion requiring regular reorienting to time, place, and event. His children and grandchildren were greatly concerned after witnessing this behavior and insisted he had been cognitively intact upon admission.

When asked about his routine food and fluid intake, the family stated he predominantly ate two well-balanced meals a day. Like many older people, his thirst mechanism had declined and drinking two or three cups of fluid per day was typical. Otherwise, the health history includes long-term hypertension, hyperlipidemia, and atrial fibrillation; all conditions are adequately controlled with medication.

> **1. Visit www.healthinaging.org/agingintheknow/chapters_ch_trial .asp?ch=57 and www.healthinaging.org/aging-and-health-a-to-z/ topic:delirium/info:causes-and-symptoms. An acronym spelling "delirium" lists multiple causes for acute confusion in the elderly. What are three possibilities for onset in Mr. Barnett?**

Based on lab work results, Mr. Barnett was found to have a urinary tract infection. He was placed on Rocephin (ceftriaxone) 500 mg IV twice a day for 6 days. His acute confusion totally cleared. A condom catheter was used until the client's discharge from the hospital. He also required transfusion of two units of packed red blood cells (PRBCs) for hemoglobin, which fell to 8.4 g.

Because of postoperative complications, the hospital's physical therapy department was not able to promote Mr. Barnett's goal of ambulating with a walker by the time of discharge. Therefore, he agreed to transfer to a rehabilitation facility, hoping the stay there would require only another week.

Mr. Barnett's first few days at the new facility went smoothly; he was highly motivated to participate in physical and occupational therapy to return home. A new problem began the evening of his third day at the rehab facility. He began having diarrhea. The frequency of needing to use a bedside commode completely exhausted him; he had an hourly bowel movement the first 12 hours after onset of the diarrhea. A stool specimen was collected and tested positive for *Clostridium difficile* (*C. difficile*).

  2. *What recent event likely contributed to Mr. Barnett's contracting C. difficile?*

  3. *Why are the elderly more at risk for this infection?*

  4. *The complication of sepsis is a concern from* C. difficile; *what pathology can lead to this?*

Mr. Barnett was placed on 0.9% sodium chloride at 75 mL/hr for the following 2 days. His family was informed of the change in his status. His daughter, Maria, came to visit and brought her father roasted cashews, a favorite treat, and told the nurse, "I am rather germ-a-phobic. What am I supposed to do when going into his room?"

  5. *How should the nurse respond to this question?*

  6. *What food restrictions are typical for individuals experiencing profuse diarrhea?*

  7. *Mr. Barnett's daughter also asks if special cleaning products are used when a* C. difficile *infection is present; what should she be told?*

Mr. Barnett was started on oral Flagyl (metronidazole) and a probiotic for the infection, which he continued to take at home when discharged. His family required careful explanation of treating a problem caused by one antibiotic with another one, but were in agreement to the plan.

  8. *Using the website http://www.medpagetoday.com/InfectiousDisease/ GeneralInfectiousDisease/35974 explain how the use of a probiotic provides hopeful treatment and prevention of* C. difficile?

Mr. Barnett had assistance from his grandson who lived with him for a month after discharge. He used a walker around his home for several weeks and gained enough strength to eventually use a cane. There were no further complications.

Suggested Resources

Bankhead, C. (2012). *Probiotics may prevent C. difficile diarrhea.* Medpage Today. Retrieved from http://www.medpagetoday.com/InfectiousDisease/GeneralInfectiousDisease/35974

Harvard Health Publications. (2010). *Clostridium difficile:* An intestinal infection on the rise. *Harvard Men's Healthwatch.* Retrieved from http://www.health.harvard.edu/ newsletters/Harvard_Mens_Health_Watch/2010/June/clostridium-difficile-an-intestinal-infection-on-the-rise

Health in Aging.org. (2012). Delerium. Retrieved from http://www.healthinaging.org/aging-and-health-a-to-z/topic:delirium/info:causes-and-symptoms

Case 8.6 ■ Herpes Zoster (Shingles)

*D*iane McAllister anticipated turning 65 years old with a positive attitude as this marked the time period she referred to as her "best third." Retirement, self-supporting adult children, and moving into a loft-style condominium were goals achieved to assist in enjoying this "last third" of her life. Several months after her birthday, an event occurred that made Diane's 65th year memorable for quite different reasons.

Sitting in a coffee shop one morning, Diane had the onset of the worst headache she ever experienced. It came on suddenly and with such intensity, she grabbed the back of her head and screamed loudly. This was followed by vomiting the cup of coffee she had just finished. Diane lost consciousness within several minutes.

In the ED of a nearby hospital, it was discovered through a CT scan that Diane experienced a subarachnoid hemorrhage (SAH) as a result of a ruptured cerebral aneurysm. In general, one third of patients who suffer an SAH will survive with good recovery, one third will survive with a disability or stroke, and one third will die (Zuccarello & Ringer, 2013).

Diane was in the intensive care unit for more than 2 weeks. She experienced moderate focal deficit with short-term memory loss, generalized muscle weakness, and difficulty swallowing. Enteral feedings through a gastrostomy tube were initiated, and she was able to ambulate with a rolling walker for support. The discharge planning nurse coordinating her care arranged for a transfer to a rehabilitation facility in a nearby town, which is scheduled for the next day.

After sitting in a recliner for several hours, Diane returned to bed and noted a burning, stabbing type pain accompanied by itching, which started at her lumbar spine area and wrapped around to her umbilicus. The area was reddened. She rated this pain as a "7" on the standard scale. Her nurse contacted the physician who ordered acetaminophen with codeine elixir, which reduced the discomfort to a "4" for an hour or so. Benadryl (diphenhydramine) liquid was also prescribed for the itching; this medicine was helpful as it promoted sleep, albeit restless.

The pain continued the next morning, which was a Friday. Her transfer to the rehab facility was postponed until Monday because new clients were not admitted on the weekend. On Sunday, Diane had patches of vesicles containing clear fluid erupt around the trunk area. Her nurse recognized this sign, and reported it as herpes zoster, commonly known as shingles.

Use a textbook or any reputable Internet source to answer the following questions, citing your reference. Find and view several images showing the virus for better understanding.

1. ***Describe the pathology associated with this condition.***

2. ***Find and report the prevalence of this infection in older adults.***

3. *What are the risk factors for herpes zoster? Diane received prednisone during her entire hospitalization for cerebral inflammation; how does this possibly contribute to the outbreak?*

4. *The staff expressed concern about being assigned to care for Diane with this infection. Which of the following nurses should avoid having contact with her?*

   a. *John, who experiences eczema on occasion.*

   b. *Carrie, who believes she may be several weeks pregnant.*

   c. *Bethany, who had a severe case of chickenpox at age 10.*

   d. *Katie, who sneezes occasionally from seasonal allergies.*

5. *What is the typical clinical course of herpes zoster?*

6. *The nurse enters Diane's room to find her crying. She states, "My neighbor has told a lot of people I have herpes and everyone thinks it's the sexual disease kind." How should the nurse respond?*

7. *Diane begins treatment immediately with Zovirax (acyclovir). Describe how this medication halts the progression of shingles, and the importance of starting it quickly after diagnosis.*

Diane achieved adequate pain control with medication and cool compresses to her affected areas. She was informed by the staff, and did some additional reading, about the potential complication of postherpetic neuralgia (persistent pain lasting longer than 6 months) following onset of the infection. She was extremely grateful that her infection cleared in about 2 weeks. During this time, she worked diligently with a speech therapist and nutritionist and was able to safely take thickened liquids by mouth. In addition, she could transfer herself in and out of bed and eventually go up and down steps with her walker. Her short-term memory loss totally cleared. She was discharged home and was finally able to carry on with her "best third."

8. *Discuss the vaccine for herpes zoster used as a preventive health measure for older adults; when should it be administered and how often?*

Suggested Resources

Centers for Disease Control and Prevention. (2011). *Shingles (herpes zoster) vaccination* Retrieved from http://www.cdc.gov/Vaccines/vpd-vac/shingles/default.htm

Centers for Disease Control and Prevention. (2014). *Shingles (herpes zoster)*. Retrieved from http://www.cdc.gov/shingles/about

Zuccarello, M., & Ringer, R. (2013). *Subaracchoid hemmorhage*. Mayfield Clinic. Retrieved from http://www.mayfieldclinic.com/PE-SAH.HTM#.VMpCz8stHug

9

The Aging Musculoskeletal System

Case 9.1 ■ Osteoarthritis

Cynthia Bausch is an RN in a geriatric practice, who has received a referral from Dr. Cobb to provide outreach to Ms. McConnell, a 68-year-old female with osteoarthritis (OA) of the right knee and hands. Dr. Cobb has asked that Ms. McConnell discontinue the ibuprofen that she has been using to treat the pain in her knee in order to prevent gastrointestinal bleeding and because her renal function has become compromised. Her serum creatinine has increased from 1.0 to 1.4 in the past 6 months. Ms. McConnell is 5 feet 5 inches tall and weighs 210 pounds. She is concerned about stopping her ibuprofen since she has been taking 600 mg every 6 hours for the past 4 years to control her arthritis pain. She has tried Tylenol without success in the past. She is worried that the pain will become disabling and interfere with her quality of life. She currently enjoys shopping with friends, going to movies, and cooking for family and friends.

Ms. McConnell was an avid skier when she was in her twenties until she injured her right knee and gave up the sport. She has not participated in any regular exercise since that time. Ms. McConnell lives alone with her dog, Max, whom she takes for short walks (about one block) daily.

Ms. McConnell's other medical conditions include hypertension and hyperlipidemia. She takes Prinzide (hydrochlorothiazide/lisinopril) 12.5/10 mg daily and Zocor (simvastatin) 20 mg every evening for these conditions.

1. *What is OA and why does its prevalence increase with age?*

2. *What risk factors for developing OA does Ms. McConnell have?*

3. *Which joints are most commonly affected by OA?*

4. *What physical exam findings should Cynthia expect to see in Ms. McConnell's right knee and hands?*

5. *Cynthia needs to calculate Ms. McConnell's glomerular filtration rate (GFR) so that she can help her to understand her physician's rationale in stopping the ibuprofen. Use the online GFR calculator found at http://nephron.com/cgi-bin/CGSI.cgi*

to calculate Ms. McConnell's GFR with the Cockcroft Gault formula.

    a. What is her GFR?

    b. With which stage of kidney disease does this GFR correspond?

    c. What factors in Ms. McConnell's history put her at risk for nonsteroidal anti-inflammatory drug (NSAID)-related renal disease?

6. *Why is Ms. McConnell's physician worried about gastrointestinal bleeding? Use this link, www.medicinenet .com/nonsteroidal_anti-inflammatory_drugs_and_ulcers/ article.htm.*

7. *Ms. McConnell is concerned about pain management without ibuprofen. What nonpharmacologic treatments can Cynthia suggest? Use the following evidence-based guideline from the American College of Rheumatology 2012 Recommendations for the Use of Nonpharmacologic and Pharmacologic Therapies in Osteoarthritis of the Hand, Hip, and Knee (Table 3, p. 469) to help you formulate your treatment plan: www.rheumatology .org/practice/clinical/guidelines/PDFs/ACR_OA_Guidelines_ FINAL.pdf.*

8. *Ms. McConnell asks what the Arthritis Foundation Self-Management is all about and what the program time commitment will be. How should Cynthia respond? Use http://patienteducation.stanford.edu/programs/asmp.html.*

9. *Ms. McConnell tells Cynthia that her friends have advised her to buy glucosamine/chondroitin. Evidence-based practice has questioned the benefits of these supplements. What should Cynthia tell Ms. McConnell about the therapeutic effectiveness and side effects associated with glucosamine/chondroitin? Use information from the National Center for Complementary and Alternative Medicine (NCCAM) found at http://nccam.nih.gov/ health/arthritis/osteoarthritis (What the Science Says).*

Suggested Resources

Hochberg, M. C., Altman, R. D., April, K. T., Benkhalti, M., Guyatt, G., McGowan, J., . . . Tagwell, P. (2012). American College of Rheumatology 2012 recommendations for the use of nonpharmacologic and pharmacologic therapies in osteoarthritis of the hand, hip, and knee. *Arthritis Care & Research, 64*(4), 465–474. Retrieved from http://www.rheumatology.org/practice/clinical/guidelines/PDFs/ACR_OA_Guidelines_ FINAL.pdf

Lozada, C. J. (2014). *Osteoarthritis.* Medscape. Retrieved from http://emedicine.medscape.com/ article/330487-overview#aw2aab6b2b4

National Center for Complementary and Alternative Medicine. (2014). *Osteoarthritis and complementary health approaches*. Retrieved from http://nccam.nih.gov/health/arthritis/osteoarthritis

Omudhome, O. (2014). *Nonsteroidal anti-inflammatory drugs (NSAIDs) and ulcers*. MedicineNet .com. Retrieved from http://www.medicinenet.com/nonsteroidal_anti-inflammatory_drugs_and_ulcers/article.htm

Case 9.2 ■ Hip Fracture

*P*earl Benson has arrived at the local hospital's ED after a neighbor, who saw her lying outside on the ground near her mailbox, called 911. Pearl is yelling out in pain and oriented to person, place, time, and event. She tells the ED nurse when asked for her pain rating, "It's the worst I've ever had in 83 years of my life."

Pearl lives alone in a rural setting and walks down the road to retrieve her mail and newspaper each afternoon. Her health has declined significantly in the past 5 years. She has lost most of her vision due to diabetes retinopathy (type 2), is treated for osteoporosis, has consistent foot pain due to peripheral vascular disease, and takes medication for gastroesophageal reflux (GERD) and hypertension. She has experienced multiple transient ischemic attacks (TIA), when she momentarily couldn't speak, and had a myocardial infarction at age 72. She is estranged from both of her adult children; they choose not to communicate due to her "abusive personality." Pearl has been divorced for several decades and has no close contacts.

In the ED, vital signs show a temperature of 98°F, heart rate 102, respirations 26, and BP 186/94. Oxygenation saturation is 90% and she is administered 2 L of O_2 per nasal cannula. Pearl is given intravenous fluids consisting of sodium chloride 0.9% at 125 mL/hr. Her electrolytes show several abnormal values: a K+ of 3.2 mEq/L, glucose 286 mg/dL, BUN 30 mg/dL, and creatinine of 1.7 mg/dL. A complete blood count revealed white blood count 11,000 cells/mcL, red blood count 4.0 cells/mcL, hemoglobin 9.8 g, and hematocrit 29%. An orthopedic consult occurred within 2 hours of her arrival; the surgeon reviewed radiology films and reported that Pearl had a femoral neck fracture of her right hip. Surgery would be required the next morning and an operative permit was signed following informed consent for a right total hip replacement (THR).

1. *At this point, which of the following medications should Pearl receive in a timely manner? Select all that apply.*

   a. *KCL in her IV fluids*

   b. *Cefazolin (Kefzol) IV*

   c. *Coumadin (warfarin)*

   d. *Morphine sulfate IV*

   e. *Regular insulin subcutaneous*

2. How common are hip fractures in the elderly?

3. What age-related physiological changes increase the incidence?

4. What risk factors contribute to hip fractures?

5. A canvas immobilizer was applied to Pearl's right leg to decrease movement. What has evidence-based practice found in regard to applying preoperative traction (e.g., Buck's) for immobilization and reducing pain for a hip fracture? Use the Cochrane Database article for your answer at http:// onlinelibrary.wiley.com/doi/10.1002/14651858.CD000168 .pub3/pdf.

Pearl undergoes a hip replacement procedure the next morning. She recovers from anesthesia and returns to her hospital room in stable condition. Nursing care focuses on preventive measures for avoidance of atelectasis (thus, pneumonia), skin breakdown (contributing to pressure ulcer), and deep vein thrombosis (leading to pulmonary embolism).

6. What specific interventions are used with the patient to prevent these complications?

7. Another important focus is avoidance of abduction of the affected hip to prevent dislocation. What measures can be used?

On the second postoperative day, Pearl's hemoglobin drops to 8.0 g. It is determined she needs to be transfused with two units of packed red blood cells. When the RN enters her room with another licensed individual, to confirm identification prior to administering the blood, an unexpected event occurs. Pearl shows her hospital wrist band and notable shaking of her hands is apparent. In addition, she is diaphoretic and looks anxious. Temperature taken within the half hour was 98°F. Her pain level with a morphine patient-controlled analgesia (PCA) pump is at "3" and other vital signs are within an acceptable range.

Pearl says to her assigned nurse, "Please get those things out of here, I can't stand them running all around. I occasionally have a mouse in my home, but I never expected a hospital room to be full of them." The experienced RN steps over to the computer, pulls up Pearl's admission nursing history, and checks under the section for alcohol consumption. It lists three servings per week. The nurse pulls up a chair next to the bed to be at eye level, and asks Pearl in a calm, pleasant tone when was the last time she had alcohol and how much?

8. What problem is the nurse assessing for at this point?

A 2 mg dose of Ativan (lorazepam) was administered IV after reporting findings to Pearl's physician. It was repeated every 6 hours for the next 24 hours, then changed to an oral route. The sedative slowed down the postoperative plan of care to have Pearl up with a walker and ambulating, transferring herself in and out of bed, and being able to go up and down several steps. Therefore, on the fifth day following surgery, she was transferred to a rehabilitation facility in stable condition.

After an additional month of therapy, Pearl was mobile again with the use of a walker. Due to her co-morbid conditions, having no social support, and living alone in a rural area, she participated in the decision to remain at the extended care facility permanently. This is a common event; the literature is replete with statistics that support the idea that half of all women having a hip fracture never return to their previous residence. Pearl made several friends at the facility, including the German shepherd that lived on the premises and was part of the "family."

> **9. For individuals who are able to return home following a hip replacement, what modifications, including equipment, are recommended for a safe recovery?**
>
> **10. What is the morbidity rate associated with a fractured hip?**

Suggested Resources

A Place for Mom. (2014). *Hip fracture in the elderly and assisted care*. Retrieved from http://www.aplaceformom.com/senior-care-resources/articles/hip-fractures-in-the-elderly

Burroughs, K. E. (2014). *Hip fractures*. UpToDate. Retrieved from http://www.uptodate.com/contents/hip-fractures-in-adults

Cheever, K. H. (2014). Management of patients with musculoskeletal trauma. In J. L. Hinkle & K. H. Cheever (Eds.), *Brunner & Suddarth's textbook of medical–surgical nursing* (13th ed., pp. 1173–1182). Philadelphia, PA: Wolters Kluwer Health.

Handoll, H. H. G., Queally, J. M., & Parker, M. J. (2011). Pre-operative traction for hip fractures in adults. The Cochrane Library. Retrieved from http://onlinelibrary.wiley.com/doi/10.1002/14651858.CD000168.pub3/pdf

Case 9.3 ■ Falls: Home Environment

*F*alls have long been defined as an occurrence in which an individual unintentionally comes to rest on the ground, the floor, or at a lower level (Tinetti, Speechley, & Ginter, 1988). Most falls take place in the home. Annually, about 2.3 million older adults are treated in the ED for fall-related injuries and more than 662,000 are hospitalized (Centers for Disease Control and Prevention [CDC], 2013). Falls are not a random event or usual result of aging. The consequences of falls for an older adult can be one of the most expensive and life-altering events associated with old age.

Some individuals have an increase in muscle weakness, loss of balance, partial loss of vision, or a change in their ability to walk. Additionally, the fear of falling can be almost as destructive as the actual event. Individuals who experience any of these factors have a higher risk of falling. Prevention of falls is especially important because a fall can result in major cuts or broken bones. Breaks of the hip or wrist are the most common, and are the cause of significant complications.

1. ***What does the Centers for Disease Control and Prevention estimate the financial cost associated with falling to be by the year 2020? Use the following link: www.cdc.gov/homeandrecreationalsafety/falls/fallcost.html.***

Consider the following case: Mary Jones is an 82-year-old woman who lives alone in her own two-story home. She has fallen once and been treated for a broken left hip at a local acute care and rehabilitation hospital this past year. Susan Smith, Mary's daughter, lives in another city that is 1,200 miles away. Susan is concerned about her mother's home environment and her chance of falling again. She wonders what she can do to help prevent her mother from falling.

2. ***Find a falls-prevention checklist for home use on the Internet and cite your source. Comment on the suggestions in relation to where you live; are any changes necessary?***

Susan chooses to contact the rehabilitation department at the local hospital in Mary's community and arranges for a home assessment targeted at preventing falls. During the initial assessment, the rehabilitation RN uncovers the following facts. Mary reports her overall health as "good." She has a strong faith in God, which helps her cope, and she goes to church on a regular basis. In the nurse's appraisal related to fall prevention, she asks about the following, because each can be a factor in causing falls.

Medication and alcohol use:

Mary takes Lopressor (metoprolol) 50 mg every morning for high blood pressure. For diabetes control, she uses Actos (pioglitazone) 30 mg in the evening, and Amaryl (glimepiride) 5 mg in the morning. She denies any side effects of the medicines or use of alcohol.

3. ***Search the Internet and choose at least one website that describes these medications and the associated side effects. Decide which, if any, of Mary's medications are a potential cause for falls.***

Vision problems:

Mary's vision with glasses is corrected to 20/20.

Neurological deficits such as balance problems, mental confusion, and faulty judgment:

There are no uncovered deficits for Mary.

Incontinence/urgency:

Mary reports no problems.

Fatigue factors:

Mary reports that she is tired. She shares that she recently had to place her husband in the Alzheimer's care unit in a VA facility 1 hour away from her home. This care is free for veterans and Mary thinks this is an important earned benefit. She drives every day to see her husband.

4. **What ideas can be offered in helping Mary visit her husband every day to help decrease Mary's fatigue?**

Fear of falling:

Mary shares that she is afraid of falling again and tells the nurse that she fell down the stairs going from her bedroom to the kitchen when she broke her hip. Although Susan calls every day at noon, Mary states that she was on the floor for what seemed like hours before she could "think" to get assistance. Fortunately, her mail carrier heard her calling for help.

5. **Risk factors for falling are divided into intrinsic, extrinsic, and situational factors. Mary has multifactoral risks. Use the article by Rubenstein (2013) at www.merckmanuals.com/professional/ geriatrics/falls_in_the_elderly/falls_in_the_elderly.html to compare and contrast these factors.**

Find the article by Anne Togher (2014) at www.lifelinesys.com/content/blog/ healthcare-professionals/falls-prevention/how-to-help-a-senior-overcome-a-fear-of-falling to answer Questions 6 and 7.

6. **What does the author recommend as the best method for reducing the fear associated with falling?**

    a. **Use of daily prayer**

    b. **Discussing feelings with a therapist**

    c. **Wearing a medical alert device**

    d. **Gaining confidence**

7. **One of many areas of teaching for Mary in relation to falls prevention in the home includes how she dresses herself. Discuss the recommendations for shoes and clothing.**

8. **Choose either (a) an exercise program to increase strength, balance, and muscle tone or (b) how to get up from a fall and briefly describe how you would begin to educate Mary.**

Suggested Resources

Baker, D. (2012). *Learn how to get up* [Video file]. Philips Lifeline. Retrieved from http://www .learnnottofall.com/content/what-if-i-fall/learn-to-get-up.jsp

Centers for Disease Control and Prevention. (2013). *Falls among older adults: An overview.* Retrieved from www.cdc.gov/homeandrecreationalsafety/falls/fallcost.html

Centers for Disease Control and Prevention. (2014). *Costs of falls among older adults.* Retrieved from http://www.cdc.gov/homeandrecreationalsafety/falls/adultfalls.html

Rubenstein, L. Z. (2013). Falls in the elderly. *The Merck manual for healthcare professionals.* Retrieved from http://www.merckmanuals.com/professional/geriatrics/falls_in_the_ elderly/falls_in_the_elderly.html

Tinetti, M.E., Speechley, M.,& Ginter, S.F. (1988). Risk factors for falls among elderly persons living in the community. *New England Journal of Medicine, 319,* 1701–1707. Retrieved from http://www.nejm.org/doi/full/10.1056/NEJM198812293192604

Togher, A. (2014). How to help a senior overcome fear of falling. *Falls Prevention.* Retrieved from http://www.lifelinesys.com/content/blog/healthcare-professionals/falls-prevention/how-to-help-a-senior-overcome-a-fear-of-falling

Wilson, S. (2012). *Try tai chi to improve balance, avoid falls.* Harvard Health Publications. Retrieved from http://www.health.harvard.edu/blog/try-tai-chi-to-improve-balance-avoid-falls-201208235198

Case 9.4 ■ Fall Prevention in a Hospital Setting

*L*aura Simpson is a 35-year-old RN who has worked part time in a pediatric office for 10 years. She is married and has three children in elementary school. Her husband lost a lucrative position as a venture capitalist due to the economic crisis in the metropolitan area where they reside. His 2-year unemployment has resulted in the couple using all savings, cashing in his retirement plan, and maxing out a credit card. Laura is making a major career change as a result; she has been hired full time at a large medical center on a gero-rehab unit. Her salary will cover the family's basic needs and provide for much needed family health and dental insurance.

The hospital provided Laura with an online, self-study course requiring 30 hours of reading and answering questions to validate understanding of the needs of geriatric clients. Topics such as age-related changes of the body systems, mental health disorders, polypharmacy concerns, and safety issues were well covered. Laura had some familiarity of the information from her several years as a medical–surgical nurse when starting her career. The focus on patient falls in health care facilities was a large section of Laura's review. She studied this section carefully and read additional material to have a better knowledge base of assessment, prevention, and the evaluation processes of patient falls. Use the following source for Questions 1 and 2: http://www.consultgerirn.com/topics/falls/want_to_know_more (Gray-Micelli & Quigley, 2012).

1. In relation to falls, what are the common causes?

2. Which of the following would be extrinsic risk factors associated with falls? Select all that apply.

a. Shoes fit properly and are in good repair

b. Bedrails do not collapse when used for transitioning or support

c. Patient gowns/clothing do not cause tripping

d. Using benzodiazepines

e. History of a previous fall

Another component of Laura's self-study course of patient care required her to review the National Patient Safety Goals (NPSG) put forth by The Joint Commission. From her years working at the pediatric office, she implemented guidelines that related to the safety of children. Now she must focus on the entire set of goals.

> 3. **Using The Joint Commission's current document, locate and document the NPSG and supportive rationale in relation to hospital falls.**

Laura devotes a good deal of time reviewing assessment tools used by health care facilities. She understands risk assessment tools fall into three categories: nursing fall risk assessments, functional assessments, and complete medical assessments.

> 4. **Which of the following are commonly used nursing fall-risk assessment tools? Select all that apply.**
>
> a. **The Morse Fall Scale**
>
> b. **The STRATIFY tool**
>
> c. **The Hendrich II Fall Risk Model**
>
> d. **Schmid Fall Risk Assessment Tool**
>
> 5. **Regardless of the fall-risk assessment tool used, what are the intrinsic risk factors most scales will assess the elderly for upon admission and regularly thereafter?**

Functional assessments measure a patient's ability to manage daily routines, such as transferring, ambulating, and bathing. Laura's self-study explains that the purpose of a functional assessment is to indicate the presence and severity of disease, measure a person's need for care, monitor change over time, and maintain an optimally cost-effective clinical operation. She is unfamiliar with the specifics of functional assessment and seeks additional information.

> 6. **Choose one of the following assessments and describe the purpose and general technique used: Timed Get Up & Go test, Tinneti Assessment Tool, or Berg Balance Measure.**

Laura reviewed the information of the falls protocol for the hospital she would be working for and found the list of interventions to be logical and relatively "easy" to implement. She also watched a video, www.youtube.com/watch?v=M30v3QhTw3U, which reviews details of an evidence-based protocol with a hospital patient.

> 7. **Review a falls protocol from a textbook, Internet source, or watch the video cited. What specific intervention(s) for prevention was new knowledge for you? Cite the reference.**

Another area relating to falls that Laura found had changed greatly since her early career in nursing pertained to interventions after a patient fall actually occurred. The policy she used more than a decade ago required filling out an incident report and continued monitoring of the patient.

8. What is involved with a "post-fall huddle"?

Although starting full-time employment in a new facility was challenging, Laura adapted well and found working with the geriatric population rewarding. In assessing and implementing the unit's falls prevention protocol, it became apparent to her that patients who had fallen previously often endured the emotional impact long after.

9. What would you expect to be common emotional outcomes for the elderly who experience a fall?

Suggested Resources

Gray-Micelli, D., & Quigley, P. A. (2012). *Nursing standard of practice protocol: Fall prevention.* Hartford Institute for Geriatric Nursing. Retrieved from http://www.consultgerirn.com/topics/falls/want_to_know_more

Morse, J. M. (2002). Enhancing the safety of hospitalization by reducing patient falls. *American Journal of Infection Control, 30*(6), 376–378.

Posiadlo, D., & Richardson, S. (1991). The timed get up & go: A test of basic functional mobility for frail elderly persons. *Journal of the American Geriatric Society, 48*(1), 104–105.

Schmidt, T. (2013). *Geriatric balance and fall prevention: Evidence-based examination and interventions.* HomeCEUConnections. Retrieved from https://www.youtube.com/watch?v=M30v3QhTw3U

The Joint Commission. (2014). *National patient safety goals.* Retrieved from http://www.jointcommission.org/assets/1/6/NCC_NPSG_Chapter_2014.pdf

Tinetti, M. E. (1986). Performance-oriented assessment of mobility problems in elderly patients. *Journal of the American Geriatrics Society, 6*(34), 119–126.

Case 9.5 ■ Immobility

Mary Allen, an 89-year-old female, has been admitted to a long-term care facility after falling and fracturing her hip 1 week ago. Prior to her admission, Mary lived in the home of one of her daughters and was able to care for herself. She was hospitalized for 4 days after the fall for surgical hip pinning. During her hospitalization, she became increasingly confused and incontinent of urine. It was determined that Mary be admitted for physical therapy. After 2 weeks at the facility, the staff and family agreed that Mary is unable to complete physical therapy related to her diagnosis of moderate level dementia with associated confusion and inability to follow commands. Her family has decided to forego physical therapy, which will mean that Mary will be wheelchair-bound and need assistance with all activities of daily living (ADL).

Mary has a history of hypertension and OA in addition to dementia of the Alzheimer's type. Mary wears glasses and has bilateral hearing aids for age-related hearing loss. Her two daughters live within 30 minutes of the long-term care facility and visit her on a daily basis. Medications include Lasix (furosemide) 20 mg every morning, aspirin (acetylsalicylic acid) 81 mg every morning, and Tylenol (acetaminophen) 650 mg every 4 hours as needed for pain. Mary has the potential to suffer complications related to decreased mobility based on her age as well as her physical health condition. As a nurse, you are aware of the potential complications of immobility and develop a plan of care that will prevent these complications.

1. *What is the impact of decreased mobility on functional status?*

2. *What are cardiovascular complications of immobility that may affect Mary?*

3. *Skin breakdown is a major complication. Because Mary is incontinent of urine and has decreased mobility, the nursing diagnosis is risk for impaired skin integrity. Identify five nursing interventions that you can implement in an independent manner to prevent skin breakdown.*

4. *In addition to the potential for skin breakdown, Mary has the potential for dehydration. Identify normal age-related changes that may predispose Mary for dehydration. What are the causes for dehydration in a long-term care setting for a patient with dementia? What assessment measures will you need to perform for a person who has the potential for dehydration? What nursing interventions must be instituted to maintain hydration status?*

As a nurse, you know that pneumonia is the fourth most common cause of death in the older adult population and is a potential complication of immobility.

5. *Mary has a decreased mobility that also may lead to the potential for pneumonia, which is a leading cause of death among the older adult population. What are normal age-related changes that may increase Mary's potential to develop pneumonia in addition to decreased mobility? Identify five nursing interventions to prevent pneumonia in an older adult who also has a decreased level of mobility.*

6. *Prior to Mary's fall, she was able to care for herself. One goal of nursing care should be to prevent a further decline in function. Discuss nursing interventions to promote function and deter premature dependence.*

Suggested Resource

Mentes, J. C. (2012). *Nursing standard of practice protocol: Oral hydration management.* Hartford Institute for Geriatric Nursing. Retrieved from http://www.consultgerirn.com/topics/hydration_management/want_to_know_more

Case 9.6 ■ Osteoporosis

*T*hree generations of women are sitting at a kitchen table having coffee following dinner. The matriarch, Violet, is 92 years old; her daughter, Lillian, is 70; and her granddaughter, Elizabeth, is 49. Violet moved in with her daughter several years ago after falling twice at her own home. She suffers from vertigo at times but, aside from bruising and soreness, she incurred no major injuries. The youngest female of the group has initiated a conversation regarding osteoporosis.

Violet makes the comment that osteoporosis was essentially unheard of during her middle adult years. She remembers seeing women with a "hump back" and certainly losing several inches in height over a span of time, which was likely associated with osteoporosis. Violet believes that her lifestyle from her early 20s through her early 70s had a favorable impact on preventing osteoporosis. She says, "Remember, I worked a dairy farm and consumed all of our products, tended a vegetable garden that fed a family of six, never smoked or partook in booze."

1. ***Translate Violet's activities as to what is currently recommended for osteoporosis prevention.***

Lillian remarks, "Well mother, you had no control over your race, body frame, and gender. We're at a higher risk than others because of these factors."

2. ***What risk factors for osteoporosis are suggested with this statement?***

Elizabeth acknowledges the healthy living of her grandmother, knowing her personal life has been quite different. She asks the two women if they have ever been tested in regards to bone density. She goes on to say her physician included this with a recent physical exam. Her mother remarks she was checked at age 65 and asks if Elizabeth having a total hysterectomy, including having her ovaries removed, was the reason for early screening.

3. ***Find a video on the Internet using Google or another source that shows the DEXA (or DXA) test available for assessing bone density and explain how it functions. Cite the source.***

4. What outcome from a hysterectomy would result in middle-age screening for osteoporosis?

The women then discuss medications related to osteoporosis as all three have drugs/supplements, but each is different. Elizabeth uses Os-Cal and a low dose of vitamin D daily. Her mother, Lillian, began using Reclast (zoledronic acid) when it came on the market and has a dose each year during her birthday week. Violet was using a bisphosphate for years, but changed to Evista (raloxifene).

5. Discuss each of these medications in relation to drug category, route/frequency, and action.

6. The nurse has provided teaching for a patient who was prescribed an oral bisphosphonate, Fosamax (alendronate), for prevention of osteoporosis. Which statement indicates further teaching is necessary?

    a. "Drinking milk while on the drug is a good idea"

    b. "Taking this med right before bedtime is recommended"

    c. "I only have to take this once a week"

    d. "This medicine should be taken on an empty stomach"

Elizabeth gets up from the table to refresh her coffee and hugs her grandmother from behind, stating, "I am so glad you moved in here with Mom. Also, that you've been agreeable with all the safety precautions recommended for elderly women with osteoporosis."

7. Discuss safety measures that can eliminate potential home hazards resulting in a fall or injury.

8. Osteoporosis has been identified as a national public health issue priority; provide a rationale for this.

Suggested Resources

American College of Preventive Medicine. (2010). *Women's health & osteoporosis time tool for nurses: A resource from the American College of Preventive Medicine.* Retrieved from http://www.acpm.org/?NurseWomOsteo_TT

Osteoporosis Canada. (2014). *Preventing falls.* Retrieved from http://www.osteoporosis.ca/ osteoporosis-and-you/living-well-with-osteoporosis/preventing-falls

Robinson, M. V. (2014). Management of patients with musculoskeletal disorders. In J. L. Hinkle & K. H. Cheever (Eds.), *Brunner & Suddarth's textbook of medical–surgical nursing* (13th ed., pp. 1141–1145). Philadelphia, PA: Lippincott Williams & Wilkins.

Stork, S. (2014). *Bone mineral density test.* Medline Plus. Retrieved from http://www.nlm.nih .gov/medlineplus/ency/article/007197.htm

Case 9.7 ■ Foot Problems in the Elderly

*B*rian Leezer has been an RN for several decades with most of his practice focused on orthopedic nursing. Once his children were in high school, he returned to college to further his education and gained an advanced nurse practitioner degree focusing in gerontology. Brian performs all physical assessments and health history exams for a medical clinic within a Veterans Administration hospital. It became apparent to him in a short time that he would continue to use his knowledge base and expertise for orthopedic nursing, as a large majority of the elderly clients he cared for reported foot problems.

During his years of practice, Brian developed a real fondness and admiration of older patients. His own parents are now in their early 80s and completely independent. They developed healthy lifestyles in their 30s that have served them well. Brian often mentions how active his mother and father are and what great role models they've served for him and his sister in regard to successful aging.

His parents are members of a senior citizens organization and both participate, as well as volunteer, for a number of activities. They asked Brian if he would prepare a presentation about common foot problems to a group that meets monthly to learn about health topics. Brian agreed and is in the process of developing his class. He decides to start with some research statistics about the prevalence of foot problems, believing it may put the audience at ease to know the high numbers of elderly affected.

> 1. *Find a statistic pertaining to the percentage of elderly people who are affected by foot problems.*

He also addresses age-related changes that can have an effect on developing pain and deformities over time.

> 2. *Age-related changes for the majority of older people include which of the following? Select all that apply.*
>
>   a. *Feet widen and flatten*
>
>   b. *The fat padding on the sole of the foot wears down*
>
>   c. *Older people's skin is dryer*
>
>   d. *Overall foot size gradually decreases*
>
> 3. *What risk factors increase one's chances for experiencing foot problems?*

When taking a history from the veterans he serves, Brian inquires about habits at home. Specifically, what types of shoes are worn inside and out in the yard, with or without socks, and the amount of support for the feet.

4. Going barefoot in the home can pose safety risks for the elderly. What specific hazards have been reported? A source can be found at www.sciencedaily.com/releases/2010/06/100623085516.htm.

When reviewing specific foot problems for the group, Brian decides to begin with problems of the toenails, as this is a common area he discovers individuals experience pain with to the point of impairing mobility. In particular, ingrown nails (onychocryptosis) are widespread among the older population. Typically, either the side of the nail or the corner piece of the nail penetrates the skin, similar to a "knife." The severity and appearance of the nail varies. This can result in an infection and the development of granulation tissue. The toe will then be red, inflamed with possible purulent drainage, and painful. Initial treatment includes antibiotics and a podiatrist to remove the embedded nail/piece, keeping a dressing over the toe, and cleansing or soaking for several days. For reoccurring ingrown nails, minor surgery may be needed to remove a portion of the nail or the entire nail.

5. What preventive measure can have the most impact on avoiding ingrown toenails?

Toenail fungus, onychomycosis, is also widespread, but the incidence is greater in older people, with men more commonly infected. Over time, nails appear very thick, with crumbly ragged edges and darkened discoloration. The nail can separate away from the tissue. Fungal infections of the nail pose the most serious health risk for people with diabetes and for those with weakened immune systems, as it can spread or result in a bacterial infection leading to cellulitis.

6. Review the medications available for fungal infections of the nails; some are topical, others systemic. Comment on a prescribed form for each route and the length of time for treatment.

Brian includes the topic of bunions in his presentation as he's frequently asked questions by clients on this topic. He relays that one often begins as a reddened area over the joint of the great toe, followed by pain throughout the small joints, but mainly at the metatarsophalangeal joint (where the toe connects to the foot). Women experience bunions more often than men; it is believed a flat foot or low arch can be a risk factor for development. In addition, wearing narrow, poor-fitting shoes with a tight shoe box around the toes is a known cause. Over time, the pain of a growing bunion can be tremendous to the point that elderly people may be unable to wear most any type of closed, supportive shoe.

7. What treatments are available for bunions other than surgical excision (osteotomy)?

Brian plans a general overview of causes for pain in the feet. He emphasizes the amount of pressure endured from standing or walking is much more than most people realize and uses the following statistic to make this point. "The feet are very small relative to the rest of the body, and the impact of every step exerts tremendous force upon them—about 50% greater than the person's body weight. During an average day the feet support a combined force equivalent to several hundred tons" (Jayson, 2014).

> **8. Briefly describe the problems and treatments for Morton's neuroma and plantar fasciitis.**

> **9. What recommendations does the American Podiatric Medical Association offer for preventing foot pain? A source is available at http://www.medicinenet.com/foot_pain/article.htm.**

Brian plans to wrap up his program by developing a written handout for each participant on the importance of daily foot care. From his years of practicing as an RN, he is aware that the ability to walk, even a short distance, is crucial for elderly people to remain at home versus institutionalized. Although foot deformities may have already occurred, or be in process, skin breakdown, infections, and other injuries resulting in immobility can be avoided at any age.

Suggested Resources

Institute for Aging Research of Hebrew Senior Life. (2010). Going barefoot in home may contribute to elderly falls. *ScienceDaily*. Retrieved from http://www.sciencedaily.com/releases/2010/06/100623085516.htm

Jayson, G. (2014). *Foot pain*. MedicineNet.com. Retrieved from http://www.medicinenet.com/foot_pain/article.htm

Koski, K. (2014). *Think foot care first!* Diamond Geriatrics, Inc. Retrieved from http://www.diamondgeriatrics.com/article-foot-care.html

Mayo Clinic Staff. (2014). *Ingrown toenails*. Mayo Clinic. Retrieved from http://www.mayoclinic.org/diseases-conditions/ingrown-toenails/basics/prevention/con-20019655

Simon, H. (2013). Foot pain prevention. *New York Times*. Retrieved from http://www.nytimes.com/health/guides/symptoms/foot-pain/prevention.html

Zagaria, M. E. (2012). Focus on the feet: Changes with age and disease. *U.S. Pharmacist*. Retrieved from http://www.uspharmacist.com/content/d/feature/c/37044

10

The Aging Neurologic System

Case 10.1 ■ Cerebrovascular Accident (CVA) (Acute Phase)

George Green, a 62-year-old African American male, is a self-employed businessman who lives alone. He is 5 feet 7 inches tall and weighs 215 pounds. Three years ago, he was diagnosed with primary hypertension (HTN). Mr. Green's family history for cardiovascular disease is unknown because he was adopted. His HTN is being treated with Tenormin (atenolol), Zestril (lisinopril), and Cardura (doxazosin), which he does not take on a regular basis. Mr. Green is ambidextrous. For approximately 1 week, he noted that he was dropping "everything" from his right hand. While working at his home computer, Mr. Green suddenly was unable to control the mouse with his right hand, as it "locked-up" and felt "strange," and the feeling began moving up his right arm. He was able to call 911 and was transported to the emergency department. Mr. Green's speech was not impaired and he remained alert the entire time.

Upon arrival at the emergency department, Mr. Green's blood pressure (BP) was 215/115. Initial diagnostic tests included blood work and a CT scan. Mr. Green received two intravenous (IV) lines and was given IV Tenormin (atenolol).

1. *What is the reason a CT scan was performed as one of the initial diagnostic procedures?*

Mr. Green is diagnosed with a hemorrhagic stroke.

2. *Based on Mr. Green's presenting symptoms:*

    a. *Which cerebral artery was most likely affected?*

    b. *What components of the National Institutes of Health Stroke Scale were most likely affected? See www.mdcalc.com/ nih-stroke-scale-score-nihss.*

3. *What risk factors does Mr. Green have for a hemorrhagic stroke? How does being adopted affect Mr. Green's evaluation of the risk factors for a stroke?*

   *4. According to statistics from the American Stroke Association, how
      does the death rate from stroke and HTN for African American
      males compare with the overall death rate for the two diagnoses?*

   5. Describe the National Stroke Association's "FAST" stroke screening.

Mr. Green is hospitalized for 3 days while his BP is regulated with medications. During
the hospitalization, he reveals that when his HTN was initially treated, he developed
edema and his medication had to be reduced.

   *6. Which of Mr. Green's medications was most likely the cause of
      the edema?*

While in the hospital, Mr. Green receives Dilantin (phenytoin).

   7. What is the reason for Mr. Green to receive Dilantin (phenytoin)?

During his hospitalization, Mr. Green is diagnosed with polycythemia vera, which is
treated with phlebotomy.

   *8. How will the diagnosis of polycythemia vera affect his future
      stroke risk?*

Mr. Green is being prepared for discharge home. His medications include the following:
   • Tenormin (atenolol) 50 mg once a day
   • Zestril (lisinopril) 10 mg once a day
   • Cardura (doxazosin) 4 mg once a day
   • Aspirin 81 mg once a day

   *9. What are special considerations for using Zestril (lisinopril) in
      the African American population?*

   *10. Because of Mr. Green's age and medications, what test will need to be
      performed on a regular basis to monitor for medication side effects?*

   *11. Review the Hartford Institute's "medication" evidence-based
      geriatric topics at http://consultgerirn.org/ for specific age-related
      medication assessment strategies for Mr. Green.*

   *12. What complementary and alternative strategies can be suggested
      to Mr. Green to help control his BP? Include the rationale and/or
      desired effect of the strategy on BP. How would you introduce the
      topic of complementary and alternative strategies to Mr. Green?*

Suggested Resources

American Heart Association. American Stroke Association. (2012). *Risk factors for stroke.*
   Retrieved from http://www.heart.org/idc/groups/stroke-public/@wcm/@hcm/documents/
   downloadable/ucm_309713.pdf

Drugs.com. (2014). *Lisinopril.* Retrieved from http://www.drugs.com/cdi/lisinopril.html

National Stroke Association. (2014). *African Americans and stroke.* Retrieved from http://www .stroke.org/site/PageServer?pagename=aamer

NIH Stroke Scale/Score. (2014). Retrieved from http://www.mdcalc.com/nih-stroke-scale-score-nihss

Zwicker, D., & Fulmer, T. (2012). *Geriatric nursing protocol: Reducing adverse drug events.* Hartford Institute for Geriatric Nursing. Retrieved from http://www.consultgerirn.com/ topics/medication/want_to_know_more

Case 10.2 ■ CVA Rehabilitation Phase

*T*erry Derstine is a 79-year-old male with a history of HTN, smoking one pack per day for 20 years, drinking an average of three beers per day, and living a sedentary lifestyle. He has never been married and lives alone in a one-bedroom apartment on the first floor. He experienced a left-sided thromboembolitic stroke resulting in right hemiplegia, dysphagia, and expressive aphasia. He is NPO (nothing by mouth) and fed through a recently inserted G-tube. Terry also has an uninhibited neurogenic bowel and bladder. He is admitted to inpatient rehabilitation after 7 days in the acute care hospital.

1. What risk factors for stroke does Terry have?

The rehabilitation nurse, Amy, completes Terry's admission assessment and finds the following:

- Hgt: 66 inches
- Wgt: 250 pounds
- BP: 184/94
- AP: 88
- R: 18
- Temp: 98.7

2. Given this assessment data, what factors will Amy emphasize when teaching Terry about reducing his stroke risk?

During the first week in rehabilitation, Terry attends physical, occupational, and speech therapy. He participates well in all of them.

3. How much therapy will Terry be expected to tolerate in this setting of care?

Terry wants to know how long he has to have a tube to feed him and when he can start eating regular food again. The barium swallow shows aspiration of thin liquids.

*4. **What should Amy explain to Terry about the need for a G-tube because of his dysphagia? How should she discuss the results of the barium swallow?***

Terry progresses well with therapies and begins a timed voiding protocol to help regain bladder control. He has problems with constipation and is ordered Colace 100 mg orally daily.

*5. **What is the purpose of a timed voiding protocol?***

*6. **What nursing instructions should be given to Terry as he takes Colace for constipation?***

Amy consults the resources at the Association of Rehabilitation Nurse's (ARN) website, www.rehabnurse.org/pubs/bowelcare.html, and reads the Practice Guidelines for the Management of Constipation in Older Adults (2002). From this document, Amy finds a list of foods high in fiber that Terry should be encouraged to eat. She implements the strategies discussed in the evidence-based guideline.

After 2 weeks, Terry has a repeat barium swallow that shows he is able to swallow safely with modifications. The speech therapist orders him to perform a chin tuck and double swallow when eating.

*7. **Why is it important for Terry to follow the protocol suggested by the speech therapist? What possible negative outcomes could result if Terry does not follow this regimen? Visit the ARN website at www.rehabnurse.org/members/content/ arn-cat.html (Association of Rehabilitation Nurses Competency Assessment Tool). Take the 10-question multiple-choice test under "dysphagia."***

Terry is going home to live alone after 3 weeks of intensive inpatient rehabilitation. He is able to ambulate with a quad cane, ankle-foot orthosis, and supervision, but may need some help initially with activities of daily living (ADL). He is continent of bowel and bladder. He has five medications to manage at home and has to check his BP weekly. His swallowing has improved, but he must still perform a modified swallow. Terry is optimistic about his future and wants to prevent any recurring stroke.

*8. **What types of services may Terry need immediately after discharge? Develop a discharge plan for Terry.***

Suggested Resources

ARN Competencies Assessment Tool. (2012). *Dysphagia*. Association of Rehabilitation Nursing. Retrieved from http://www.rehabnurse.org/members/content/arn-cat.html

Association of Rehabilitation Nurses. (2002). *Practice guidelines for the management of constipation in adults*. Rehabilitation Nursing Foundation. Retrieved from http://www.rehabnurse .org/pdf/BowelGuideforWEB.pdf

Case 10.3 ■ Parkinson's Disease

*B*randi Kohler is a geriatric care manager for a large geriatric practice. She is visiting Mary Reed and her daughter, Susan, in response to Susan's concerns that her mother may be suffering from dementia. Mary's primary care physician has asked Brandi to obtain a comprehensive health history and to perform some cognitive testing before Mary's scheduled physician visit. Susan repeats her concerns about her mother's memory, stating that Mary is struggling to keep track of her medications and appointments and often repeats the same stories and comments multiple times in a conversation. Mary smiles and says, "Well, what do you expect from an 86-year-old?"

Brandi notices a distinct pill-rolling, resting tremor in Mary's left hand and asks about it. Both Mary and Susan note that it has been present for years and her daughter adds that Mary has become "clumsy" and drops items regularly. In addition, she has struggled to double click with the mouse when playing Solitaire on the computer, button her blouse, and thread a needle. They both attributed these problems to normal aging. Mary also tells the nurse she has to wake her body up in the morning before getting started; she describes the fact that her mind seems to awaken before her body can respond, and that her body feels stiff in the morning.

Brandi gathers the following data:

Past medical history:

Osteoporosis, right hip fracture following a fall on icy driveway last year, hypothyroidism, and gastroesophageal reflux disease (GERD).

Medications:

- Fosamax (alendronate) 70 mg weekly
- Calcium + vitamin D 600 mg/400 IU twice a day
- Pepcid (famotidine) 20 mg
- Synthroid (levothyroxine) 88 mcg daily
- No over-the-counter or herbal medications

Review of systems:

General: No weight loss, some feelings of fatigue daily, appetite good, sleeping well at night.

Head, ears, eyes, nose, and throat (HEENT): Denies headaches, able to read newspaper with glasses, able to hear TV at normal volume, no ear pain, no tinnitus, dentures fit well, no oral sores, able to eat all foods without problem, clear nasal discharge when eating, denies dry mouth or sour taste in mouth, no difficulty swallowing or episodes of coughing while eating, denies visual blurring or diplopia, last dental exam 2 months ago, last eye exam 6 months ago

Cardiovascular (CV): Denies chest pain, denies palpitations, able to walk several blocks without dyspnea or fatigue, no syncope, no dizziness or orthostatic symptoms

Respiratory: No dyspnea, no cough

Abdomen: Constipation—bowel movement every 2 to 3 days with straining and hard stool, denies abdominal pain, no nausea, vomiting, or diarrhea, no reflux symptoms

Genitourinary: Urgency with occasional incontinence for several years, wears Depends, especially at night, no loss of urine with coughing or laughing, no dysuria, sexually inactive since spouse died 10 years ago, no vaginal discharge or burning

Skin: Denies rashes or skin lesions

Extremities: No edema

Musculoskeletal: Frequent falls due to loss of balance, stiffness in entire extremity not confined to single joint, feels unsteady with walking but, once she gets going, can walk several blocks without difficulty

Neurologic: Resting tremor 10 years, no paresthesias, overall weakness not confined to any particular area, no dysphasia or dysarthria

Psychological: Denies hallucinations or depression

Social history: Lives with daughter who works full time. Daughter sets up pill box, does shopping and meal preparation, and provides transportation. Retired school teacher. Taught 4th grade, retired 21 years ago. Widowed 10 years ago. Moved in with daughter 1 year ago after fall and hip fracture.

Health practices: Denies smoking, alcohol use, or street drugs

Functional and cognitive assessments:

- ADL: independent but avoids clothing with buttons and uses Velcro closure on shoes, has tub bench
- Lawton instrumental activities of daily living (IADL) scale: 5/8 0 score in areas of medication management, shopping, and food preparation
- Folstein's Mini-Mental Status Exam (MMSE): 23/30–8/10 orientation, missed date and day; 3/3 registration; 3/5 attention and calculation; 1/3 recall; language 8/9—unable to copy design
- Geriatric Depression Scale: 4/30

1. Brandi suspects that Mrs. Reed may have Parkinson's disease. What symptoms led to this suspicion?

2. How is Parkinson's disease diagnosed?

3. Lewy body dementia can present with Parkinson-like symptoms. How are these conditions clinically distinguished from each other?

Use the following website to answer the next two questions prepared by Harvath and McKenzie (2012): www.consultgerirn.com/topics/depression/want_to_know_more.

4. Interpret the Geriatric Depression Scale score obtained by Brandi.

5. *What other assessments may be helpful in this case?*

6. *It is obvious to you that Susan has become fairly overwhelmed with the thought of continuing to care for her mother who is becoming increasingly dependent. What can you do to help Susan?*

7. *What nonpharmacologic strategies can slow the progression and decrease complications associated with Parkinson's disease?*

8. *Susan asks if you can recommend any dietary suggestions for her mother in order to help keep her bones strong and weight up to protect her from complications of future falls. What can you suggest to Susan?*

Suggested Resources

Glass, J. (2012). *Adapting your home for Parkinson's disease*. WebMD. Retrieved from http://www.webmd.com/parkinsons-disease/guide/parkinsons-home-safety?page=2

Harvath, T. A., & McKenzie, G. L. (2012). *Geriatric nursing protocol: Depression in older adults*. Hartford Institute for Geriatric Nursing. Retrieved from http://consultgerirn.org/topics/depression/want_to_know_more

Holden, K. (n.d.). *Ten nutrition tips for living well with Parkinson's disease*. Retrieved from www.parkinson.org

Parkinson's Disease Foundation. (2014a). *Caring in Parkinson's*. Retrieved from http://www.pdf.org/en/caregiving_fam_issues

Parkinson's Disease Foundation. (2014b). *What is Parkinson's disease?* Retrieved from http://www.pdf.org/en/about_pd

Case 10.4 ■ Alzheimer's Disease

Annie Kraft and her 74-year-old mother, Marguerite Taylor, arrive for their appointment with you, a geriatric care manager. Marguerite is retired and lives alone in her single-family house. There is no mortgage on the home and Marguerite is financially comfortable with her husband's pension and Social Security income.

Annie tells you that she scheduled this appointment after becoming aware that her mother has been having trouble keeping up with her daily responsibilities. She lives about 3 hours away from Marguerite and assumed her mother was getting along okay until she received a phone call from the local police asking her to pick her mother up from the station. Apparently, Marguerite had planned a trip to Annie's house by a route that she often takes, but became confused and ended up about 100 miles away from her destination. She was picked up by police after neighbors called to report that she had been circling their neighborhood for hours. Annie was dismayed and surprised to find her mother looking disheveled and confused. Marguerite had no idea where she was or what day it was, and she kept repeating that she did not deserve to be arrested, despite assurances that she was not in trouble. She struggled to make herself understood; she was rambling and forgetting words. Marguerite's generally calm demeanor was gone; she was accusing everyone of conspiring to make her look stupid and denied that she had been lost. She said she had been out on a sightseeing trip. Annie brought her mother home and found bills and collection notices stacked on the dining room table. Her mother had always been a fastidious house cleaner but the house was dusty and cluttered. Molded food was found in Tupperware containers in the refrigerator, where there was also silverware stored. Empty medication bottles were discovered in the bathroom cabinets.

1. *Go to the following American Academy of Neurology website, www.alz.org/alzheimers_disease_10_signs_of_alzheimers.asp, and review the 10 Warning Signs of Alzheimer's Disease. Which of these warning signs are apparent in Marguerite's case?*

2. *Is Marguerite struggling with ADL, IADL, or both? Which of these are generally compromised first? If you are unfamiliar with these terms, use the online Merck Manual website to help: www.merck.com/mkgr/mmg/sec3/ch30/ch30a.jsp.*

Annie tells you that Marguerite's husband died 2 years ago. Following his death, Marguerite withdrew from friends and family but is always pleased when Annie calls and visits. They have spoken by phone weekly and arranged monthly outings since his death. Annie had assumed that her mother was coping well until this incident.

Marguerite's past medical history includes insomnia, osteoarthritis, GERD, and hypothyroidism. She takes Tylenol P.M., Vicodin (hydrocodone/acetaminophen), Prilosec (omeprazole), and Synthroid (levothyroxine) for these disorders.

You perform a Folstein's MMSE and Marguerite, a college graduate, scores a 22/30. She missed 3 points on orientation questions, 3 points on delayed recall, and 2 points on calculation and reasoning.

Marguerite is calm now that her driving ordeal is over. She tells you that she has been struggling to keep track of appointments and bills. She has been worried that she may be "losing her mind." She has several friends with dementia and never wants to be a burden on Annie. She tells you about her friend's husband who needed to go to a memory unit in a nursing home and lost his ability to swallow. "He became a vegetable, kept alive with a feeding tube. I would never put myself or my daughter through that," Marguerite says.

3. *Interpret this MMSE score. Use information on the following website to help: www.brown.edu/Courses/BI_278/Other/ Clerkship/Didactics/Readings/THE%20MENTAL%20STATUS%20 EXAMINATION.pdf.*

4. *What disorders present similar to Alzheimer's disease?*

5. *Which of Marguerite's medications may be contributing to her confusion?*

6. *What screening tests are done to rule out reversible causes of dementia?*

7. *What is the difference between dementia and Alzheimer's disease?*

8. *If a diagnosis of Alzheimer's disease is made by Marguerite's primary care provider, what medications will likely be started?*

9. *How do these medications work?*

10. *Explain the difference between conservator, guardian, medical power of attorney, and durable power of attorney. See www.caring.com/articles/difference-power-attorney-guardianship-conservatorship.*

11. *Has Marguerite demonstrated the capacity for decision making?*

12. *What care options should be discussed with Annie and Marguerite?*

Suggested Resources

Alzheimer's Association. (2014). *Alzheimer's management and patient care.* Retrieved from http://www.alz.org/health-care-professionals/medical-management-patient-care.asp

House, P. M. (n.d.). *The mini-mental status exam.* Retrieved from http://www.brown.edu/Courses/BI_278/Other/Clerkship/Didactics/Readings/THE%20MENTAL%20STATUS%20EXAMINATION.pdf

Kemisan, L. (2014). *Activities of daily living: What are ADLs and IADLs.* Caring.com. Retrieved from http://www.caring.com/articles/activities-of-daily-living-what-are-adls-and-iadls

Rosenblatt, C. L. (2014). *What is the difference between a power of attorney and a conservatorship or guardianship?* Caring.com. Retrieved from http://www.caring.com/articles/difference-power-attorney-guardianship-conservatorship

Case 10.5 ■ Dizziness/Vertigo

*M*rs. Santo is a 70-year-old female who visits the senior clinic with a complaint of dizziness that has occurred several times during the past week. She states that the first episode occurred when she was grocery shopping. She reports looking up and reaching for a cake mix on the top shelf at the grocery store and becoming so dizzy that she had to hold onto the shelf to keep from falling. She also became nauseated and felt like the room was spinning with this episode. Mrs. Santo states that she stood very still, looking straight ahead, and the dizziness passed after about 3 minutes. She reports another event occurred this morning when she attempted to get out of bed; she rolled onto her right side and became so dizzy, lightheaded, and nauseated that she had to lie back down. It took several attempts, but after approximately 1 hour she was able to carefully get out of bed. She states that she is concerned these may be stroke symptoms so she had her friend drive her to her appointment.

Mrs. Santo's past medical history is negative for stroke, head injury, cardiac arrhythmia, or carotid artery disease. She has HTN and osteoporosis, which have been in good control. Her home medications are as follows: Diovan HCT (hydrochlorothiazide/valsartan) 12.5/80 mg one tablet orally daily; Fosamax (alendronate) 70 mg one tablet orally once weekly; calcium with vitamin D tablets 500 mg one tablet three times daily. She reports an allergy to penicillin, which causes a "full body rash." The nurse inquires about similar episodes of dizziness in the past and recent illnesses. Mrs. Santo states that she recalls having a very short episode of dizziness approximately 3 years ago, but that it "went away on its own." She denies recent cold symptoms, earache, or change in speech, coordination, or strength.

The nurse inquires about Mrs. Santo's living arrangements and social history. She reports that she retired from a clerical job at a trucking company. She has been a widow for 3 years and resides in her own one-story condominium; she has one daughter who is married and lives 2 hours away with her husband and children.

The nurse asks about problems with mobility and driving. Mrs. Santo states that she walks without assistive devices, is independent in ADL and IADL, and she continues to drive. She states that she is very independent and is afraid that this dizziness may change her lifestyle. She reports being active, going to the senior center weekly with friends for lunch, and engaging in church activities every Wednesday and Sunday. She states that once a month she drives to her daughter's house and spends the weekend. Mrs. Santo states, "But I'm not doing any of these things now . . . I'm afraid to drive with these episodes of dizziness. I don't know when they are going to come on."

1. What are some safety concerns that can be identified in this case?

2. Could medications be a cause of this patient's dizziness?

The nurse performs a physical assessment and finds: BP 130/85, heart rate 72/min, respirations 20/min, and temperature 98.0. Mrs. Santo gets up to change into a gown, becomes very dizzy, and grabs onto the nurse's arm.

3. What action should the nurse take?

4. What observations/assessments are important to make during this episode of dizziness?

The nurse assists Mrs. Santo to a lying position on the examination table with her head elevated to 45 degrees. She provides reassurance, rechecks vital signs, and performs a quick neurologic examination noting no change in speech or movement, but observes that Mrs. Santo's eyes appear to be jerking. She stays with the client and uses the call system to request assistance.

The nurse practitioner arrives and quickly reviews the history, performs a physical examination, and uses a special procedure called the Dix-Hallpike maneuver. She positions the examination table flat, and then moves the patient's head 45 degrees to the right while tipping her head back quickly over the end of the examination table. She notes that after 20 seconds in this position, dizziness and rotary nystagmus are present.

5. ***What is the purpose of the Dix-Hallpike maneuver? Use the video at www.youtube.com/watch?v=kEM9p4EX1jk for assistance.***

6. ***What is rotary nystagmus? Cite your source.***

The nurse practitioner explains to the patient that her symptoms appear to be caused by benign paroxysmal positional vertigo (BPPV), a condition caused by small calcium particles located in the inner ear that float into a structure of the inner ear (the semicircular canal) and cause the sensation of dizziness. She explains that this is a common and self-limiting condition that occurs more often in older adults. The nurse practitioner instructs that this condition can be helped by performing exercises called Epley's maneuver.

7. ***How is Epley's maneuver performed? The video at www.youtube .com/watch?v=ja-0DHpBfqk may be helpful to learn about this technique.***

Mrs. Santo is placed through the maneuvers three more times and her symptoms resolve while she is in the office. She is told she must rest in the office before leaving and sleep in a recliner chair at 45 degrees for at least 2 consecutive days following this procedure. She is given a patient teaching handout on how to perform the exercises and referred to physical therapy for gait and balance evaluation and BPPV exercises.

8. ***How can this patient benefit from a physical therapy referral?***

9. ***What other guidelines or referrals might you provide?***

Suggested Resources

Ham, T. C. (2014). *Dizziness in older people.* Dizziness-and-imbalance.com. Retrieved from http://www.dizziness-and-balance.com/disorders/age/Dizziness%20in%20the%20Elderly.htm

Seller, R. H. (2007). *Differential diagnosis of common complaints* (5th ed.). Philadelphia, PA: Saunders/Elsevier.

Wedro, B. (2014). *Benign paroxysmal positional vertigo.* emedicine health. Retrieved from http://www.emedicinehealth.com/benign_positional_vertigo/article_em.htm

11

The Aging Cardiovascular System

Case 11.1 ■ Coronary Artery Disease: Living With Chronic Stable Angina

*M*elissa Jacobs works in a cardiac rehabilitation center monitoring patients referred for managing their cardiac conditions. She is beginning work with 71-year-old Marilyn Banks, recently released from the hospital following observation for chest pain and discomfort. Melissa reviews the following in the client's chart. Marilyn lives alone but has a son who lives nearby and checks in on her frequently. She was shopping at the mall with her friend when she experienced chest pain and some discomfort, which radiated down her left arm. She was brought by ambulance to a local hospital. She described the pain as a squeezing sensation and indicated that she had previously experienced episodes where she felt short of breath. She is a noninsulin-dependent diabetic; she is 5 feet 5 inches tall and weighs 205 pounds. She describes herself as relatively active but does not participate in a regular exercise program. She is a nonsmoker and has an occasional glass of wine. Her father died of a heart attack at age 66 and her brother had angioplasty with a stent at age 60. She indicates that she never really worried much about heart disease because it is an "old man's disease."

Prior to the incident, Marilyn was taking the following medications: Lipitor (atorvastatin calcium) 40 mg orally daily and metformin HCl (glucophage) 850 mg twice a day. She has always had borderline high blood pressure (135/85), and when she arrived at the hospital, her blood pressure was 153/98. Blood tests revealed the following: troponin, creatine kinase, and myoglobin levels were all normal. B-type natriuretic peptide was also normal. Her total blood cholesterol was elevated at 260 mg/dL with LDL 189 mg/dL and HDL at 40 mg/dL. Her triglycerides were 220 mg/dL and her glucose levels were normal. During the hospital stay, the following tests were completed. Marilyn's EKG was normal but a stress test indicated a prolonged Q-T interval after 5 minutes of exercise on a treadmill. Subsequent assessment with coronary angiography indicated a blockage of approximately 50% in the coronary artery.

She was discharged with orders to implement lifestyle changes, hence the visit with the cardiac rehabilitation center, and to return for a follow-up visit in 2 weeks. Upon discharge, the doctor increased the dosage of the Lipitor (atorvastatin calcium) to 80 mg orally daily and prescribed Lopressor (metoprolol tartrate) 100 mg orally daily. He also prescribed Nitrostat (nitroglycerin) 0.3 mg tablets to be used in the event of a subsequent attack of chest pain and daily use of low-dose aspirin (81 mg).

1. *What are the risk factors for coronary artery disease (CAD) that Marilyn has in her patient history?*

2. *What is the common pathophysiology of CAD?*

3. *Evaluate the blood work results for Marilyn.*

4. *Evidence indicates that the presence of a substance called C-reactive protein is correlated with the risk of CAD. Explain this correlation.*

5. *Is heart disease just an "old man's disease?" Explain your thoughts.*

6. *Evaluate the results of the EKG and stress test.*

7. *Why did Marilyn's physician initiate changes in her Lipitor (atorvastatin calcium) dosage?*

8. *What purposes do the specific medications listed serve?*

9. *Consult a website, such as the one maintained by the American Heart Association. If you were counseling Marilyn, what lifestyle changes would you help her try to achieve?*

Suggested Resources

American Heart Association. (2012). *Choose a healthy lifestyle.* Retrieved from http://www.heart .org/HEARTORG/Conditions/Diabetes/PreventionTreatmentofDiabetes/Choose-a-Healthy-Lifestyle_UCM_313880_Article.jsp

Maddox, T. M. (2012). *Heart disease and C-reactive protein (CRP) testing.* WebMD. Retrieved from http://www.webmd.com/heart-disease/guide/heart-disease-c-reactive-protein-crp-testing? page=2

National Heart, Lung and Blood Institute. (2012). *What is coronary artery disease?* Retrieved from http://www.nhlbi.nih.gov/health/dci/Diseases/Cad/CAD_WhatIs.html

Singh, V. N. (2014). *Coronary heart disease.* emedicine health. Retrieved from http://www .emedicinehealth.com/coronary_heart_disease/article_em.htm

Texas Heart Institute. (2013). *Long Q-T interval.* Retrieved from http://www.texasheartinstitute .org/HIC/Topics/Cond/longqts.cfm

Case 11.2 ■ Congestive Heart Failure

Madeline Brunner is an 84-year-old woman that you are visiting in her facility for wound care. She developed a pressure ulcer during her hospitalization for a left total hip replacement. She also has osteoarthritis (OA) in her right hip and is planning a right hip replacement in the near future. The wound and her hip are doing well but she complains that she is not feeling well today and thinks she is "coming down with a cold." She has had a nonproductive cough with increased shortness of breath for the past 2 days and has needed to sleep in her recliner because she is uncomfortable lying in her bed. Her appetite has been poor, which she attributes to the fact that she has been constipated with the narcotic prescribed after her surgery. She has been able to take ample quantities of beef and chicken broth only for the past few days due to an upset stomach. Normally, Madeline is able to walk up and down her hall with the physical therapist without difficulty, but yesterday she could only walk about 10 feet before needing to rest due to shortness of breath. Madeline lives alone in an assisted living facility and has two adult daughters who provide social support and manage her finances. She manages her own medications and shows you her pill box is correctly set up; and Madeline is able to explain the purpose for each of her medications. She does not smoke. Her past medical history includes the following:

- CAD with myocardial infarction (MI) in 2007
- Congestive heart failure (CHF)
- OA hips s/p left hip replacement 6 months ago
- Hypertension (HTN)
- Hypercholesterolemia

Current medications taken orally include the following:

- Lasix (furosemide) 40 mg every morning
- K-Dur (potassium chloride) 20 mEq every morning
- Lopressor (metoprolol) 25 mg, 0.5 tablets twice a day
- Prinivil (lisinopril) 10 mg every morning
- Vicodin (acetaminophen/hydrocodone) 500/5 mg, 1 tablet three times a day
- Aspirin 81 mg daily
- Zocor (simvastatin) 20 mg every evening
- Advil (ibuprofen) 400 mg three times a day

Seasonal flu shot was given in late October last year. On exam, you take the following vital signs:

BP 110/62; pulse 102; respirations: 22; O_2 sat 92%

You also document:

- Heart sounds: S1S2 with S3 gallop, no murmurs or rubs
- Lung sounds: rales in bases
- ABD: soft, nontender, distended with positive hepatojugular reflex; bowel sounds normal in all four quadrants
- Extremities: capillary refill less than 2 seconds, 2+ edema bilaterally

1. What do you suspect may be causing Madeline's symptoms?

2. What are the pertinent positive findings on your physical exam? Explain the pathophysiology of each of these findings.

3. *What may have precipitated this problem?*

4. *Does Madeline demonstrate symptoms of right- or left-sided heart failure, or both? Explain. The American Heart Association (AHA) website, www.heart.org/HEARTORG/ Conditions/HeartFailure/AboutHeartFailure/Types-of-Heart-Failure_UCM_306323_Article.jsp, will assist you with your answer.*

5. *Into which New York Heart Association functional class does Madeline normally fit? Into which American College of Cardiology (ACC)/AHA stage of heart failure does she fit?*

6. *How is CHF diagnosed?*

7. *Does Madeline's current treatment program comply with ACC/ AHA guidelines?*

8. *What action should you take at this point?*

9. *Madeline's primary care physician orders a B-type natriuretic peptide (BNP), chest x-ray, EKG, and echocardiogram and increases the dose of her Lasix (furosemide) and K-Dur (potassium chloride). What is the purpose of these diagnostic tests?*

10. *How can you help Madeline to prevent future CHF exacerbations and hospitalizations related to this condition? A "Congestive Heart Failure Zones for Management" guideline, found at www .improvingchroniccare.org/downloads/rygchf_copy1.doc, may be a helpful source.*

Suggested Resources

American Heart Association. (2012). *Types of heart failure.* Retrieved from http://www.heart .org/HEArTorG/Conditions/HeartFailure/AboutHeartFailure/Types-of-Heart-Failure_ UCM_306323_Article.jsp

Cleveland Clinic. (2011). *B-type natriuretic peptide (BNP) blood test.* Retrieved from http:// my.clevelandclinic.org/heart/diagnostics-testing/laboratory-tests/b-type-natriuretic-peptide-bnp-bloodtest.aspx

Congestive Heart Failure Zones for Management. (n.d.). *Improving chronic illness care.* Robert Wood Johnson Foundation. Retrieved from http://www.improvingchroniccare.org/ downloads/rygchf_copy1.doc

Emory Healthcare. (2014). *Heart failure stages and functional classifications.* Retrieved from http://www.emoryhealthcare.org/heart-failure/learn-about-heart-failure/stages-classification.html

Yancy, C. W., Jessup, M., Bozkurt, B., Butler, J,. Casey, D. E., Drazner, M. H., . . . Wilkoff, B. L. (2013). 2013 ACCF/AHA guideline for the management of heart failure. *Journal of the American College of Cardiology, 62*(16). Retrieved from http://content.onlinejacc.org/article .aspx?articleid=1695825

Case 11.3 ■ Chronic Atrial Fibrillation

*M*artha Snow is an RN working in a rehabilitation/subacute facility and is passing out morning medications. She is approached by a patient in a wheelchair, Mrs. Ellen Smith, who reports "feeling funny . . . like my heart is racing" and asks Martha to check her heart.

Ellen Smith is a 76-year-old Caucasian female who was admitted to the rehabilitation facility for physical therapy and occupational therapy following hospitalization for a fall and right hip contusion. She was negative for hip fracture, and a CT scan of the head showed no ischemic or hemorrhagic stroke or intracranial bleed. She has a past medical history of HTN, type 2 diabetes, osteoporosis, and chronic atrial fibrillation. Her current medications are as follows: Zestoretic (hydrochlorothiazide/lisinopril) 12.5/10 mg orally daily, Cordarone (amiodarone) 100 mg orally daily, Glyburide 5 mg orally daily, Actonel with calcium (risedronate/calcium carbonate) 35/1,250 mg one tablet orally once a week, and Coumadin (warfarin) 3 mg one tablet orally every evening.

1. Discuss the epidemiology associated with atrial fibrillation and cite the source.

Social history shows that Martha is married, lives in a one-story home with her husband, is a retired legal secretary, and has two adult children and three grandchildren who all live in close proximity. Her functional status prior to hospitalization was independent in all activities of daily living (ADL) and instrumental ADL, ambulatory without assistive device, and continues to drive. In relation to advance directives, she is her own medical decision maker; her husband has durable power of attorney medical in case of incapacity. She is full-code status.

2. In evaluating Mrs. Smith's complaint of "racing heart," what further assessment should the nurse perform?

3. What are some key precipitating or aggravating factors for the presence of arrhythmia the nurse should explore?

4. What are three pathophysiological changes in atrial fibrillation that result in common symptoms?

Martha assists Mrs. Smith to return to her room and get in bed to complete further assessment. The nurse asks Mrs. Smith when she first noticed her symptoms, what she was doing at that time, how long the symptoms have lasted, and how severe the symptoms are on a scale of 0 (not noticeable) to 10 (severe). She also inquires whether there are any additional events other than the palpitations. Mrs. Smith reports that the symptoms began this morning when she was in the bathroom washing her face and brushing her teeth. She reports going to the dining room and eating breakfast, thinking that "they would stop on their own." She continues to say the symptoms have lasted about 1 hour and remained the same intensity (5/5), but she is concerned that they have not stopped on their own, and it is time for her to go to therapy and exercise. Mrs. Smith denies dizziness or faint-like feelings, shortness of breath, chest pain, nausea, or anxiety. She states, "My heart sometimes does this. My doctor told me to rest when this happens." Martha asks Mrs. Smith whether she took all of her medication yesterday and she reports, "I took everything they gave me." The nurse reviews the medications with Mrs. Smith and finds that she reports taking amiodarone 200 mg one tablet orally daily at home. Martha notes that the amiodarone order from the hospital is for 100 mg—one tablet orally daily.

Physical examination findings show blood pressure of 130/80, irregular pulse with a heart rate of 90 bpm, respirations 20 per minute, pulse oximetry at 93% on room air, and the prebreakfast accucheck at 110. A quick physical assessment resulted in the following findings:

- HEENT: within normal limits, oral mucosa moist
- Respiratory: nonlabored breathing, lungs clear to auscultation, no wheeze or crackles
- Cardiovascular: irregular rate and rhythm, apical heart rate: 95 bpm, no jugular venous distention at 45°, extremities: slight pedal edema with 2+ pulses bilaterally, right hip bruise
- Neurologic: alert, oriented to person, time, and place, no motor or speech deficits

5. Which of the physical findings should the nurse be concerned about?

6. What are the goals of care for patients with persistent or chronic atrial fibrillation?

Martha reviews Mrs. Smith's latest laboratory reports, which are within normal limits with a therapeutic international normalized ratio (INR) of 2.5. The nurse discusses her findings with Mrs. Smith, explaining that her blood pressure is stable but her heart rate is slightly elevated. She relays that she will contact the client's health care provider based on the controversy of the amiodarone dosage. She recommends that Mrs. Smith rest and call for assistance if she experiences increased palpitations or new complaints (e.g., chest pain, shortness of breath). She also asks Mrs. Smith whether she would like her husband notified about this complaint and the current actions being taken. Mrs. Smith replies that she would very much appreciate her husband being contacted.

7. What orders or interventions can the nurse anticipate?

After contacting the primary care provider, Martha obtains the following orders: (1) ECG today, (2) increase amiodarone to 200 mg, one tablet orally daily, (3) vital signs once per shift and as needed, and (4) notify with occurrence of chest pain, shortness of breath, persistent complaint of palpitations, heart rate less than 60 or greater than 95. In addition, continue Coumadin 3 mg one tablet orally daily and obtain a PT (prothrombin)/INR twice weekly. The nursing staff should notify the primary care provider if the INR is less than 2.0, or greater than 3.0. The nurse informs Mrs. Smith of the discussion.

8. What is the rationale for increasing the PT/INR to twice weekly?

When the nurse reassesses Mrs. Smith, she reports that she is feeling "better since resting . . . the palpitations are gone." Repeat vital signs show Mrs. Smith's blood pressure to be 118/80, heart rate 80 and irregular. The nurse continues to assess the client's symptoms throughout the day. Mrs. Smith participates in physical therapy in the afternoon without symptom reoccurrence.

9. What are other medication options in addition to Coumadin that have come onto the market in recent years?

10. Atrial fibrillation is referred to as the "burden of the future" in some health care literature. How would you interpret this label and what could be the cause? (Hint: Consider prevalence and economics of the disease.)

Suggested Resources

Casey, P. E. (2014). Management of patients with dysrhythmias and conduction problems. In J. L. Hinkle & K. H. Cheever (Eds.), *Brunner & Suddarth's textbook of medical–surgical nursing* (13th ed., pp. 703–705). Philadelphia, PA: Lippincott Williams & Wilkins.

Doheny, K. (2013). *Comparing the new blood thinners to Coumadin.* WebMD. Retrieved from http://www.webmd.com/heart-disease/atrial-fibrillation/news/20130528/new-blood-thinners-compared

Forgoros, R. N. (2014). *Atrial fibrillation—A comprehensive overview.* About.com Heart Disease. Retrieved from http://heartdisease.about.com/od/atrialfibrillation/a/afib_overview.htm

Sanoski, C. (2009). Clinical, economic, and quality of life impact of atrial fibrillation. *Journal of Managed Care Pharmacy, 15*(6 Suppl. b), S4–S9. Retrieved from http://www.amcp.org/data/jmcp/1003.04-09.pdf

Case 11.4 ■ Peripheral Vascular Disease

*L*ois Rogers works in a community health center. She is visiting with Gordon Toguid, a 67-year-old African American man. Gordon complains of recent onset of intermittent leg pain when he is out walking his dog and says that his feet always feel cold. The pain, which is generally localized to his calves, subsides when he is able to sit down and rest for a bit, but he says that his legs will feel "like lead" for a while. Lois takes the following history. Gordon lives alone, is divorced for several years, and does not have children. Gordon has normal weight for his height. He is a smoker and estimates that he smokes about a pack of cigarettes every day. He drinks occasionally. He has taken medication for elevated cholesterol, Zocor (simvastatin) 20 mg per day for 3 years. He indicates that he takes Advil (ibuprofen) 400 mg when his leg pain is bad.

> **1. List some of the side effects of the cholesterol-lowering medication that Gordon is using. Could the medication be the cause of Gordon's issues?**
>
> **2. What is intermittent claudication?**
>
> **3. What are common risk factors for peripheral vascular disease?**
>
> **4. What is the common pathophysiology of peripheral vascular disease?**

Lois examines Gordon and notes the following physical findings. His resting pulse rate is 71 bpm. His blood pressure is high, 143/92, and she notes that she has spoken to him about his blood pressure before, but he refused to be medicated. She notes a diminished pulse in his dorsalis pedis arteries, more so in his right than left, but does not discern weakness in the popliteal pulses, although his legs are muscular. The skin on his feet appears mottled and dry, and his lower extremities are cool to the touch. She notes bruits in the iliac and femoropopliteal arteries. Measurement of ankle-brachial index (ABI) indicates a measurement of 0.78 in his right leg and 0.89 in his left leg.

> **5. What are bruits?**
>
> **6. Using the Hartford Institute for Geriatric Nursing website, http://Consultgerirn.org (Coke, 2010), what is a measurement of the ABI? Why can it be helpful to assess an ABI during a routine exam of elderly patients?**
>
> **7. What lifestyle changes might you recommend to Gordon?**
>
> **8. What medications might Gordon benefit from using?**
>
> **9. What signs should Gordon watch for to indicate that the disease may be progressing?**

Suggested Resources

Agency for Healthcare Research and Quality. (2013). *Evidence-Based Practice Center Systematic Review Protocol. Treatment strategies for patients with peripheral artery disease*. Retrieved from http://effectivehealthcare.ahrq.gov/ehc/products/368/948/Peripheral-Artery-Disease-Amended-Protocol_130131.pdf

Coke, L. A. (2010). *Vascular risk assessment of the older cardiovascular patient: The ankle-brachial index (ABI)*. Hartford Institute for Geriatric Nursing. Retrieved from http://consultgerirn.org/uploads/File/trythis/try_this_sp4.pdf

National Heart, Lung and Blood Institute. (2014). *What is peripheral arterial disease?* Retrieved from http://www.nhlbi.nih.gov/health/dci/Diseases/pad/pad_what.html

Society of Interventional Radiology. (2014). *Peripheral arterial disease*. Retrieved from http://www.sirweb.org/patients/peripheral-arterial-disease

U.S. Food and Drug Administration. (2013). *FDA drug safety communication: New restrictions, contraindications, and dose limitations for Zocor (simvastatin) to reduce the risk of muscle injury*. U.S. Department of Health and Human Services. Retrieved from http://www.fda.gov/drugs/drugsafety/ucm256581.htm

Case 11.5 ▪ Hyperlipidemia

*M*r. Adam Nightwolf, a 65-year-old American Indian male, is retired from military service and lives with his daughter. Mr. Nightwolf was diagnosed with CAD and type 2 diabetes 5 years ago. He has come to the new tribal community health clinic for an annual examination. Steve Andrews, clinic admissions nurse, is taking a health history and performing an initial physical exam.

Mr. Nightwolf has a history of angina and smokes four cigarettes a day. On physical examination, his body mass index (BMI) is 28.6, his waist circumference is 40 inches, and his blood pressure is 142/88 mmHg. His radial pulses are 2+, and his dorsalis pedis pulses are 1+.

His current medications are as follows:

- 10 mg of Glucotrol (glipizide) and 1,000 mg of Glucophage (metformin) twice a day
- 50 mg of Tenormin (atenolol) daily
- 20 mg of Prinivil (lisinopril) daily
- 40 mg of Zocor (simvastatin) daily
- 325 mg of aspirin daily

Admission lab results for Mr. Nightwolf:

- Total cholesterol: 172 mg/dL
- Triglycerides: 330 mg/dL
- HDL-cholesterol: 38 mg/dL
- LDL-cholesterol: 130 mg/dL
- Serum glucose level: 180 mg/dL
- Hemoglobin A1c: 8.3%
- Blood urea nitrogen: 24 mg/dL
- Creatinine: 1.4 mg/dL

Steve notes that Mr. Nightwolf is short of breath walking down the hall to the exam room. This dyspnea subsides after 5 minutes of rest, but Mr. Nightwolf says, "I can't walk or do as much as I used to. I was able to run 5 miles when I was 40."

1. ***What history, laboratory results, or physical examination findings should be of the greatest concern to the admissions nurse? What might these findings represent?***

2. ***What changes seen in Mr. Nightwolf's physical exam might be due to common age-related changes? Use the Hartford Institute for Geriatric Nursing evidence-based practice guidelines (Smith & Cotter, 2012), www.consultgerirn.com/topics/normal_aging_ changes/want_to_know_more, and identify age-associated cardiovascular changes shown by Mr. Nightwolf.***

3. What other tests should the nurse expect to be carried out for Mr. Nightwolf? What assessments should the nurse perform?

Steve is a new nurse at the tribal health clinic and does some research on cardiovascular disease risk factors in the American Indian population.

4. Why is Mr. Nightwolf at greater risk for a cardiovascular event, such as a cerebrovascular accident (stroke) or myocardial infarction (heart attack)? Go to the following website, www.heart.org/idc/groups/heart-public/@wcm/@sop/@smd/documents/downloadable/ucm_319569.pdf, and identify at least four statistics that explain Mr. Nightwolf's risks.

Mr. Nightwolf says, "I am not much of a cook, and my daughter works long hours. I eat a lot of frozen dinners and food from cans."

5. What can Steve suggest to Mr. Nightwolf to reduce the fat and salt in his diet? Identify at least five dietary changes that Mr. Nightwolf could make that would reduce his risk of stroke and heart attack.

Mr. Nightwolf says, "I heard that exercise can help lower cholesterol. I want to be more active. Is there anything I can do?"

6. What information could Steve give to Mr. Nightwolf to safely allow him to exercise?

Mr. Nightwolf returns to the clinic in 3 months. He reports that he is walking once a day and is cooking one meal a day for himself. He has not stopped smoking, but tells Steve, "I want to quit."
Lab results for Mr. Nightwolf:

- Total cholesterol: 182 mg/dL
- Triglycerides: 250 mg/dL
- HDL-cholesterol: 39 mg/dL
- LDL-cholesterol: 110 mg/dL
- Serum glucose level: 148 mg/dL (fasting)
- Hemoglobin A1c: 7.2%
- Blood urea nitrogen: 21 mg/dL
- Creatinine: 1.1 mg/dL

7. What improvements can Steve identify in Mr. Nightwolf's lab tests? What do they represent?

At the end of the visit, Steve talks to Mr. Nightwolf about the "Life's Simple 7" guideline to remind him of factors that can reduce the risk of stroke and heart disease.

8. Find an online source for "Life's Simple 7" and discuss each element; cite the source used.

Suggested Resources

American Heart Association. (2014a). *Life's Simple 7/Eat better*. Retrieved from http://www .heart.org/HEARTORG/GettingHealthy/Lifes-Simple-7-Eat-Better_UCM_449577_Article.jsp

American Heart Association. (2014b). *Make the effort to prevent heart disease with Life's Simple 7*. Retrieved from http://www.heart.org/HEARTORG/GettingHealthy/Make-the-Effort-to-Prevent-Heart-Disease-with-Lifes-Simple-7_UCM_443750_Article.jsp

Dressler, D. K. (2014). Management of patients with coronary vascular disorders. In J. L. Hinkle & K. H. Cheever (Eds.), *Brunner & Suddarth's textbook of medical–surgical nursing* (13th ed., pp. 732–734). Philadelphia, PA: Lippincott Williams and Wilkins.

Go, A. S., Mozaffarian, D., Roger, V. L., Benjamin, E. J., Berry, J. D., Borden, W. B, . . . Woo, D. (2013). Heart disease and stroke statistics—2013 update: A report from the American Heart Association. *Circulation, 127*, e6–e245. Retrieved from http://www.heart.org/idc/groups/ heart-public/@wcm/@sop/@smd/documents/downloadable/ucm_319569.pdf

Smith, C. M., & Cotter, V. T. (2012). *Nursing standard of practice protocol: Age-related changes in health*. Hartford Institute for Geriatric Nursing. Retrieved from http://www.consultgerirn .com/topics/normal_aging_changes/want_to_know_more

Case 11.6 ■ Abdominal Aortic Aneurysm

Vincent Dufrane is sitting at his dining room table with a small group of friends and family members helping him celebrate his 75th birthday. They have enjoyed a wonderful meal, and now he is preparing to open gifts brought to him by the guests. Most people would find this a fun, perhaps exciting, time yet Vincent dreads it. Background on the family dynamics will better explain his trepidation.

Vincent married his wife, Jaquelyn, in his early 50s after living alone for a decade following a divorce. Jaquelyn was a coworker who was widowed with a teenage daughter. The couple married after Jaquelyn's daughter, Jennifer, graduated from high school and left home to attend the state university; her plan was to obtain a bachelor of science degree in nursing.

Jennifer accomplished this goal and worked 5 years in critical care at the university medical center. She then decided to return to graduate school. Looking ahead in her career, she believed advanced practice in gerontology would be an excellent route to best use her skills. She is passionate about her role in promoting health and encouraging successful aging. This passion carries over to Vincent; she has constantly persuaded him to seek medical evaluation and screenings, change his lifestyle behaviors, and live with a positive outlook about getting older.

Vincent knows Jennifer means well and loves him unconditionally, yet her zealous personality related to health promotion has become irritating. He repeatedly receives gifts from her with what he terms a "hidden agenda," trying to enforce him to take better care of his physical and emotional well-being. For example, in the basement sits an exercise bicycle, a treadmill, expensive athletic shoes, and loads of books related to successful aging. In addition, she has given him certificates for massage, and gift baskets full of vitamin supplements, nicotine patches, herbal lotions, and sun block products for his very pale skin. When Vincent is handed Jennifer's package to open tonight on his birthday, he takes a deep breath and hopes he can show some degree of appreciation regardless of the contents.

What Jennifer chose this year for her stepfather was a prepaid ultrasound of his carotid arteries and aorta. The exam has been scheduled in 2 days at a free-standing vascular health center. She tells Vincent, "This is a painless, quick and very important procedure; as a bonus, I'm taking you to lunch afterward." Jennifer selected this medical exam based on her knowledge of Vincent's risk factors and recommended screening for abdominal aortic aneurysm (AAA).

1. What risk factors does Vincent present for AAA?

2. What does the U.S. Preventive Services Task Force (2014) recommend as a screening for AAA?

Vincent's health history is positive for cardiovascular disease. He has been hypertensive for 25 years and takes three medications to keep his blood pressure under control. These include oral prescriptions for Atenolol (tenormin), Prinivil (lisinopril), and Hydrodiuril (hydrochlorothiazide). For hyperlipidemia, Lipitor (simvastatin) is used nightly. At the age of 62, he underwent triple coronary artery bypass graft surgery. After that procedure, significant lifestyle behavior changes were attempted.

Vincent worked for a major tobacco company most of his adult life. Nearly everyone at the plant smoked, as cigarettes were provided free to all employees. From the age of 25, until he was diagnosed with HTN at age 50, Vincent smoked three packs a day. He reduced that amount to one pack per day, which he still uses, despite full awareness of the dangers.

3. Calculate Vincent's total lifetime dose (also referred to as pack-year history) of nicotine intake.

In addition, a major change has occurred with Vincent's daily nutrition. He was a "meat and potato" man for many years. Coffee intake was immeasurable; he had a pot brewing at all times following retirement. The other preferred food group was desserts. Vincent consumed several gallons of ice cream a week, enjoying it primarily before bedtime. Breakfast was always something sweet; from doughnuts, to a piece of pie, cookies, or even a candy bar.

Following his bypass surgery, Jennifer provided postoperative care at home for several weeks. She saw his vulnerable physical and emotional state as the perfect opportunity to begin encouraging and teaching him about healthy choices. She and her mother love him dearly for his easygoing, generous spirit, and protective nature toward them; thus, they want him as healthy as possible. Although Vincent has consistently complained about making these lifestyle choices, he has cooperated fully with Jennifer's recommendations, other than remaining a smoker.

The vascular center exam took less than 30 minutes. The ultrasound technician asked whether Vincent and his daughter could wait another hour for the vascular specialist to discuss the results. Jennifer knew at this point an abnormal finding was discovered. She remained calm and countered with the idea of them having lunch nearby and returning within an hour. Dr. Olsen delivered the news that afternoon that a 5.8-cm AAA was discovered just below the renal arteries. He arranged an appointment for Vincent with his cardiac surgeon for further evaluation and treatment plans.

Use the following article to assist in answering Questions 4 through 8 found at www
.uptodate.com/contents/abdominal-aortic-aneurysm-beyond-the-basics (Mohler, 2014).

4. *As a nurse, how would you describe what an AAA is to a client?*

5. *Vincent's wife is amazed and quite frightened when informed of
the AAA. She exclaims, "I don't understand, he has no symptoms
whatsoever of this thing growing in him!" What would be your
response to this statement?*

6. *From her nursing background, Jennifer is focused on the fear of
rupture of the aneurysm prior to treatment. Based on the size of
her stepfather's aneurysm, what is the percentage of risk?*

After further evaluation, including a complete physical exam, a CT scan, and multiple
lab studies, Vincent is scheduled for surgical repair of his AAA. He phones a former
coworker to share the news and is quite confused when this gentleman shares that
he also has an AAA and has undergone "watchful waiting" of his aneurysm for several
years rather than having surgery.

7. *What is the current evidence-based practice for determining
whether surgical intervention is necessary based on the size of
an AAA?*

The cardiovascular surgeon met with Vincent and Jennifer and stated he would like
one further diagnostic procedure prior to scheduling a repair of the aneurysm. An
angiography was performed to view the iliac arteries. The outcome was positive; no
torsion, calcification, or thrombi were present. Based on these findings, endovascular
grafting was determined as the approach to use for the infrarenal AAA repair. Jennifer
called her mother to report, "I have good news. They are able to fix the aneurysm
without having to use the standard open surgical repair; it will be done by a specially
trained radiologist rather than a heart surgeon."

During the days following the angiogram, Jennifer wanted to inspect Vincent's
abdomen several times a day; she respectfully did not do so. View the brief YouTube
video at www.youtube.com/watch?v=_7Regw_HEq8, to see what potential assessment
finding worried Jennifer.

8. *Should an AAA rupture, it is considered a medical emergency
with a very high mortality rate. What type of symptoms might
precede this event?*

9. *Compare and contrast the advantages of using endovascular
grafting versus open surgical repair of an AAA.*

Vincent has the procedure the following week and spends one night at the hospital.
He returns home and for 2 weeks does not participate in driving, lifting more than
5 pounds, or any type of strenuous house or yard work. He expresses his gratitude to
Jennifer for her nursing knowledge and insights that led to the discovery of his aneurysm. He tells her, "In return for this special gift you gave me, I'm wearing a nicotine

patch and enrolling in a smoking cessation program through the American Cancer Society. I can't make any promises, but I will give it my best try."

Suggested Resources

Cooper, M. M. (2013). *Abdominal aortic aneurysm*. MedLine Plus. Retrieved from http://www.nlm.nih.gov/medlineplus/ency/article/000162.htm

Mohler, E. R. (2014). *Patient information: Abdominal aortic aneurysm (beyond the basics)*. UpToDate, Wolters Kluwer Health. Retrieved from http://www.uptodate.com/contents/abdominal-aortic-aneurysm-beyond-the-basics

Society of Interventional Radiology. (2014). *Interventional radiologists treat abdominal aneurysms nonsurgically*. Retrieved from http://www.sirweb.org/patients/abdominal-aortic-aneurysms

U.S. Preventive Services Task Force. (2014). *Screening for abdominal aortic aneurysm*. Summary of recommendation. Retrieved from http://www.uspreventiveservicestaskforce.org/uspstf/uspsaneu.htm

Case 11.7 ■ Anemia

*M*r. Brown is an 83-year-old male with a past medical history that includes HTN, CAD, congestive cardiomyopathy, and coronary artery bypass grafting (at age 73). He was recently diagnosed with anemia by his primary care provider and was referred to a specialist. He is being seen by a hematologist/oncologist who performed blood tests and a bone marrow biopsy and diagnosed myelodysplastic syndrome (MDS). Mr. Brown has been sent to the infusion center at the hospital for a blood transfusion. He is accompanied by his son and wife. After Mr. Brown completes check-in, he receives his identification bracelet, and the nurse verifies orders for the blood transfusion. The nurse brings Mr. Brown and his family into a treatment room at the infusion center and proceeds with the transfusion center treatment protocol.

Upon interviewing Mr. Brown for the infusion center initial assessment, the nurse learns that the patient reports a 3-month history of fatigue and occasional palpitations, which he attributed to his heart condition. He states he would often rest in the afternoon; napping a couple of hours would make him feel better, then he would have enough energy to get through the rest of his day. He reports the symptoms got worse about 4 weeks ago; he began to feel dizzy whenever he would get up after sitting for any length of time, and he felt that he was becoming too weak. His wife interjects, "He was so weak when he stood up that he almost fell a couple of times. So I insisted he make an appointment to see the doctor." This prompted him to schedule an appointment with his primary care provider. The physician examined him in the office and informed him that he may have anemia and that he needed laboratory studies to evaluate for this condition.

1. *What symptoms does Mr. Brown report that may be experienced with anemia?*

2. *Is anemia a common occurrence in older adults? What co-morbid conditions can increase the incidence?*

The primary care provider ordered a complete blood count, thyroid-stimulating hormone (TSH), iron studies, serum B12, folate, and comprehensive metabolic panel and found the following abnormal results: hemoglobin 8.5, hematocrit 26, platelet count 110,000; MCV 104, peripheral smear showed increased blasts and ringed sideroblasts; BUN 22, creatinine 1.1; serum B12, folate, iron, and TSH within normal limits.

3. *Which of Mr. Brown's laboratory values confirm the diagnosis of anemia?*

Mr. Brown's primary care provider refers him to a specialist promptly. One week later, he followed up with the hematologist/oncologist and had additional outpatient blood work and a bone marrow aspiration. His hemoglobin dropped to 7.0, requiring a blood transfusion.

4. *What is MDS? What are the overall goals for treatment?*

The hematologist instructed Mr. Brown to go to the infusion center at the hospital where he would have additional blood drawn for typing and cross matching and subsequently receive two units of packed red blood cells. Mr. Brown reports to the nurse that the hematologist also explained other medical interventions that he could have for treatment of this condition, which included "shots to make my body produce more blood cells, vitamins, chemotherapy, or bone marrow transplant." Mr. Brown states, "I decided to have the blood transfusion. . . . I don't know if I will do anything else after this."

5. *What patient teaching should the nurse provide regarding the procedure of a blood transfusion?*

6. *What should Mr. Brown's comment, " . . . I don't know if I will do anything else after this" prompt the nurse to do?*

The nurse reviews Mr. Brown's home medications, allergies, and history of past blood transfusions and any reactions experienced. He denies any known allergies and reports that the only blood transfusion he has had in the past was when he had his open heart surgery, and he did not have any reaction or complication. Mr. Brown states that he took his medications this morning with the exception of a baby aspirin as directed by his physician.

The nurse completes further assessment and finds the following: Mr. Brown denies chest pain or shortness of breath. He states, "I get winded if I do any walking." He denies abdominal complaints and reports he has a little swelling of his feet and ankles " . . . but I have that all the time . . . elevating my legs makes it go down." He denies any dizziness, headache, or chills.

Physical examination: BP 140/80, heart rate 88 per minute, respirations 18 per minute, temperature 98.7; pulse oximetry 94% on room air. Skin, pale; HEENT, conjunctiva pale; respiratory, lungs clear to auscultation; cardiovascular, regular rate and rhythm; no jugular venous distention; trace edema of feet and ankles bilaterally; pedal pulses +2 = bilaterally.

7. *What is the purpose of the nursing assessment prior to the blood transfusion? Does Mr. Brown appear to be stable for this procedure?*

8. *Put the following steps in correct order for transfusing blood according to standard protocol.*

    a. *Collect a set of vital signs 15 minutes after the transfusion has started.*

    b. *Assure a large bore angiocath or central line intravenous access is available.*

    c. *Set the IV pump to allow for a 3-hour time period of infusion.*

    d. *Obtain the packed red blood cells (PRBCs) from the blood bank.*

    e. *Validate the patient's identification, blood type, donor type, and expiration of the blood product at the bedside with another licensed professional.*

Mr. Brown receives his first unit of blood without reaction and actually naps through most of the transfusion. While receiving the second unit of blood, the nurse notes that Mr. Brown's blood pressure has increased to 150/90, his pulse is somewhat bounding, his temperature remains normal (98.6), and pulse oximetry remains good on room air (98%). The nurse checks for other signs and symptoms. Mr. Brown denies chest pain, dizziness, fever, chills, cough, or headache. Physical examination shows: respiratory, lungs clear; cardiovascular, regular rate and rhythm; edema of lower extremities remains the same.

9. *What may these symptoms represent? What action should the nurse take?*

10. *Briefly review various types of transfusion reactions a patient may experience with blood products.*

Two weeks later, Mr. Brown and his wife visit the oncologist/hematologist's office for a routine follow-up. They have discussed further treatment options and have made the decision to continue with supportive care. Use the website Myelodysplastic Syndromes at www.cancer.gov/cancertopics/pdq/treatment/myelodysplastic/Patient/page3 to answer Question 11.

11. *Under the category of "supportive treatment," what other options besides transfusion therapy and antibiotics are available?*

12. *If Mr. Brown uses one of these options, why might a community health nurse be required to administer the drug?*

Suggested Resources

Artz, A. S. (2013). *Anemia in the elderly.* Medscape. Retrieved from http://emedicine.medscape
.com/article/1339998-overview#aw2aab6b4

National Cancer Institute. (2014). *PDQ® myelodysplastic syndromes treatment.* Bethesda, MD:
National Cancer Institute. Retrieved from http://cancer.gov/cancertopics/pdq/treatment/
myelodysplastic/Patient

Thomas, M. L. (2014). Management of patients with non-malignant hematologic disorders. In
J. L. Hinkle & K. H. Cheever (Eds.), *Brunner & Suddarth's textbook of medical–surgical
nursing* (13th ed., pp. 900–902). Philadelphia, PA: Lippincott Williams and Wilkins.

Case 11.8 ■ Pacemaker Implantation

Grayson Beecher is a 74-year-old African American male who has just been
informed of the need for a permanent pacemaker. He has a long-term history
of HTN that has required a lot of medication adjustments for over two decades. His
family history was strong for cardiac disease. What were not strong among his siblings were efforts toward health promotion insofar as lifestyle changes. Specifically, at
age 50 Mr. Beecher quit smoking after doing so since he was a teenager, has two or
three servings of alcohol per month, and maintains a 1,200 calorie healthy heart diet
consistently. He also has diabetes (type 2), diagnosed in his 40s, has kept physically
active, takes his Glucotrol XL (glipizide) as ordered, and is monitored every 3 months
by his internist in order to remain noninsulin dependent. All of his five siblings have
died due to cardiac and/or renal implications.

A month ago, Mr. Beecher's Prinivil (lisinopril) was increased from 60 mg orally
daily to 80 mg. In addition, he takes a thiazide diuretic and a calcium channel blocker
with the goal of maintaining a systolic pressure of 130 mmHg or less. The first antihypertensive drug group he used years ago was beta-blockers. Several different brands
at various doses were not effective in controlling his blood pressure as the sole antihypertensive. Therefore, his physician went to Steps 2 and 3 using the stepped-care
approach for managing high blood pressure.

1. What does the literature report about antihypertensive use in African Americans?

Mr. Beecher experienced lightheadedness and dizziness consistently with the higher
dose of his ACE inhibitor. At home, he knew to rise very slowly from the sofa or
his bed to avoid falling or passing out. It was his part-time job that presented a
challenge. Mr. Beecher works 4 hours a day, Tuesday through Saturday at the local
Walmart store as a greeter. At times, he bends over to give customers a basket for
their purchases, and this activity became very hazardous as he stumbled when rising and almost fell daily.

Following a physical exam, 12-lead electrocardiogram, lab work, and an overnight stay on a telemetry unit, it was determined Mr. Beecher was experiencing a third-degree AV-block with bradycardia averaging 45 bpm. His cardiologist gave him a quick review of the need for a permanent pacemaker, stating "you'll be back to your old self in no time at all after we slip this in your chest." Mr. Beecher wasn't necessarily afraid of having the procedure, but he was disappointed. He had been so compliant with life-style changes as a middle-age adult to the present, and associated the pacemaker with failure of taking care of himself properly. A patient education video, www.youtube .com/watch?v=hu0qVXLjM7M, was shown to Mr. Beecher. He signed the informed consent and had the procedure.

2. *What is the purpose of a pacemaker? Describe the various types and speculate which one the patient would require.*

3. *Briefly describe the surgical procedure used for pacemaker insertion.*

4. *What are potential complications of pacemaker use? Identify a minimum of five.*

5. *Describe the home care for the incision site and activity restrictions.*

6. *What benefits does a wireless remote pacemaker (FDA approved in 2009) offer a patient?*

Mr. Beecher stayed overnight on a telemetry unit at the hospital following the pacemaker implant. He had soreness around the operative site the next morning, but otherwise no complaints. After breakfast, he was visited by Susan Clark, a cardiac nurse practitioner, who provided a physical exam and discharge teaching. Although contemporary pacemakers are less susceptible to interference than older models, electromagnetic energy can interfere in some cases. Therefore, Susan started to review safety measures, in particular related to avoidance of certain electromagnetic devices, and Mr. Beecher became very upset. Susan discussed a list of items from the patient brochure, which included walking quickly through doors at places of business that contained antitheft devices. Mr. Beecher stated, "I stand at the doorway of Walmart 20 hours a week that has this type of contraption built in. I cannot give up this job; the workers and regular customers are all the family I've got. Plus, the extra money I make as a greeter helps pay for all of my medicine. The doctor should have told me this before the procedure."

7. *What other electromagnetic devices should a patient with a pacemaker implant use caution around to avoid deactivating of the device? Select all that apply.*

   a. *Microwave oven*

   b. *Battery-operated radio*

   c. *Airport security scanner*

   d. *Electric blanket*

   e. *Cell phone*

8. Do you agree Mr. Beecher should have been informed preoperatively of items he would have to avoid? How might the nurse help with his present state of despair?

A 1-month checkup found Mr. Beecher's vital signs within normal range, no postoperative complications, and without further dizziness or lightheadedness. He was provided with a permanent identification card listing the physician's name, model and type of device, manufacturer's name, and the hospital used for insertion. He was still employed at his job and due to return the following day. Rather than a role as a greeter, he was inside the store stocking items in the pharmacy section; this was not as enjoyable for him, but allowed him to see his "family" of coworkers and customers, as well as provide needed income.

Suggested Resources

Flack, J. M., Sica, D. A., Bakris, G., Brown, A. L., Ferdinand, K. C., Grimm Jr, R. H., . . . Jamerson, K. A. (2011). *Management of high blood pressure in Blacks*. American Heart Association. Retrieved from http://hyper.ahajournals.org/content/56/5/780.abstract

Olshansky, B., & Hayes, D. L. (2014). *Patient information: Pacemaker (beyond the basics)*. UpToDate. Wolters Kluwer Health. Retrieved from http://www.uptodate.com/contents/pacemakers-beyond-the-basics

Schiariti, M., Cacciola, M., & Puddu, P. E. (2011). *Complications of pacemaker insertion*. Intech open.com. Retrieved from http://cdn.intechopen.com/pdfs-wm/13785.pdf

12

The Aging Pulmonary System

Case 12.1 ■ Pneumonia

*C*assie Cornwell is a 20-year-old part-time nursing assistant on a busy hospital unit working 12-hour shifts each weekend. In addition, Cassie is enrolled as a full-time nursing student at a state university. She really enjoys this particular unit as there is a variety of patients, and she learns a lot from the RNs assigned there. In particular, patients with respiratory conditions are an interest as she has grown up with and been exposed to chronic lung disease in her parents' home. Her younger brother was diagnosed with cystic fibrosis as a toddler. Nebulizers, inhalers, peak flow meters, and so on, are common items around her household.

Today's assignment entails five patients for whom Cassie will provide personal care, mobility, vital signs, assisting with meals, measuring intake and output, and so forth. The group includes a 70-year-old male (Mr. Dooley) and an 81-year-old female (Mrs. Lee), both diagnosed with pneumonia. She recently finished the respiratory system in her pathophysiology course and is thinking about the content in relation to these two individuals.

> ### 1. What physiological age-related changes contribute to a higher incidence of pneumonia in the elderly? What risk factors may increase the incidence?

The last weekend Cassie worked, she spent quite a bit of time with an elderly woman admitted with pneumonia from a nursing home, providing personal care and offering reassurance with her breathing struggles, as the woman had no visitors. Cassie learned today that the patient died a few days later. She was surprised as most of the unit deaths are related to cardiac or renal disease.

> ### 2. What is the mortality rate for pneumonia? Cite your source.

The RN responsible for the care of Cassie's patients briefly explains to her there are many types of pneumonia. Mr. Dooley has community-acquired pneumonia (CAP) and was admitted from home, while Mrs. Lee has been on the unit for over a week, initially admitted for uncontrolled diabetes; she is classified as having hospital-acquired pneumonia (HAP).

3. Compare and contrast these two classifications. Include the most common organisms associated with each type.

After obtaining both patients' vital signs and speaking with them briefly, Cassie notes major differences between the findings, appearance, and complaints of each person. Mr. Dooley, with a streptococcal source of pneumonia, states he has chest pain when attempting to deep breathe or cough. Mrs. Lee's only pain-associated symptom is a frontal headache. Both patients are pale, very weak, and without an appetite. Cassie is informed that Mrs. Lee's pneumonia is viral.

4. Compare and contrast the expected differences in vital signs with these types of pneumonia.

In addition to a headache, Mrs. Lee has nasal congestion, a sore throat, and complaints that her chest feels "tight." Upon auscultation, breath sounds are diminished in the bilateral upper lobes. Blood cultures were negative, white blood cell count was 8,500, and a chest film showed patchy infiltrates. A sputum specimen for culture and sensitivity was ordered over 24 hours ago. Mrs. Lee has been unable to provide this due to minimal coughing and stating, "I'm too weak to try to spit something up."

5. What measures might be helpful in thinning the mucus to allow for specimen collection?

Mr. Dooley has coarse crackles upon auscultation; copious rusty, blood-tinged sputum; and his chest film showed bilateral lobar infiltrates. He experiences orthopnea, chills, and continuously looks anxious.

6. What specific treatment does this patient need that would not be anticipated for Mrs. Lee?

Although the cause, type, and symptoms are different in these two cases of pneumonia, both patients have similar nursing interventions identified for their care plans. Goals include the following:

- Improving airway patency
- Promoting rest and conserving energy
- Promoting fluid intake
- Maintaining nutrition
- Promoting the patient's knowledge

7. Create specific interventions for how the nurse can accomplish these goals.

On a lunch break with the RN responsible for Cassie's assignment, she comments again about the patient she cared for last weekend who died as a result of her pneumonia. She worries that when she returns to work next Saturday, she might discover a similar outcome for Mr. Dooley or Mrs. Lee. The RN reviews with Cassie common occurrences, which can contribute to mortality.

8. Identify a minimum of five complications associated with pneumonia.

Several days later, Cassie was in her nursing student role at a community health promotion fair. She was excited (and a bit anxious) as her focus that morning was to administer vaccines for both pneumonia and influenza. As part of her preparation the night prior to clinical, she studied details of both types of vaccines.

9. Discuss the pneumococcal vaccine in relation to the Centers for Disease Control (CDC) recommendations.

Suggested Resources

Guimarães, C., Lares Santos, C., Costa, F., & Barata, F. (2011). *Pneumonia associated with health care versus community acquired pneumonia: Different entities, distinct approaches.* Retrieved from http://www.elsevier.pt/en/revistas/revista-portuguesa-pneumologia-320/ artigo/pneumonia-associated-with-health-care-versus-community-acquired-90024834

Mayo Clinic Staff. (2013). *Pneumonia—Complications.* Mayo Clinic. Retrieved from http://www .mayoclinic.org/diseases-conditions/pneumonia/basics/complications/con-20020032

National Center for Immunization and Respiratory Diseases at the Centers for Disease Control and Prevention. (2014). *Pneumococcal vaccines—CDC answers your questions.* Retrieved from http://www.immunize.org/catg.d/p2015.pdf

Schaffner, W. (2014). *Why the elderly are more susceptible to pneumonia.* AgingCare.com. Retrieved from http://www.agingcare.com/Articles/Pneumonia-and-Elders-Why-they-are-more-susceptible-136822.htm

Scrib.com. (2009). *Nursing process of pneumonia.* Retrieved from http://www.scribd.com/ doc/18990725/Nursing-Process-of-Pneumonia

Thompson, E. G. (2013). *Pneumonia—Topic overview.* WebMD. Retrieved from http://www .webmd.com/lung/tc/pneumonia-credits

Case 12.2 ■ Lung Cancer

*M*ary Lou Ellis is leaving a retirement party, given in her behalf, with one of the biggest "life secrets" thus far in her 65 years. She received word yesterday that testing confirmed the diagnosis of lung cancer; she chose not to share this information at the party. Her main reaction when speaking to the pulmonary specialist in the office was that of embarrassment; not fear, anxiety, or shock, as might be expected.

Mary Lou has been an RN since she was 22 years old, and her career has been varied. She worked at a local hospital as a staff nurse for a decade, served as a clinical instructor the following 10 years, and for over 20 years has been an advanced nurse practitioner for an internal medicine group. The majority of her patients are in the elderly population, and she witnessed many lung cancer diagnoses, as well as death that followed. All but several of the many persons affected were smokers, confirming her knowledge of a high rate of association of tobacco and the disease.

A long-term life secret Mary Lou has kept is being a smoker herself. She started with cigarettes in nursing school, as did many of her classmates, as a stress-relief measure. After starting her first nursing position, many coworkers smoked, and she noted how they were "looked down on" from peers that did not. Taking more frequent smoke breaks, regardless of how busy the unit was, became a source of conflict. Over time, smoking was prohibited in various public buildings (including hospitals), social venues, restaurants, and so forth. Mary Lou never complained about these restrictions as she was a "closet smoker"; she used her car and home smoking privately for decades.

One afternoon at the office, Mary Lou had a new patient to work up who was a female and close to her own age. When she walked into the exam room, the smell of tobacco was strong in the air, as well as on the patient's hair, skin, and clothing, during the physical exam. During the health history, the woman denied being a current smoker, or ever having smoked in her life. Mary Lou asked whether she lived with smokers, and the patient stated she lived alone. Although Mary Lou checked all the "no/never" boxes on the form, she wrote under the comment section, "reeks of cigarette smoke."

This encounter had a profound effect on Mary Lou; she literally saw herself in this woman, as she had denied being a smoker every time when asked her entire life. Prior to a doctor or dental visit, Mary Lou always showered at the last minute, put on a fresh change of clothes, brushed her teeth twice, and used cologne and breath mints in order to maintain her "secret." She felt like such a hypocrite that day and was ashamed of herself to the point she quit smoking on the spot at age 55.

1. *What is the rate of smoking for the county in which you live? Use the website www.countyhealthrankings.org to compare the county rate with the rate stated overall. Then compare your county with any from the state of Utah (lowest percent of smokers in the United States). Comment on the results.*

2. *What are other risk factors, besides tobacco use, for lung cancer?*

She went to a physician following two upper respiratory infections several months apart and requested a chest film. It was obtained and an area of suspicious density was seen in the upper left lobe. Mary Lou was diagnosed with nonsmall cell lung carcinoma (NSCLC) following diagnostic testing.

3. *Distinguish small cell from NSCLC as to prevalence and the cell types associated.*

4. *What further diagnostic testing may have been used in order to confirm the diagnosis?*

5. *What is the most frequent symptom of lung cancer? If it were pain, do you think a difference in the timing of the diagnosis, thus the overall outcome, might be different for those with lung cancer?*

Mary Lou's appointment with a thoracic surgeon is 4 days away. She has been going over and over the possibility of metastasis of her adenocarcinoma of the left upper lung lobe, which won't be known until the actual procedure. She was raised in the Christian faith and has been praying multiple times a day: silently and out loud while walking around her house. What she repeats is: *"Please God, let them remove all the cancer and have it not be in my lymph or surrounding tissue. I will come clean with my 35-year smoking history and volunteer my time working with the homeless, at the food shelter, in the prison, or with any other group you lead me to, if you can just let me live longer."*

6. What stage of Elisabeth Kübler-Ross's stages of grieving is Mary Lou demonstrating?

Mary Lou used the Internet and came across a study of personal interest. She is African American and is intrigued, but saddened, by statistics she discovers.

Brigham and Women's Hospital provides an extensive report on women and lung cancer (2010) at www.brighamandwomens.org/departments_and_services/womenshealth/connorscenter/images/womenandlungcancerfinal-april22,2010pdf.pdf. Use this source for the remaining questions.

7. Find the table, "Lung Cancer Incidence in Men and Women by Race." Compare and contrast the statistics for African American women with females from the other races listed.

The study also addresses that lower lung cancer survival rates may be attributable to disparities in access to health care, as well as different patterns of treatment for the disease.

8. Identify a minimum of five disparities/patterns for African American women with lung cancer.

Mary Lou underwent a video-assisted thoracoscopic surgery (VATS) procedure resulting in a left upper lobectomy the following week. Lymph node dissection was negative for cancerous cells, and no local or regional spread was detected.

9. Advantages for the VATS include which of the following? Select all that apply.

a. Less pain medication required postoperatively

b. Local anesthesia is all that is necessary

c. Fewer perioperative complications

d. Shorter hospital stay

On a follow-up visit with the surgeon, she was commended for asking for the chest film due to having the respiratory infections close together, since her cancer was a Stage IB, and many are more progressed. The surgeon also discussed how imperative receiving an honest, accurate health history in relation to smoking history is for overall planning and treatment. On that topic, Mary Lou knew if she recovered from surgery and was able to forego chemotherapy and/or radiation, what her volunteer "prayer project" mentioned earlier would entail. She connected with the American Cancer Society and reached out to adolescent African American girls to provide teaching, information, and support about the dangers of smoking. What inspired this topic was material in the "Out of the Shadows" report.

> ***10. Report and comment on the section related to marketing menthol cigarettes to the African American female community.***

Suggested Resources

American Lung Association. (2014). *Lung cancer fact sheet.* Retrieved from http://www .lung.org/lung-disease/lung-cancer/resources/facts-figures/lung-cancer-fact-sheet .html#other_Causes

Brigham and Women's Hospital. (2010). *Out of the shadows: Lung cancer.* Mary Horrigan Connors Center for Women's Health and Gender Biology. Lung Cancer Alliance.org. Retrieved from http://www.brighamandwomens.org/departments_and_services/womenshealth/ connorscenter/images/womenandlungcancerfinal-april22,2010pdf.pdf

National Cancer Institute. (2014). Small cell lung cancer treatment (PDQ®). Retrieved from http:// www.cancer.gov/cancertopics/pdq/treatment/small-cell-lung/healthprofessional/page1

Case 12.3 ■ Chronic Obstructive Pulmonary Disease

*M*rs. Virginia Wade is a 74-year-old African American woman with a 22-year history of chronic obstructive pulmonary disease (COPD). She has been admitted to a medical unit for an acute onset episode of her disease. Her social history includes being married with one son who visits weekly and several siblings who visit her annually. Mrs. Wade is retired from a plastics factory. She lives with her spouse in a third-floor apartment located in an urban setting. Mrs. Wade no longer smokes but had a 42-pack-year history. There is no use of alcohol or illegal drugs. It is her third admission in the past 8 months. Her medications while hospitalized are as follows:

- $D_5$1/2 NS at 125 mL/hr
- Solumedrol (methylprednisolone sodium succinate) 125 mg IV every 6 hours
- Ipratropium bromide and Combivent (albuterol sulfate) inhalation aerosol every 4 hours as needed for shortness of breath
- Spiriva Handihaler (tiotropium) 18 mcg inhaled daily
- Fluticasone propionate 250 mcg and Advair 250/50 (salmeterol 50 mcg) one inhalation twice a day
- Humibid (guaifenesin) 300 mg orally daily
- Prinivil (lisinopril) 20 mg daily

- Lasix (furosemide) 40 mg, oral twice a day
- Novolin R insulin coverage, subcutaneous every 6 hours according to sliding scale
- Prilosec (omeprazole) 40 mg tablet orally daily
- Xanax (alprazolam) 0.25 mg, oral every 6 hours as needed for anxiety

Mrs. Wade's vital signs are temperature 99°F, heart rate 100, respiration 27, blood pressure 132/74. Chest film is clear with evidence of hyperinflation and enlarged right ventricle. Urine output is adequate with greater than 400 mL per shift. Mrs. Wade states she routinely drinks 5 to 6 glasses of water or juice daily. No significant weight loss has occurred over the past month (she is 5 feet 4 inches tall, and weighs 172 pounds). Her lab tests were predominantly within normal range. The serum glucose was 208 mg/dL and WBC 7,600/μL.

- Respiratory therapy orders are as follows:
- O_2 at 3 L per nasal cannula continuously with humidification
- Pulmonary function tests
- Arterial blood gases (ABG)
- Chest film repeated in the morning

1. What are Mrs. Wade's risk factors for developing COPD?

One piece of data from the patient's pulmonary function test was a forced expiratory volume (FEV) of 55%. Best practice guidelines are created from the Global Initiative for Chronic Obstructive Lung (GOLD). This is a collaboration between the National Institutes of Health and the World Health Organization.

2. Use the GOLD criteria to evaluate what stage of COPD Mrs. Wade is experiencing. Go to www.goldcopd.org/uploads/users/files/ GOLD_Report_2014_Jun11.pdf.

3. What expected age-related changes have contributed to the COPD?

4. What are three psychosocial-oriented nursing diagnoses Mrs. Wade might be experiencing?

5. Mr. Wade is worried about taking his spouse home and wants to know what preparations he should make. There is portable oxygen available at home with 50 feet of tubing. What safety precautions can you discuss with Mr. Wade?

6. Mrs. Wade says she does not have diabetes and wonders why she is getting insulin as needed, based on glucometer assessments. How do you explain this to her?

7. You auscultate and percuss Mrs. Wade's lungs. What do you expect to hear?

Mrs. Wade's ABGs are as follows:

- pH: 7.36
- CO_2: 66
- pO_2: 58

- HCO_3: 35
- SaO_2: 88%

8. Interpret her blood gas result; is this compensated or uncompensated?

9. What is the impact of age on arterial blood gas interpretation?

10. Utilize the article, "Best Practices in COPD" to find what recommendations are most important for prevention of COPD. Go to http://journals.lww.com/tnpj/Fulltext/2011/05000/ Best_Practices_in_Chronic_Obstructive_Pulmonary.6.aspx.

Suggested Resources

Garvey, C. (2011). Best practices in COPD. *Nurse Practitioner, 36*(5), 16–22. Retrieved from http://journals.lww.com/tnpj/Fulltext/2011/05000/Best_Practices_in_Chronic_Obstructive_Pulmonary.6.aspx

Johnson, K. (2012). GOLD criteria for COPD. *WebMD*. Retrieved from http://www.webmd.com/lung/copd/gold-criteria-for-copd

Smith, C. M., & Cotter, V. T. (2012). *Geriatric nursing protocol: Age-related changes in health*. Hartford Institute for Geriatric Nursing. Retrieved from http://www.consultgerirn.com/topics/normal_aging_changes/want_to_know_more#item_5

Case 12.4 ■ Tuberculosis

Mary Alice Ray is a 75-year-old Caucasian woman, who for the past year has been living with her daughter and son-in-law in a nice suburb of a small southern town. She was diagnosed with COPD 10 years ago. Shortly before moving in with her family, Mary Alice's condition declined.

She was a 160-pack-year Lucky Strike smoker from age 7 until age 74. This past year, her weight declined from 110 pounds to 88 pounds. She is 5 feet 1 inch tall. Her serum albumin decreased from 3.5 to 2.8, and her total lymphocyte count declined from 1,200–1,500 cells to 700–800. Her emphysema requires her to have 1 to 2 L/min of oxygen via nasal cannula.

Kate, a home health care nurse, completes a home evaluation, as Mary Alice's symptoms have worsened. In her health history intake, she finds out that when Mary Alice was a teenager, she tended to her mother who had tuberculosis (TB). She did not have a clinically significant case of TB at that time. With her current decline due to the emphysema and impaired immune system, Kate suspects a reactivation of a latent TB case. Kate establishes a care plan with Mary Alice's primary care provider to confirm her suspicion of TB.

1. *What additional symptoms should Kate inquire of Mary Alice?*

2. *In what order are diagnostic steps taken to confirm TB?*

    a. *Positive medical history of exposure, positive sputum test for acid-fast bacillus, purified protein derivative (PPD) (two-step), chest x-ray*

    b. *Positive medical history of exposure, PPD (two-step), chest x-ray, positive sputum test for acid-fast bacillus*

    c. *Chest x-ray, PPD (two-step), positive medical history of exposure, positive sputum test for acid-fast bacillus*

    d. *Positive medical history of exposure, positive sputum test for acid-fast bacillus, chest x-ray, PPD (two-step)*

3. *A PPD test should be administered as a*

    a. *Skin scratch*

    b. *Intramuscular (IM) injection*

    c. *Subcutaneous injection*

    d. *Subdural (raised wheal)*

4. *Why do you believe that older persons may be at a greater risk for contracting TB? Some ideas are available at www.helpage.org/blogs/prakash-tyagi-869/challenges-of-dealing-with-tb-in-older-people-300.*

The family voices concern to the nurse and asks her to explain more about why Mary Alice has TB now, but did not have it as a teenager. Kate explains that, with age, the T-cell mediated immune response wanes, allowing latent TB to become active.

5. *What risk factors does TB include for developing or reactivating?*

6. *How is TB transmitted?*

7. *What organs can become infected with TB?*

The family asks what treatment options are available, because they have concern for her recent difficulty breathing and worry about her comfort.

8. *Take the visual tour of drug therapies used for TB to answer the following questions. It is located at www.niaid.nih.gov/topics/tuberculosis/Understanding/WhatIsTB/VisualTour/pages/mdr-tb.aspx.*

    a. *What are the first-line drugs (all used for over 40 years)?*

    b. *What are several major concerns about the second-line drugs?*

    c. *What developments in treatment are in process?*

9. *What function test should be closely monitored in the elderly to prevent further complications?*

Kate knows that successful treatment of TB is dependent on medication adherence due to the long course of treatment and side effects. Mary Alice is immediately admitted to the hospital. She quickly develops a secondary pneumonia.

10. *What precautions do hospitals take with patients who have a known active infection of TB?*

Sadly, on the fifth day of her admission, Mary Alice dies from the complications of her pneumonia and impaired respiratory function. Kate knows prevention is essential with TB. The relatives caring for Mary Alice all have a follow-up two-step PPD and test negative for TB.

Suggested Resources

American Lung Association. (2014). *Tuberculosis*. Retrieved from http://www.lungusa.org/lung-disease/tuberculosis/?gclid=CKOd0NOXzZ8CFRednAody3RE0g

Centers for Disease Control and Prevention. (2012). *Basic TB facts*. Retrieved from http://www.cdc.gov/tb/topic/basics/risk.htm

Centers for Disease Control and Prevention. (2014). *Tuberculosis: An overview*. Retrieved from http://www.cdc.gov/nchhstp/newsroom/docs/TB-overview-FactSheet.pdf

National Institute of Allergy and Infectious Diseases. (2012). *Tuberculosis*. NIAID website. Retrieved from http://www.niaid.nih.gov/topics/tuberculosis/Understanding/WhatIsTB/VisualTour/pages/firstline.aspx

Tyagi, P. (2011). *Challenges of dealing with TB in older people*. HelpAge. Retrieved from http://www.helpage.org/blogs/prakash-tyagi-869/challenges-of-dealing-with-tb-in-older-people-300

Case 12.5 ▪ Pulmonary Embolism

*M*artha Stanley is a 72-year-old female on her third postoperative day from a right total knee replacement. The procedure was elective and scheduled several months ago. Mrs. Stanley has been a physically active woman her entire life but because of pain had to curtail daily walks, playing golf, and senior travel tours, which she enjoys and misses. Her overall health status is considered "good." All preadmission lab work (complete blood count, platelets, chemistry, and urinalysis) was within normal limits. She takes Lisinopril (prinivil) for hypertension, Zocor (simvastatin) for hyperlipidemia, Premarin (conjugated estrogen) for postmenopausal hormone replacement, and Boniva (ibandronate) for osteoporosis protection. The previous surgeries include a caesarean section in 1968, carpal tunnel repair in 1978, and bladder suspension in 1990.

Her postoperative course has been uneventful thus far. She has worked well with physical therapy and uses a walker to ambulate, she has a continuous passive motion

(CPM) machine for the right leg (2 hours on and 2 hours off, when awake), adequate urine output, and vital signs within normal range. Mrs. Stanley's main concern with surgery was pain management. She has a lifelong needle phobia and worried that the only route for narcotics would be injections. Prior to having her lab work, she was given a dose of oral Valium (diazepam), and the antecubital space was anesthetized with topical cream. Her husband had to hug her tightly with her face turned away from seeing the syringe and lab tubes. Intravenous access was obtained in the operating room after she inhaled several breaths of nitrous oxide.

Mrs. Stanley is due to be discharged later today. Physical therapy must work with her on stair climbing. She has three steps to reach the front door of her home. Occupational therapy also wants to review getting dressed and some general safety measures for home.

Kye Lewellyn is, and has been, Mrs. Stanley's nurse. Kye has finished obtaining change-of-shift report. The nursing assistant working on her team reports that when obtaining vital signs, Mrs. Stanley's pulse oximetry reading showed an oxygen saturation of 88%. As Kye is walking to her room, she is interrupted by a physician needing information and then sees another patient on the floor beside his bed, so another 5 minutes or more passes until she reaches Mrs. Stanley.

Upon entering the room, Kye observes Mrs. Stanley in bed, supine with the CPM machine on the right leg. The patient looks anxious, has her hand over her chest, and states, "I can hardly breathe."

1. Which of the following should be the nurse's first action?

a. Obtain a blood pressure

b. Remove the CPM machine

c. Listen to breath sounds

d. Elevate the head of the bed

After applying supplemental oxygen at 3 L/min per cannula, Kye recorded the following vital signs: T 98°F, HR 108, RR 30, and BP 145/90. The oxygen saturation dropped to 84%. Pulmonary assessment revealed symmetric chest excursion without use of accessory muscles, respiratory rate regular, with moderate depth and labored. Course crackles with diminished breath sounds were found throughout the anterior and posterior chest, without friction rub, increased voice resonance, or tactile fremitus. Mrs. Stanley's surgeon comes to her room and determines she needs an immediate work-up for the potential of pulmonary embolism (PE). He explains she had some risk factors, but it is a difficult disease to diagnose and a missed diagnosis can be fatal. In addition, presenting signs and symptoms mimic other conditions such as myocardial infarction and pneumonia.

2. What is the incidence of PE in the elder population?

3. What are three noninvasive diagnostic tests that can be used for diagnosis supported by evidence-based practice?

Mrs. Stanley hears the doctor mention acquiring a certain lab test and reminds him of her needle phobia and starts to cry. The surgeon responds, "We'll hold off on that, it's not a very helpful test with older people anyway."

> **4. Explain why the D-dimer test may be ineffective for diagnosing PE in the elderly person.**
>
> **5. What risk factors from the patient's history coincide with the development of PE?**

Following confirmation of a deep vein thrombosis (DVT) located in the operative leg, the orthopedic surgeon reviews Mrs. Stanley's medications in order to begin anticoagulant therapy.

Being on Premarin (conjugated estrogen) is of concern for the hypercoagulability properties, but another discovery is more of an issue to the physician. It is noted that every postoperative dose of Lovenox (enoxaparin) 40 mg subcutaneous was not given. When asked about the reason, Kye responds, "She refused because needles send her into a panic attack."

> **6. How should this situation have been handled differently to promote patient safety?**
>
> **7. What nursing measures can be used postoperatively to prevent DVT formation?**

Mrs. Stanley has been receiving daily doses of Coumadin (warfarin) 2 mg orally since surgery. This is increased to 3 mg along with initiation of a continuous weight-based Heparin infusion. She and her husband are advised of the need for additional hospital days, as well as for regular serum tests, to assess her clotting times.

> **8. What lab tests are used to monitor the anticoagulant therapies and what is the desired range?**
>
> **9. What measures could be offered to assist the patient with her needle phobia when it is crucial she has up to several sticks a day for appropriate monitoring?**
>
> **10. A PE can occur from sources other than a DVT (blood); what are several examples?**
>
> **11. Create three priority nursing diagnoses for the patient with a PE.**

Three days later, Mrs. Stanley is to be discharged home. She is very fatigued, primarily from the emotional turmoil experienced. She can transfer independently and has progressed to a three-point cane. There is no dressing over the operative knee; half of the staples have been removed and replaced with steri-strips. Vital signs are within normal range, and she uses an oral pain medication every 6 hours, which is effective. Her husband will be with her at home continuously, along with several neighbors bringing food and offering assistance as needed. She will remain on Coumadin (warfarin) for another several months.

> **12. Focusing on safety, what teaching will be provided in relation to this medication?**

Suggested Resources

Brooks, J. A. (2014). Management of patients with chest and lower respiratory tract disorders. In J. L. Hinkle & K. H. Cheever (Eds.), *Brunner and Suddarth's textbook of medical–surgical nursing* (13th ed., pp. 600–603). Philadelphia, PA: Lippincott Williams & Wilkins.

Ensz, S. (2014). *Needle phobia (Trypanophobia)*. International Scleroderma Network. Retrieved from http://www.sclero.org/support/emotional-adj/needle-phobia/a-to-z.html

Newman, J. H. (2013). Pulmonary embolism. *Merck Manual*. Retrieved from http://www.merckmanuals.com/professional/pulmonary_disorders/pulmonary_embolism/pulmonary_embolism.html

Urban, K., Kirley, K., & Stevermer, J. J. (2014). It's time to use an age-based to D-dimer. *Journal of Family Practice, 63*(3), 155–158. Retrieved from http://www.jfponline.com/fileadmin/qhi/jfp/pdfs/6303/JFP_06303_PURLS.pdf

Case 12.6 ■ Influenza Prevention in the Elderly

*M*addy Carlton is feeling overwhelmed with physical and mental fatigue as she leaves her shift at Valley View Extended Care Campus. Maddy serves as the facility's director of education and development. In addition to her usual roles with employee orientation, in-service, and credentialing, she has spent a lot of time on the topic of influenza (the "flu") of late. Her e-mail is flooded with messages from a variety of sources warning of a pandemic; similar information is on the news when she watches television, and the nursing staff has repeatedly questioned her for insights.

In addition to this increased stress at work, Maddy oversees the health care for her 77-year-old mother and 80-year-old mother-in-law. Both women are single and live alone but increasingly need assistance with decision making. Her mother is aware of the public concern over a flu pandemic and has stated she will not leave her home to take any chance of exposure for the upcoming 4 months. Maddy's mother-in-law had to be hospitalized several years ago due to developing pneumonia as a complication of the flu and refuses vaccination as "it sure didn't help me in the past."

Since taking the position at the extended care facility, Maddy has a new challenge to contend with: mandatory flu vaccines for employees. Although there has always been encouragement and the vaccine is provided free to all employees, it has now become the law in her state. She cannot remember an issue that has created more controversy among staff throughout her career, and simply cannot understand "what is the big deal"? Maddy is planning on developing a program focused on flu prevention for her own employer, which also could be repeated at the local senior citizen center and her church. Despite her fatigue, she realizes she needs to put together this education offering quickly, for it to be most effective.

Read the brief article found at www.advisory.com/daily-briefing/2013/11/04/facing-penalties-hospitals-take-hard-line-on-employee-flu-shots to answer the first three questions.

1. *What does the American Hospital Association propose to health care facilities of 100 beds or more as a "penalty" for noncompliance with reporting influenza vaccination rates among health care personnel under Medicare's quality-reporting program?*

2. *What goal has the Centers for Disease Control set for percentage of flu vaccines administered to health care workers by the year 2020?*

3. *What is an alternative action for health care workers to prevent flu transmission should they not be vaccintated?*

Maddy is preparing a handout to use for her flu prevention in-service. Questions 4 through 8 pertain to material she wants to share with the attendees.

4. *In regards to an overview of influenza, when would be an ideal time (month of the year) for this in-service to be presented?*

5. *What two types of influenza viruses cause epidemic disease?*

6. *Describe the pathophysiology associated with transmission.*

7. *What age-related factors increase an elderly person's risk for influenza?*

8. *What are two antiviral drugs approved by the Food and Drug Administration for preventing the flu? Many strains have become resistant to the original two influenza antivirals; what are these? Use the website www.fda.gov/drugs/drugsafety/ informationbydrugclass/ucm100228.htm.*

9. *What teaching could you provide to elderly persons who state they will isolate themselves to avoid flu exposure (for example, Maddy's mother)?*

Suggested Resources

Advisory Board Company. (2013). *Facing penalties, hospitals take hard line on employee flu shots.* The Daily Briefing. Retrieved from http://www.advisory.com/daily-briefing/2013/11/04/facing-penalties-hospitals-take-hard-line-on-employee-flu-shots

Centers for Disease Control and Prevention. (2013a). *How flu spreads.* Retrieved from http://www.cdc.gov/flu/about/disease/spread.htm

Centers for Disease Control and Prevention. (2013b). *What you should know and do this flu season if you are 65 years and older.* Retrieved from http://www.cdc.gov/flu/about/disease/65over.htm

U.S. Food and Drug Administration. (2013). *Influenza (flu) antiviral drugs and related information.* Retrieved from http://www.fda.gov/drugs/drugsafety/informationbydrugclass/ucm100228.htm

World Health Organization. (2014). *Influenza (seasonal).* Retrieved from http://www.who.int/mediacentre/factsheets/fs211/en

13

The Aging Endocrine System

Case 13.1 ■ Diabetes Mellitus (Screening)

*T*he home health care nurse, Gene Gilmore visits Carol Spivey to complete a home assessment. Mrs. Spivey's husband suffers from Alzheimer's disease, and she reports caregiver exhaustion. Her husband is napping while the assessment takes place. Their two-bedroom apartment is well kept and organized. Mrs. Spivey is a welcoming, warm 82-year-old woman, who presents with a bright affect. She states she cannot understand why she recently has had no energy. Mrs. Spivey reports she is trying to watch her water intake, because she is up all night going to the bathroom and then cannot get enough sleep after caring for her husband all day. She is 5 feet 4 inches and weighs 190 pounds.

1. Go to www.nhlbi.nih.gov/health/educational/lose_wt/BMI/ bmicalc.htm and calculate her body mass index.

Mrs. Spivey relays that, over the past month, she has lost 12 pounds without trying, and lately she feels like she needs to have her eyes rechecked, because sometimes things look cloudy. Mrs. Spivey asks whether her recent urinary tract infection is really what is causing her fatigue.

2. Gene suspects that the cause could be one of the following:

a. Mrs. Spivey is suffering from depression

b. Mrs. Spivey did not take her antibiotics correctly

c. Mrs. Spivey has a need for additional screening for type 2 diabetes

d. She is complaining to seek attention because she is overwhelmed by her husband's care

Gene completes a finger stick and finds her blood sugar to be 250.

3. He knows that type 2 diabetes mellitus is the most prevalent form of diabetes in all age groups and results from one of the following:

a. B-cell destruction resulting in a lack or underproduction of insulin

b. *A normal process of aging*

c. *Eating too much sugar*

d. *A combination of insulin resistance and insulin secretory defect.*

4. *What additional screening should the nurse complete?*

5. *What are the risk factors for the development of type 2 diabetes mellitus? Go to the National Diabetes Education Program (n.d.) at www.ndep.nib.gov/am-i-at-risk/index.aspx and list the possible risk factors.*

6. *What additional educational information could the nurse include to improve household safety and management of Mrs. Spivey's diabetes?*

Gene contacts Mrs. Spivey's primary care provider and makes an appointment for her tomorrow. The nurse also makes an appointment for her husband to attend a local adult day care group, and asks whether this might be a viable option for her to take breaks from time to time. Mrs. Spivey agrees to this initial care plan. Mrs. Spivey asks what she should expect for her visit tomorrow with her primary care provider.

7. *What lab tests would be recommended for follow-up with her primary care physician or nurse practitioner?*

8. *Gene understands that poor glycemic control could cause what complications?*

Carol thanks Gene profusely for the time and attention she received during the home visit. She shares her financial concerns about having a potential chronic illness as Mr. Spivey's Alzheimer's disease has added a number of expenses. Gene attempts to reassure her based on his knowledge of Medicare.

9. *Use the weblink www.nia.nib.gov/health/publication/diabetes-older-people#medicare to document what assistance may be available via Medicare.*

Suggested Resources

American Diabetes Association. (2014). *Standards of medical care—diabetes.* Retrieved from http://care.diabetesjournals.org/content/37/Supplement_1/S14.full

National Diabetes Education Program. (n.d.). *Diabetes risk factors.* U.S. Department of Health and Human Services. Retrieved from http://www.ndep.nih.gov/am-i-at-risk/DiabetesRiskFactors.aspx

National Institutes on Aging. (2014). *Diabetes in older people—A disease you can manage.* Retrieved from http://www.nia.nih.gov/health/publication/diabetes-older-people

Case 13.2 ■ Diabetes Mellitus and Medication

Sybel Young is an 83-year-old woman who has been widowed for 9 years. She lives in a very small town in the same home she has occupied for the past 55 years. She enjoys walking to the senior center every day to socialize with her friends as well as receive a hot lunch given by the center. Sybel does not cook much for herself since her husband passed away. Sybel lived independently in her home until recently when she hurt her leg due to a fall in the backyard; she now lives in her home with the rotating assistance of her three daughters. Due to the fall and subsequent decline in her physical ability to walk, a home health nurse will be evaluating her need for home services. Sybel reveals to the nurse that she has had several falls within the past 3 months but isn't sure how many. Upon review of her medical history, Sybel states she was diagnosed with type 2 diabetes at the age of 36. She has been overweight since early adulthood and currently weighs 236 pounds with a height of 5 feet 8 inches. Sybel has taken various diabetes medications over the years to control her disease. She currently takes Glucophage (metformin) 1,000 mg orally, twice daily, and Glucotrol (glipizide) 10 mg orally daily for diabetes, timolol ophthalmic solution 0.25% twice daily for glaucoma, and Prinivil (lisinopril) 40 mg orally daily for hypertension. Sybel has experienced diabetic neuropathy in her legs and feet for at least 5 years, but she reports that it has "gotten worse over the past several months," which seems to correlate with the increase in falls. The nurse asks her to document her blood sugar levels with a new meter every morning for a month. Sybel tells the nurse that her blood sugar has been an average of 110 with her older meter; however, after a month with the new meter Sybel's blood sugar levels have actually averaged 170. Lab work shows that her hemoglobin A1C level is 7.7%. The nurse suggests that Sybel have her medication reevaluated in order to better control her blood sugar level.

At the next home health visit, Sybel reports to the nurse that she went to her family physician and he changed her diabetes medication from Glucotrol (glipizide) to Actos (pioglitazone) 45 mg orally daily in order to better control her blood sugar levels. Further, her doctor scheduled a physical therapist to come into her home twice a week.

The home health nurse reviews a nutrition program that will help Sybel to maintain lower blood sugar levels. Sybel changed her eating habits after her husband passed away, but she reports a more balanced and healthy diet, since her daughters have been cooking for her.

1. *What are considered normal ranges for blood sugar levels and hemoglobin A1C levels?*

2. *The nurse counseled Sybel on her blood sugar levels and a nutrition program. What other areas can the nurse counsel her on to maintain or improve well-being?*

3. *What are some common side effects of diabetes medications?*

4. *Compare and contrast three diabetes medications for dosage, drug mechanism, interactions, and side effects.*

5. *Name some diabetes resources that would help Sybel review new guidelines and ideas concerning diabetes as a disease, medications, nutrition programs, and so forth.*

6. *Although Sybel has a long medical history of diabetes, support groups specifically for individuals with diabetes may help her better manage her disease as she gets older. Find out if your community has diabetes support groups and management programs.*

7. *When is it necessary to consider changing from an oral diabetes medication to insulin injections?*

8. *What are some issues associated with starting insulin injections in an older adult?*

Suggested Resources

Khardori, R. (2014). *Type 2 diabetes mellitus medication.* Medscape. Retrieved from http://emedicine.medscape.com/article/117853-medication

Porter, L. (2014). *Transitions: Moving from oral medications to insulin.* OneTouch. Retrieved from http://www.onetouch.com/articles/transitionspart2

Case 13.3 ■ Diabetes Mellitus and Nutrition

*D*ave Blankenship is a 66-year-old male who has been divorced for 10 years. He lives independently in a condominium in the heart of a major metropolitan area. Although he recently retired from his career as an architect, he continues to provide consulting on small local architect jobs and volunteers at the local Veterans Administration hospital 2 days a week.

Dave has always been relatively healthy and has had no major concerns other than a slightly elevated cholesterol level, until recently when he started feeling excessively tired after his daily exercise routine. He has also noticed a feeling of excessive thirst and has increased his daily water intake. Concerned about his health status, Dave visited his family physician today and received a diagnosis of type 2 diabetes. While at the physician's office, Marcia Moore, the head clinic nurse, suggests to Dave that he should join the Living With Diabetes management program that provides education information and training on diabetes as a disease, nutrition plans, medication information, and support groups. Marcia works as the RN alongside a registered dietician in the nutrition educational portion of the Living With Diabetes management program and feels that Dave will greatly benefit from the program.

The following week, Dave attends his first session in the Living With Diabetes management program. Marcia asks the group of new participants to provide a detailed account of how they perceive their current nutrition status and what they generally consume in a typical week. She then instructs them to keep a detailed daily record of what they consume including how many items fit into each food group, proportion sizes, restaurant visits, and an average calorie count. After 2 weeks of recording all requested information, Dave returns to the program to talk with Marcia about his nutritional intake. Dave tries to eat a healthy balanced diet and exercises regularly, but upon closer inspection, Marcia highlights some areas of concern in his nutritional intake.

Dave enjoys eating at restaurants with friends about five times a week, because he is single and doesn't enjoy cooking for just himself. When he eats at restaurants, Dave tends to choose meals high in calories, fat, and sodium such as ribeye steak with garlic butter sauce; a baked potato loaded with butter, sour cream, and cheese; and the special crescent rolls with cinnamon butter. Marcia counsels Dave to make healthier choices from the menu items such as baked chicken with sautéed onions and peppers, steamed broccoli with a spray of butter, and a side of fruit. She also suggests exercising, going to the movies, and doing other activities with friends to maintain the social contacts he enjoys instead of always going to restaurants.

At home, Dave usually makes meals consisting of cereal, sandwiches, salads, various vegetables and fruits from the local farmers market, pasta, various breads, and all varieties of meat. He very rarely eats cakes, ice cream, or any sugary snacks, but uses pure sugar in his morning coffee. Marcia suggests that Dave visit the American Diabetes Association (ADA) website concerning food and fitness at www.diabetes.org/food-and-fitness to read about food options and exercise programs. Marcia counsels Dave on choosing healthier meal options including chicken, fish, and lean red meat such as sirloin steak instead of meats with a higher fat content including veal, ground chuck hamburger, and ribeye steak. She further counsels Dave on lowering his consumption of carbohydrates including breads, cereals, and pasta, which currently make up a large portion of Dave's daily menu. She suggests greatly reducing his carbohydrate intake, but a small daily portion would be fine as long as Dave switches from white breads and pastas to 100% whole wheat and whole grain options. Marcia suggests switching from regular sugar to a sugar substitute in Dave's morning coffee and any cola consumption should be switched to diet varieties. Marcia suggests that Dave cut his vegetables and separate meats into single servings after grocery shopping to make fixing meals for just himself less time consuming, which may reduce his desire to eat at restaurants so frequently. Marcia provides Dave with the following sample menu:

Breakfast: Egg white omelet with onions and peppers, two slices of turkey bacon

Lunch: Tuna salad with low-fat mayonnaise on a bed of lettuce, whole wheat crackers, side of fruit

Dinner: Baked tilapia fish with lemon, spaghetti squash, salad with a couple sprays of light vinaigrette salad dressing

1. *What are some ways to maintain a healthy diet for diabetes disease management?*

2. *Some examples of diabetes nutritional resources include www.diabetes.org/food-and-fitness/food/what-can-i-eat www.ndep.nih.gov. Can you find three other resources that would be beneficial?*

3. *Some people believe they can eat what they want as long as they take a diabetes medication. Why is nutrition so important, if medication is available to manage diabetes?*

4. *How does proper nutrition work to stabilize blood sugar levels?*

5. *With proper diet and exercise, can a person eventually not need to take diabetes medication?*

6. *Name the three main types of carbohydrates and give examples of each type.*

7. *How can you prepare for eating healthy when going to restaurants?*

8. *The ADA has come out with a list of 10 diabetes superfoods. Try to make your own list of foods you think would be a diabetes superfood, then compare your list to the ADA's list at www .diabetes.org/food-and-fitness/food/what-can-i-eat/making-healthy-food-choices/diabetes-superfoods.html.*

Suggested Resources

Arathuzik, G. (2014). *An overview of diabetes meal planning.* Nutrition Close-up. Retrieved from http://www.eggnutritioncenter.org/wp-content/uploads/2012/04/Winter-2014-Close-Up.pdf

Castle, K. J. (2014). *Basic foods for elderly diabetes patients.* LIVESTRONG.com. Retrieved from http://www.livestrong.com/article/67158-basic-foods-elderly-diabetes-patients

National Diabetes Information Clearinghouse (NDIC). (2014). *What I need to know about eating and diabetes.* Retrieved from http://diabetes.niddk.nih.gov/dm/pubs/eating_ez

14

The Aging Genitourinary System

Case 14.1 ■ Transient Urinary Incontinence

Working in a busy women's health clinic has been an enjoyable position for Angela McCormick, who joined the group as a nurse practitioner a decade ago. She has studied and focused on female urinary problems in recent years, and obtained certification in geriatrics. Today, Angela is precepting Travis Cook, a third-year medical student, who has a 2-week rotation at the clinic. The first client is new to the practice and was referred by her sister. Dolly Phan is a 75-year-old Vietnamese woman who made an appointment due to "leaking urine." Dolly came to the United States in 1989 as a refugee. Her sister married a GI who served in the Vietnam War and arrived two decades earlier; all other nuclear and extended family members remain in their country of origin.

Angela begins by introducing herself and Travis and explaining the need for a medical history followed by a physical examination. Travis has never interacted with anyone from Vietnam and enthusiastically participates with the interview and exam. He makes several observations about Dolly, which spur his curiosity. After the visit is complete, he asks his preceptor the following questions related to the Vietnamese culture.

1. ***Why was there minimal eye contact made by Miss Phan during the visit? Why did she smile the entire time, regardless of the questions being asked?***

2. ***When performing her physical exam, you mentioned the red streaks observed on her back were due to "coining therapy"; what exactly does that mean? Use the website www.mybesthealthportal .net/health/natural-medicine-healing/coining-therapy-for-health .html, which includes a photo.***

Miss Phan reports a 2-week history of incontinence, described specifically as, "Urine comes out unexpectedly even if I've emptied my bladder within the hour." She states this occurs a minimum of five times a day. She has noticed no change in the color, clarity, odor, or amount of output. When asked to attempt to quantify the amount of urine involuntarily loss, Miss Phan says it ranges from drops to enough to soak her clothing. Her vital signs were within normal range with the exception of a low-grade fever of

99.3°F. She is 62 inches tall and weighs 157 pounds. She rates her pain as a "2" on a standardized scale, reporting a dull ache to her low back.

Prescription medications include Prilosec (omeprazole), Lipitor (atorvastatin), Plendil (felodipine), and Actonel (risedronate). In addition, she uses diphenhydramine (Benadryl) a couple times a week to induce sleep and, in the past week, Sudafed (pseudoephedrine) for a pronounced cold.

3. What age-related changes can affect the ability to control urination?

Use the Hartford Institute for Geriatric Nursing websites for the following questions: http://consultgerirn.org/topics/urinary_incontinence/want_to_know_more (Dowling-Castronovo & Bradway, 2012) and http://consultgerirn.org/uploads/File/trythis/try_this_11_1.pdf (Dowling-Castronovo, 2013).

4. What criteria are assessed using either the DIAPPERS or TOILETED mnemonic for transient incontinence?

5. What benefits can the use of a bladder diary offer?

6. Avoiding medications that may contribute to urinary incontinence is an evidence-based nursing care strategy. What, if any, of Miss Phan's drugs should be further investigated?

7. Two nursing care strategies suggested for overflow urinary incontinence are a post-voiding residual and Crede's maneuver. Briefly describe both.

Miss Phan was seen again 3 days later. Her urine culture showed moderate growth of bacteria. Her bladder diary was completed and through self-report she stated, "things have gotten a little better, I've had some leakage once or twice a day and it's maybe a spoonful of urine." Angela explains that the urinary tract infection and possibly multiple doses of her cold medicine were likely the cause for the transient incontinence. In addition to an antibiotic prescription, she gave Miss Phan a patient teaching brochure about preventing urinary tract infections. After she left, Travis, the medical student, made the comment, "Incontinence is a part of getting old that will eventually affect everyone, right?"

8. How would you respond to this statement?

Suggested Resources

A Place for Mom. (2013). *Elderly urinary incontinence.* Retrieved from http://www.aplaceformom.com/senior-care-resources/articles/elderly-urinary-incontinence

Behar, J. (2012). Coining therapy for health. *Natural Medicine.* Retrieved from http://www.mybesthealthportal.net/health/natural-medicine-healing/coining-therapy-for-health.html

Conforth, T. (2014). What is transient incontinence? *About.com Women's Health.* Retrieved from http://womenshealth.about.com/od/bladdercontrol/f/transient_incontinence.htm

Dowling-Castrovono, A. (2013). Urinary incontinence assessment in older adults part I—Transient urinary incontinence. Hartford Insititute for Geriatric Nursing. Retrieved from http://consultgerirn.org/uploads/File/trythis/try_this_11_1.pdf

Dowling-Castronovo, A., & Bradway, C. (2012). Nursing standard of practice protocol: Urinary incontinence (UI) in older adults admitted to acute care. Hartford Institute for Geriatric Nursing. Retrieved from http://consultgerirn.org/topics/urinary_incontinence/want_to_know_more

National Association for Continence. (2014). *How medications affect your bladder*. Retrieved from http://www.nafc.org/bladder-health/medications/

Resnick, N. M., & Yalla, S. V. (1985). Management of urinary incontinence in the elderly. *New England Journal of Medicine, 313*, 800–804.

Vietnam Culture. (n.d.). *Vietnamese non-verbal communication*. Retrieved from http://www.vietnam-culture.com/articles-55-6/Non-verbal-communication.aspx

Case 14.2 ■ Benign Prostatic Hypertrophy

*N*ancy Gilbert is 71 years old and is in a loving, married relationship with Henry, her husband of 50 years. She is visiting with her nurse practitioner, Cheryl, for an annual checkup at a local free clinic in their community. As they are finishing her appointment, Cheryl asks whether Nancy has any additional questions. Nancy indicates that she is worried about Henry, who has been rising frequently at night to urinate and experiencing sudden urges to urinate. She has seen lots of commercials on TV about enlarged prostate, and she is concerned for Henry's well-being. He seems embarrassed to talk about the problem and Nancy is wondering whether there might be a "gentlemen practitioner" for him to visit. Cheryl gives Nancy a referral to a urologist.

1. Why is it common for people to feel uncomfortable talking about prostate issues? What assurances/advice can Cheryl offer Nancy?

Three months later, Cheryl receives a call from Nancy who indicates that she and Henry would like to come speak with her and get more information on a problem with Henry's prostate gland. They have additional questions and Nancy has assured Henry that Cheryl is easy to talk to and that they should take advantage of the free clinic. They would like to seek her opinion on the treatment options offered by the urologist.

After visiting with Henry and Nancy for awhile, Cheryl asks what prompted Henry to visit with the urologist. Henry indicated that he found himself unable to urinate one day after taking a dose of Benadryl (diphenhydramine) to control his allergy symptoms. This alarmed him, and he finally called the urologist whom Cheryl had recommended to Nancy. At this point, Cheryl asks Henry some additional questions and inquires about his medication history. Henry is 71 years old, in overall good health, 5 feet 11 inches, and 175 pounds. Henry indicates that he takes Lipitor (atorvastatin calcium) 40 mg orally daily to keep his cholesterol levels under control. He says that he read that the side effects can cause renal impairment and asks whether the Lipitor might have caused him to retain the urine.

2. *How might you explain the difference between renal impairment and urinary retention to this patient?*

3. *Why might the use of over-the-counter decongestants result in the inability to urinate?*

Cheryl asks Henry to cite other symptoms that he had been suffering from prior to the emergency visit with the urologist. He indicates that in addition to frequently rising at night to urinate, he had experienced a weak stream and hesitancy to start elimination of his bladder. In addition, the urologist performed a digital rectal exam (DRE) and took blood to do a prostate-specific antigen (PSA) test. The results of the DRE were that he had an enlarged prostate, but the PSA was within a normal range. The urologist recommended ultrasound of the rectum and a prostate biopsy. Nancy and Henry are seeking help from Cheryl to interpret the results of the tests and discuss the need for the biopsy.

4. *What information would you share with Nancy and Henry about the data that can be derived from a DRE and the PSA test?*

5. *Why might the urologist be recommending the ultrasound and prostate biopsy?*

Cheryl concurs with the doctor and explains why it will be helpful to have the biopsy.
Two weeks later, Cheryl calls Nancy and Henry to see how they are doing. Henry is excited to share that the biopsy was negative and that the diagnosis is benign prostatic hypertrophy. He indicates that for now the doctor has put him on a medication, Flomax (tamsulosin) 0.4 mg, taken every day one half hour after breakfast. He is very pleased not only with the results, but he was concerned that he might have to have surgery and is relieved that he will not have to do so.

6. *What are some of the medication options available to patients with benign prostatic hypertrophy? What are the mechanisms of their action? Cite the source of your information.*

7. *What herbal remedy is proposed as an option for men with benign prostatic hypertrophy?*

8. *Henry and Nancy are in a loving relationship that includes an active sex life. Why is Henry concerned about surgical intervention for his benign prostatic hypertrophy in relation to sexual performance?*

Suggested Resources

National Cancer Institute. (2014). *Prostate-specific antigen (PSA) test—National Cancer Institute—Comprehensive cancer information*. Retrieved from http://www.cancer.gov/cancertopics/factsheet/Detection/PSA

National Kidney and Urologic Diseases Information Clearinghouse. (2012). *Prostate enlargement: Benign prostatic hyperplasia*. Retrieved from http://kidney.niddk.nih.gov/kudiseases/pubs/prostateenlargement

Case 14.3 ■ Functional Incontinence

Ralph Carson, 81 years old, is admitted to a medical–surgical unit in the local hospital after a visit to his physician's office. He was at his physician's office for a routine physical when it was discovered that his blood pressure was 210/100. Mr. Carson's physician wanted him admitted for further evaluation of his hypertension.

Mr. Carson's health status has been relatively stable in the past. He has a history of spinal stenosis, which has progressively led to an unsteady, slower gait. He currently lives alone, which concerns his daughter, who also lives in town. At her suggestion, he recently began using a three-pronged cane to ambulate. He does maintain his driver's license, yet he limits his driving to short trips during the day.

The nurse admitting Mr. Carson finds him to be pleasant and talkative but unsure as to why he was being admitted. He reports that he has never had "pressure problems" before, but he is hopeful that this problem will be resolved. His current home medications include Neurontin (gabapentin), Cymbalta (duloxetine), Flomax (tamsulosin), and Ambien (zolpidem). He denies using any over-the-counter medications but does state that he has an "occasional" beer or glass of wine in the evenings. The nurse concludes the interview, orients Mr. Carson to the call light and the location of the bathroom, and starts IV fluids of normal saline. Before she leaves the room, she instructs Mr. Carson to call for assistance prior to getting out of bed by using the call light.

Mr. Carson's daughter visits him in the hospital, bringing him a cheeseburger and sweet tea from his favorite restaurant. She tells him again that she is concerned that he lives alone and asks him to consider moving in with her upon discharge from the hospital. Mr. Carson's daughter leaves, much to his relief, as he had been waiting to get up to use the restroom. He presses the call light and waits for a response, but does not receive one. Not wanting to bother his nurse, he decides to ambulate to the bathroom without assistance. He has some difficulty managing the IV pole and works to untangle it from the side rail. He feels the need to void, and rushes to the bathroom, but trips over the IV pole and falls to the floor. The nurse arrives in the room, finding Mr. Carson on the floor after having fallen and urinated on himself.

1. *Define functional incontinence. How would the nurse know that Mr. Carson experienced functional incontinence and not some other type?*

2. *What factors in Mr. Carson's environment contributed to his incontinence?*

3. *What factors in Mr. Carson's diet contributed to his incontinence?*

The nurse wants to obtain an order for an indwelling urinary catheter for Mr. Carson to avoid this problem occurring again. She speaks with the nurse on charge about contacting the physician. The charge nurse explains to Mr. Carson's nurse that an indwelling Foley is not the best option.

4. *Why is an indwelling urinary catheter not the best treatment for functional urinary incontinence?*

5. *According to the Hartford Institute for Geriatric Nursing's standard of practice protocol, what nursing care strategies should be implemented to care for Mr. Carson's incontinence? (See the website http://consultgerirn.com with authors Dowling-Castronovo & Bradway, 2012.)*

Two days later, Mr. Carson is being discharged. He will stay with his daughter temporarily. In addition to his previous medications, he has now been prescribed Cardizem (diltiazem) for his hypertension. Mr. Carson tells the nurse that he is worried that he will have another episode of incontinence at his daughter's house.

6. *Create a discharge plan for Mr. Carson that addresses his concerns about his incontinence.*

Mr. Carson has a home health nurse who visits twice a week to monitor his blood pressure and his overall condition. The home health nurse is concerned that Mr. Carson's blood pressure is 140/82 while sitting, but drops to 110/58 when standing. She is also concerned that Mr. Carson is limiting his fluid intake in order to prevent incontinence.

7. *Why is orthostatic hypotension a concern in someone with functional incontinence?*

8. *Using the information on functional incontinence from the website http://consultgerirn.org, what interventions should the home health nurse implement in order to help Mr. Carson with his incontinence?*

Suggested Resources

Dowling-Castronovo, A., & Bradway, C. (2012). *Nursing standard of practice protocol: Urinary incontinence (UI) in older adults admitted to acute care.* Hartford Institute for Geriatric Nursing. Retrieved from www.consultgerirn.org

Ratini, M. (2012). *Functional incontinence*. WebMD. Retrieved from http://www.webmd.com/urinary-incontinence-oab/functional-incontinence?page=2

Resnick, N. M., & Yalla, S. V. (1985). Management of urinary incontinence in the elderly. *New England Journal of Medicine, 313,* 800–804.

Case 14.4 ■ Acute Renal Insufficiency

*M*ike Harris is a 65-year-old White male (weight, 245 pounds; height, 66 inches) with a history of kidney stones (urolithiasis). He was admitted to the medical–surgical unit with severe left flank pain, painful urination, hematuria, and nausea that had been present for 3 days. On admission, his blood pressure is 140/90, heart rate is 88 bpm, and respirations are 24 per minute.

Unit nurse Marcia Long completes an admission history. Mr. Harris states that he takes Advil (ibuprofen) 800 mg four times a day for knee pain. He also uses Tums (calcium carbonate USP) frequently for heartburn. He reports that he is a retired truck driver and lives alone. Mr. Harris states, "I don't like to cook. I eat a lot of fast food, and drink about a gallon of coffee with cream every day." Further questioning reveals that Mr. Harris has no health insurance, other than Medicare, and has not seen his primary care provider since his last episode of kidney stones, 18 months ago.

In addition, Marcia completed the Hospital Admission Risk Profile (HARP) for Mr. Harris. She determined the client to be at low risk for functional decline while hospitalized, using this evidence-based practice assessment tool. The Hartford Institute for Geriatric Nursing website provides access to the HARP instrument in its *How to Try This* series at http://consultgerirn.org/resources (Graf, 2008).

1. What is the purpose of the HARP assessment tool? What areas of function are measured?

In the emergency department (ED), Mr. Harris had intravenous pyelography performed; it showed a kidney stone in the left ureter. Marcia instructs Mr. Harris to strain all urine and walk with assistance as much as possible; she also administers intravenous analgesic ordered by the primary care provider.

2. What risk factors does Mr. Harris have for the development of kidney stones?

Within 24 hours, the kidney stone has not passed out of the ureter. It is determined that the stone will be removed by the use of ureteroscopy. The procedure was successful with the urologist using an ultrasound device to fragment and remove a 2-cm stone. A stent was placed in the left ureter. Analysis showed that Mr. Harris had a calcium stone.

The day after the procedure, Mr. Harris is being discharged. Marcia Long is planning discharge teaching for Mr. Harris.

3. *What is most important for Marcia to include in discharge teaching?*

4. *Should Marcia instruct Mr. Harris to stop the use of calcium-rich foods or calcium supplements?*

One month after his ureteral stent was removed, Mr. Harris comes to the emergency room with left flank pain, swelling of his hands and feet, and a heart rate of 100 bpm, BP 150/100, respirations 24 per minute. A CT scan of the abdomen shows a 1-cm kidney stone obstructing the urethra.

On admission, his BUN is 48 mg/dL, and his serum creatinine is 2.8 mg/dL. Catherine Sandlin, the ED nurse, takes an admission history. Mr. Harris states that he continued to take Advil for pain, and did not increase his water consumption as instructed, because "it hurt to pee."

5. *What history, laboratory results, or physical examination findings should be of the greatest concern to the admissions nurse? What might these findings represent?*

6. *What risk factors did Mr. Harris have for developing acute renal insufficiency (ARI)?*

Mr. Harris is admitted to the intensive care unit. On his first hospital day, Mr. Harris has a urine output of 500 mL over a 24-hour period. His BUN is 55 mg/dL, and his serum creatinine is 3.1 mg/dL.

7. *What other lab tests should the nurse monitor on Mr. Harris? What assessments should the nurse perform?*

On day 4, his urine output increases to 1,000 mL in 24 hours. Mr. Harris has multiple medications that are ordered to be given intravenously.

8. *What are special nursing considerations for administering IV medications to Mr. Harris?*

Gradually, Mr. Harris shows improvement in kidney function. His average output is 2 L per day, and his edema has decreased significantly. On discharge, his BUN is 24 mg/dL, and his serum creatinine is 1.3 mg/dL.

9. *What dietary instructions should the nurse give Mr. Harris? Give five examples of foods that Mr. Harris should limit or eliminate from his diet.*

Suggested Resources

Diet Health Club. (2014). *Diet for acute renal failure.* Retrieved from http://www.diethealthclub .com/health-issues-and-diet/acute-renal-failure/acute-renal-failure-diet.html

Graf, C. (2008). *The Hospital Admission Risk Profile (HARP).* Hartford Institute for Geriatric Nursing. Retrieved from http://www.nursingcenter.com/pdf.asp?AID=807029

Mayo Clinic Staff. (2012). *Acute kidney failure*. Mayo Clinic. Retrieved from http://www
.mayoclinic.org/diseases-conditions/kidney-failure/basics/symptoms/con-20024029

Case 14.5 ■ Pelvic Organ Prolapse

*I*n the waiting room of a public health clinic for low-income families sits 72-year-old Sarah Yoder with her youngest of five children, Elizabeth. The pair is a part of a community of Amish families living a few miles away. Elizabeth came to the clinic several days ago to ask for an appointment for her mother, as no telephone is owned by the family. Her mother had been seen a decade ago when she had stomach pain and diarrhea, which wouldn't clear using complementary medicine suggested by other Amish acquaintances. This appointment was scheduled for a "woman's problem," and Elizabeth requested a female practitioner.

Sarah has only known the Amish culture and is very satisfied with her life. She attended school until the 8th grade and had to stop when her mother became quite ill and later died from childbirth complications. She married at 17 and deeply loved her husband, who died 5 years ago from a myocardial infarction. Four of her five children live in the community; the oldest chose to leave and sends his mother a letter every month or so. Her culture does not permit photographs to be taken, and she often wonders whether her son resembles his late father.

It is a warm summer day and Sarah is dressed in her usual Amish attire: a long-sleeved cotton blouse, full length skirt, and bonnet covering her hair. She does not like to leave her community for any reason, particularly for something so terribly personal. At the other Amish women's urging, she agreed to be checked and see whether something could help her "woman's problem." For over a month, when Sarah sits on the toilet, there is something bulging out from her vagina. There is no pain per se, but her fear is part of her internal organs are going to fall out and she may die as a result.

Sarah and her daughter enter an exam room with the nurse practitioner, Kathleen Prentice, a long-time employee who is very familiar with the Amish community and visits their area twice a year to give immunizations to the young children. She attempts to take a health history but most questions are answered by Elizabeth on her mother's behalf with minimal information. She discovers Sarah has never had a pelvic exam in her life; all children were home-birthed with the assistance of a midwife. Elizabeth asks whether her mother has to be checked "down there" as she's dreading, and Kathleen explains why it is necessary, emphasizing she will be gentle and as brief as possible to obtain a thorough assessment.

> **1. Explain the recommendations from the American College of Obstetricians and Gynecologists (ACOG) on routine pelvic examination and cervical cytology screening for a woman over 65 years of age.**

2. What alterations in a typical pelvic examination could be provided to promote psychosocial comfort for this client? Include the information from the following source with your ideas: www .ncbi.nlm.nih.gov/pmc/articles/PMC3101979.

Kathleen chooses to perform the pelvic exam first, and then assess the other systems. She talks to Sarah and explains what she is doing throughout the exam, along with asking her questions about her everyday life to show interest and promote a trusting relationship. Kathleen knows not to touch Sarah any more than necessary and does not have her disrobe; she lifts her shirt to assess breath/cardiac sounds, put her hands under her clothing briefly to assess peripheral pulses, and so forth. She finishes her physical assessment and tells Sarah and her daughter that her bladder has "slipped down into her vagina," which is known as a cystocele. She then prints off a sagittal view of a drawing of a female's pelvis from the computer to better explain this condition.

3. Describe the pathophysiology and age-related changes associated with cystocele.

4. What are the typical symptoms?

It was difficult to obtain information about urinary dysfunction from Sarah or her daughter as they both seemed very uncomfortable with the topic. Kathleen shares that incomplete emptying of the bladder could lead to infection, and it is most important to be treated if symptoms arise. She is fully aware that elective surgery is rarely agreed to by Amish patients, so she mentions it briefly in the context of the cystocele eventually enlarging. At this point, the nurse practitioner would classify Sarah's pelvic organ prolapse as mild to moderate.

5. What are two nonsurgical treatments for mild to moderate cases such as this?

6. Find a photo of a pessary(s) on the Internet or in a textbook. Develop a brief teaching guide for proper use.

7. Is hormone replacement therapy an option for treatment? A website addressing this topic can be found at www .emedicinehealth.com/pelvic_organ_prolapse-health/ page13_em.htm.

Kathleen approached the use of a pessary very matter-of-factly with Sarah after she confirmed the client had never inserted a tampon, diaphragm, or any medications vaginally. She chose the correct size based on her exam and used another picture to show the pessary in place. Typically, she would have a woman insert it into her body right in the exam room to demonstrate understanding. With Sarah, she walked her to the restroom and suggested she raise one leg higher onto a step stool or the toilet seat, if capable, to facilitate insertion. She then checked her very quickly back in the exam room to find the pessary was supporting the bladder exactly as intended.

Elizabeth agreed to return with her mother for a 1-week follow-up visit and every several months thereafter to be assessed for vaginal erosion or ulcers, which can be a complication. When preparing to leave, she handed Kathleen a square package wrapped in brown paper. "We are without money at the present time and hoped very much you would accept this for our payment instead." Kathleen unwrapped the item to find a beautiful handmade quilt, similar to ones she had seen in upscale gift shops in the nearby city for $400 or more. She was momentarily overwhelmed and then commented on the intricate, meticulous stitching and vibrant colors of the quilt as she carefully looked it over.

Accepting gifts from patients has presented a long-term ethical dilemma to the point corporate guidelines have been developed addressing the issue at some facilities.

Review the article by Abvier (2010) found at www.americannursetoday.com/beyond-a-box-of-chocolates-2 on this topic.

8. *What are your thoughts on the nurse accepting a gift such as this for payment of services? Should she keep it, return it, or do something else with the quilt?*

Suggested Resources

Abvier, A. R. (2010). Beyond a box of chocolates. *American Nurse Today*. Retrieved from http://www.americannursetoday.com/beyond-a-box-of-chocolates-2

Bates, C. K., Carroll, N., & Potter, J. (2011). The challenging pelvic exam. *Journal of General Internal Medicine*, *26*(6), 651–655. Retrieved from http://www.ncbi.nlm.nih.gov/pmc/articles/PMC3101979

Marshall, S. (2011). *Pelvic organ prolapse*. emedicine Health. Retrieved from http://www.emedicinehealth.com/pelvic_organ_prolapse-health/page13_em.htm

Pagano, T. (2014). *The pelvic exam and menopause*. WebMD. Retrieved from http://www.webmd.com/menopause/menopause-pelvic-exam

University of Chicago Medical Center. (2014). *Female pelvic organ prolapse*. Retrieved from http://www.ucurology.org/areas-of-specialization/female-pelvic-organ-prolapse

Case 14.6 ■ Catheter-Associated Urinary Tract Infections

*L*inda Keller is an RN who graduated with a BSN degree in 2000. She began her career on a medical–surgical nursing unit at a large teaching hospital in Oklahoma City. Over the next 4 years, she married and gave birth to twin boys. In 2005, her life changed dramatically. The marriage ended and her mother experienced a severe cerebral vascular accident. Due to financial problems and a sense of obligation as the only child with health care experience, Linda and her young sons moved to her previous hometown of Louisville, Kentucky, to live with her mother.

Linda settled into a very regimented lifestyle over the next 3 years. Due to right hemiplegia, her mother required essentially around-the-clock care. She had a gastrostomy tube for feeding and medication administration, an indwelling urinary catheter, and the need for vigilant skin care to prevent breakdown. She was transported by ambulance every 3 months to her primary health care provider for a routine visit. Linda looked forward to attending these visits, although for a rather selfish reason . . . the physician and office staff always commented on the excellent care her mother received. Linda took pride in keeping her mother at home; she had one brief hospitalization for treatment of a pneumonia.

In 2008, Linda's mother died in her sleep. Linda chose to remain living in her hometown. She needed to gain employment as there was no inheritance from her mother and the sale of her home resulted in minimal financial gain when shared with her siblings.

Linda decided to return to acute care nursing. She required a month-long orientation period due to her absence of practice in this type of setting. A number of changes were of great surprise to Linda insofar as regulations put forth in 2008. In particular, the avoidance of using indwelling urinary catheters for postoperative or incontinent patients was puzzling. In orientation, she was provided with a document that listed many hospital-acquired conditions (HACs) that Medicare/Medicaid would no longer reimburse hospitals for occurrence of while hospitalized.

Review the document listing the HACs at www.cms.gov/Medicare/Medicare-Fee-for-Service-Payment/HospitalAcqCond/Hospital-Acquired_Conditions.html, which was updated in 2012 (no additions are planned in 2014–2015).

1. Are there any events you were not aware of on this list? If so, please comment.

Among the HACs selected by the Centers for Medicare & Medicaid Services, catheter-associated urinary tract infection (CAUTI) has been designated a high priority due to the high cost and high incidence, and because it can be reasonably prevented through application of accepted evidence-based prevention guidelines.

2. This case study focuses on CAUTI. Provide a definition and a statistic estimating the number of CAUTIs annually in our nation. Document the source.

Use the evidence-based resource on the Hartford Institute for Geriatric Nursing related to this topic found at http://consultgerirn.org/uploads/file/trythis/try_this_11_1.pdf provided by Dowling-Castronovo and Bradway (2012) to answer Questions 3 through 6.

3. The Centers for Disease Control and Prevention (CDC) has developed explicit surveillance criteria for CAUTI. What are they?

4. What percent of CAUTIs are deemed preventable using evidence-based practice? What alternates are suggested in place of indwelling catheters?

5. You have received an order to insert an indwelling catheter; what size would you choose for an adult?

6. *Does a catheter made of latex have less risk of causing an infection?*

7. *There has been a tremendous focus on strategies to prompt removal of unnecessary urinary catheters. What are some interventions used for this purpose? Describe what a "stop order" entails.*

8. *Linda listened carefully during hospital orientation about information contained in all of these questions. She made the following comment to the nurse educator conducting the session, "This all seems like a lot more work for the nursing staff; having to give a bedpan or urinal frequently, assist persons to the bathroom, and provide hygiene for those who are incontinent. I think I will have to really adjust my planning for patient care." What are your thoughts about Linda's comments?*

Suggested Resources

Centers for Medicare & Medicaid Services. (2014). *Hospital acquired conditions.* Retrieved from http://www.cms.gov/Medicare/Medicare-Fee-for-Service-Payment/HospitalAcqCond/Hospital-Acquired_Conditions.htmlom

Dowling-Castronovo, A., & Bradway, C. (2012). *Urinary tract infection prevention geriatric nursing protocol: Prevention of catheter-associated urinary tract infection.* Hartford Institute for Geriatric Nursing. Retrieved from http://consultgerirn.org/topics/prevention_catheter-associated_uti/want_to_know_more

15

Nutrition and the Aging Gastrointestinal System

Case 15.1 ■ Mealtime Difficulties

*A*n interdisciplinary health team meeting is taking place at Trinity Healthcare, a long-term care facility that is family owned and operated. The focus is discussing how to meet the nutritional needs of a resident, Kathryn Kelty, who was admitted from a local hospital several weeks ago. Mealtime difficulties have been consistent for this resident and she has lost a pound per week since arriving.

Mrs. Kelty is 86 years old and a widow of 2 years. She has a son who lives an hour away and visits on the weekends; most of her friends, neighbors, and husband's family have died, leaving a minimal support group. Her health history includes macular degeneration with approximately 50% of residual vision; osteoarthritis affecting the hands, knees, and spine; atrial fibrillation with a pacemaker insertion at the age of 78; and moderate-stage dementia. Mrs. Kelty sleeps very poorly at night; thus, she is drowsy and fatigued for most of the day.

1. *What age-related physiological changes can affect nutrition of the elderly?*

Use the article by Tonarelli (n.d.) located at http://seniors-health-medicare.suite101 .com/article.cfm/mealtime-tips-for-dementia-caregivers, for the next two questions.

2. *In addition to weight loss, what other potential, negative consequences are results of poor nutrition in the elderly population? Select all that apply.*

a. Anemia

b. Dehydration

c. Infections

d. Aspiration pneumonia

e. Pressure ulcers

3. Individuals with dementia may demonstrate dangerous eating habits; identify four examples.

The staff at Trinity has adopted the use of the most current evidence-based practice in working with mealtime difficulties of their residents. At the discussion today, Mrs. Kelty's physician, a nurse manager, a speech pathologist, a dietician, and a social worker are present. The nurse reports the resident has been observed closely at meals and is unable to take food to her mouth, chew, and swallow without regular cues and prompts. The speech pathologist notes a swallowing study completed before admission showed no structural or mechanical issues resulting in dysphagia. The social worker's history from Mrs. Kelty's son relayed a lifelong history of meals being taken with others and the enjoyment she experienced from cooking and setting an attractive table, regardless of the time of year or event. Her physician adds that no new medication has been introduced for over a year, which could affect appetite. The blood urea nitrogen and serum creatinine levels are at a high normal; increased fluid intake is recommended before renal involvement occurs.

Review the evidence-based protocols for mealtime difficulties (Amella & Aselage, 2012) from the Hartford Institute for Geriatric Nursing located at http://consultgerirn .org/for the following three questions.

4. Noting the premeal assessment criteria, what activities does your own family have in relation to rituals, blessings, culture, or food prohibitions?

Using the Edinburgh Feeding Evaluation in Dementia Scale found at http://consult-gerirn.org/uploads/File/trythis/try_this_d11_1.pdf (Amella & Lawrence, 2007), Mrs. Kelty scored an 8 overall; specifically, 2 points for the first 4 of 11 items assessed. On the Katz Index for Functional Ability (Wallace & Shelky, 2007), her score was a 3: eating (1 point), dressing (1 point), and bathing (1 point). Mrs. Kelty continues to be relatively independent with getting in and out of the bed or a chair, using the toilet, and controlling her bladder and bowels.

5. Interpret the scores for each of these assessments.

6. Taking into account Mrs. Kelty's physical and cognitive health, what evidence-based interventions may be most helpful for her during mealtimes?

The dining experience in nursing homes was the focus of an article by Speroff, Davis, Dehr, and Larkins (2005). Review the article found on pages 292–295 for the next two questions (www.ncmedicaljournal.com/wp-content/uploads/NCMJ/jul-aug-05/ Fullcopy.pdf).

7. Discuss the Dining With Dignity program. Would you recommend this approach for Mrs. Kelty?

8. Positive outcomes for the recommended changes in dining experiences include which of the following? Select all that apply.

a. Reduced need for supplements

b. Noticeable increase in energy

c. Less weight loss

d. Less waste of food

e. Fewer resident complaints

Suggested Resources

Amella, E. J., & Aselage, M. A. (2012). *Nursing standard of practice protocol: Assessment and management of mealtime difficulties.* Hartford Institute for Geriatric Nursing. Retrieved from http://consultgerirn.org/topics/mealtime_difficulties/want_to_know_more

Amella, E. J., & Lawrence, J. F. (2007). *Try this: Eating and feeding issues in older adults with dementia: Part II: Interventions.* Hartford Institute for Geriatric Nursing. Retrieved from http://consultgerirn.org/uploads/File/trythis/try_this_d11_1.pdf

Anderson, J. E., & Prior, S. (2014). *Nutrition and aging.* Colorado State University Extension. Retrieved from http://www.ext.colostate.edu/pubs/foodnut/09322.html

Shelky, M., & Wallace, M. (2012). *Try this: The Katz index of independence in activities of daily living.* Hartford Institute for Geriatric Nursing. Retrieved from http://consultgerirn.org/uploads/File/trythis/try_this_2.pdf

Speroff, B.A., Davis, K. H., Dehr, K. L., & Larkins, K. N. (2005). The dining experience in nursing homes. *North Carolina Medical Journal.* Retrieved from http://www.ncmedicaljournal.com/wp-content/uploads/NCMJ/jul-aug-05/Fullcopy.pdf

Tonarelli, L. (n.d.). Mealtime tips for dementia caregivers. *Suite101®.* Retrieved from http://seniors-health-medicare.suite101.com/article.cfm/mealtime-tips-for-dementia-caregivers

Wood, D. (2011). Enjoyable dining—Can we build an evidence base? *Leading Age Magazine, 1*(6). Retrieved from http://www.leadingage.org/magazine/feature.aspx?id=3764

Case 15.2 ■ Oral Health

*C*indy Shuppert is the clinical services director at a 100-bed long-term care (LTC) facility. She began working with the geriatric population several years after becoming an RN, and plans to continue to do so. As a current graduate student, Cindy is seeking a nurse practitioner certification. For a class assignment, Cindy developed and presented an in-service for the staff where she is employed on the topic of oral health for the elderly.

She began her program emphasizing the need for a thorough assessment, including the lips, oral mucosa, and tongue. Cindy uses an evidence-based assessment tool for screening the residents in relation to oral health. It is the Kayser-Jones Brief Oral Health Status Examination (BOHSE), found at http://consultgerirn.org/uploads/File/trythis/try_this_18 (Taub, 2012).

1. What additional components should be assessed using a tool such as this?

Cindy used a recent admission to the LTC facility as an example for assessing oral health using the BOHSE. Mr. Briggs, an alert and oriented 80-year-old male, had developed osteomyelitis in the residual limb of an amputated lower leg, and needed 6 weeks of intravenous antibiotic therapy. He was able to self-feed and provides his own oral hygiene. He had eight natural teeth remaining on top, and a lower denture plate. He scored a 1 on all categories except assessment of gums, which were documented as follows: swollen and bleeding gums, redness at border around seven of eight upper teeth, four loose upper teeth, and generalized redness of gums under artificial teeth.

2. What would the recommendation be based on these findings?

Care strategies were covered in detail; Cindy emphasized the mechanical action of a toothbrush to remove plaque from teeth was the best practice, compared with a foam swab, which is recommended for cleaning the oral mucosa only. A new employee mentioned a facility where she once worked that used lemon glycerin swabs regularly, and she was curious why none were available at this one.

3. What are negative effects caused by using lemon glycerin swabs/swabsticks?

Xerostomia, or dry mouth, is a common problem with the elderly. When asking the audience for causative factors, nurses stated medications, chemotherapy/radiation for cancer, and chronic disease states, which are correct. Cindy stated, "One article I read on this topic said that dry mouth is "the rule rather than the exception among the elderly" and that "the consequences can be catastrophic" (Fletcher, 2014).

4. What are a minimum of five drug groups known to cause xerostomia?

Cindy reviews findings from an article that offers several recommendations for treatment of xerostomia and drugs to stimulate hyposalivation, found at www .dimensionsofdentalhygiene.com/print.aspx?id=12293.

5. Use this source or another of your choice to discuss treatment options for older people.

Denture care was also a topic covered at the in-service. Whether the resident has a full set, upper or lower dentures only, or a partial plate, staff should consistently give proper care.

Watch the 1-minute video related to dentures and nutrition, and review the information on denture care provided by the American Dental Association at www .mouthhealthy.org/en/az-topics/d/Dentures.

6. Which of the following are best practice guidelines when caring for dentures? Select all that apply.

a. *Denture care should be provided once a day, every morning or evening.*

b. *Remove the lower plate by pulling down and lift forward and out.*

c. *Brush dentures with toothbrush/toothpaste using an up-and-down motion.*

> d. *Clean the grooved area of the denture, which fits against the gum.*
>
> e. *Brush the resident's tongue.*

An experienced RN attending the in-service stated at one point, "It seems as though many older people think that a decline in their oral health is a normal part of aging." Cindy acknowledged this myth, but added, "With the coverage of services offered by Medicare, it's no wonder."

> **7. *What information can you find regarding dental health coverage and Medicare?***

Lastly, the body image and social implications for oral health problems were addressed. Loss of teeth, decayed teeth, poor fitting dentures, xerostomia, and malodorous breath can have negative outcomes for an elderly person.

> **8. *Develop two psychosocial-based nursing diagnoses related to poor oral health.***

Suggested Resources

Dalhousie University. (2011). *Brushing up on mouth care.* Retrieved from http://www.ahprc.dal.ca/projects/oral-care/pdfs/iS-oralSwabs.pdf

Fletcher, J. (2014). *Dry mouth in the elderly can be overlooked by caregivers.* AgingCare.com. Retrieved from http://www.agingcare.com/Articles/dry-mouth-in-elderly-147642.htm

Janson, E. (2014). *Medications that may cause xerostomia (dry mouth).* Dentistry.com. Retrieved from http://www.dentistry.com/conditions/mouth-problems/medications-that-may-cause-xerostomia-dry-mouth

Noble, W. H., Aziz, K., Edwards, K., & Salmon, E. (2012). Xerostomia from A to Z. *Dimensions of Dental Hygiene.* Retrieved from http://www.dimensionsofdentalhygiene.com/print.aspx?id=12293

O'Connor, L. (2012). Oral health care. In E. Capezuti, D. Zwicker, M. Mezey, & T. Fulmer (Eds.), *Evidence-based geriatric nursing protocols for best practice* (4th ed., pp. 411–412). New York, NY: Springer Publishing Company.

Taub, L. M. (2012). Try this: Best practices in nursing care to older adults. *The Kayser-Jones Brief Oral Health Status Examination (BOHSE).* Hartford Institute for Geriatric Nursing. Retrieved from http://consultgerirn.org/uploads/File/trythis/try_this_18.pdf

Case 15.3 ■ Diverticular Disease

*J*ane Schmidt is an advanced practice nurse working in the gastroenterology department at a major university hospital. John Shepherd is a 73-year-old man who is visiting with Jane for follow-up after a routine colonoscopy. In the screening paperwork,

Jane notes that Mr. Shepherd indicated intermittent episodes of constipation and diarrhea, both accompanied by lower abdominal discomfort and excessive flatulence. When Jane asks about these symptoms, he says that the episodes usually subside and that he really does not think much of it, "just part of getting old, probably something I'm eating at my new place." Mr. Shepherd is 5 feet 9 inches and 225 pounds. He has been widowed for several years and has recently moved to an independent living facility where his meals and housekeeping are provided. The meals he is complaining of generally consist of a meat choice, a starch, and a side of vegetables. He says that he usually eats breakfast in his apartment, a bowl of cornflakes and milk. John indicates that they rarely have fresh fruits and vegetables and that he does not like the canned vegetables very much. He takes the following medications: Zocor (simvastatin) 40 mg orally daily and Pepcid (famotidine) 20 mg orally as needed to control heartburn episodes. He is not allergic to any medications. His blood pressure (BP) is 130/80. He is able to take care of his own daily needs and is relatively active, but does not like to participate in many of the activities offered in his facility. His colonoscopy findings are negative for any large masses. A polyp was removed, and pathology reports indicated that it was benign. The report indicates the presence of several diverticula with some mild inflammation noted.

For the following questions, consult an online resource, such as:

- American College of Gastroenterology, www.acg.go.org
- American Gastroenterology Association, www.gastro.org
- American Society of Colon and Rectal Surgeons, www.fascrs.org
- International Foundation for Functional Gastrointestinal Disorders, www.iffgd.org
- National Digestive Diseases Information, http://digestive.niddk.nih.gov

1. *Explain the findings of the colonoscopy indicating the presence of diverticula.*

2. *What is the difference between diverticulosis and diverticulitis?*

3. *Would you say that Mr. Shepherd is suffering from diverticulosis or diverticulitis?*

4. *Is Mr. Shepherd right when he says that diverticulosis is just part of getting old? Explain your rationale.*

5. *Can diet play a role in the incidence of diverticular disease?*

Using a tool for evidence-based management of diverticular disease, such as the online journal *Clinical Evidence*, or by consulting information from the previously listed organizations, answer the following.

6. *What is the most beneficial diet for a patient with diverticular disease?*

7. *Would you recommend a course of antibiotics for Mr. Shepherd? Explain your answer.*

8. **What signs or symptoms should you recommend Mr. Shepherd be aware of that might indicate escalation of the disease?**

9. **When might surgery be proposed as an option for treating diverticular disease?**

Suggested Resources

National Digestive Diseases Information Clearinghouse. (2012). *What I need to know about diverticular disease.* Retrieved from http://digestive.niddk.nih.gov/ddiseases/pubs/diverticu

National Digestive Diseases Information Clearinghouse. (2013). *Diverticulosis and diverticulitis.* Retrieved from http://digestive.niddk.nih.gov/ddiseases/pubs/diverticulosis

Rafferty, J. (2014). *ASCRS: Diverticulitis.* American Society of Colon and Rectal Surgeons. Retrieved from www.fascrs.org/physicians/education/core_subjects/2005/diverticultis

Reinhard, T. (2014). Diverticular disease—A re-examination of the fiber hypothesis. *Today's Dietician, 16*(3). Retrieved from http://www.todaysdietitian.com/newarchives/030314p46.html

Shahedi, K. (2014). *Diverticulitis treatment & management.* Medscape. Retrieved from http://emedicine.medscape.com/article/173388-treatment

Case 15.4 ■ Chronic Constipation

George Grady is an 84-year-old retired police officer who lives with his wife of 66 years. They both reside in a retirement community and receive their primary care from a nurse practitioner in their local Veterans Administration health services program. George has been assigned to a nurse case manager, Geneva, an RN, for coordination of his care.

George was diagnosed with benign prostatic hyperplasia (BPH) about 15 years ago and has been treated with a number of different agents that all caused increasing cognitive impairment. He has restricted his fluid intake, thinking this will help with his sense of urinary urgency. His bowel movements have become less and less frequent from about one to three per week to one every other week.

1. **How is constipation defined?**

2. **What is the most probable cause of George's constipation?**

   a. **A normal process of aging**

   b. **BPH**

> c. **Dehydration and cognitive impairment**
> d. **Little access to health care services**
>
> 3. **What are additional causes of constipation?**

George's wife, Carol, appears puzzled and asks which types of medications could cause constipation and, over time, what harm may result. Geneva offers a reply.

> 4. **List examples of medication classes known to cause constipation.**
>
> 5. **What are complications of chronic constipation?**

George has had four Fleet enemas over the past month. The nurse practitioner started George on 70% sorbitol, but he cannot tolerate the taste, so he is switched to polyethylene glycol 70% suspension and seems to be responding to this course of treatment.

> 6. **What are treatments for constipation?**
>
> 7. **What types of nonmedicinal recommendations can the nurse encourage for this patient?**

Because George is very focused on having regular bowel movements, his BPH has not been treated adequately; consequently, he is started on oxybutynin chloride 10% gel topically as Gelnique for overactive bladder (OAB). His prostate-specific antigen (PSA) is currently between 7.0 and 9.0 ng/mL, and his urologist is evaluating him to decide whether or not to start him on Lupron (leuprolide acetate) and Casodex (bicalutamide).

In the interim, his constipation has gotten worse due to not drinking sufficient fluids, so Miralax (polyethylene glycol) is started. George is having one to three stools a week, but he is getting up four to five times during the night, and he has reported falling three times in the past month. As a consequence, the nurse practitioner evaluates using Milk of Magnesia (MOM) every other night, between 45 and 60 mL. In the past, he has refused MOM, but states the mint flavor form would be his preference to the generic unflavored kind. He now has a bowel movement every other day.

> 8. **What nursing recommendations should Geneva make to the family for the management of George's constipation with MOM?**

Suggested Resources

Basson, M. D. (2014). *Constipation in adults*. emedicine Health. Retrieved from http://www.emedicinehealth.com/constipation_in_adults/article_em.htm

Johanson, J. F. (2011). *Clinical factors and complications of constipation in the elderly*. e-iMPaCCT. Retrieved from http://www.cmecorner.com/portal/topic_detail.asp?id=elderlyconstipation.org&cid=38

Khan, A., & Morley, J. E. (n. d.). *Constipation in the elderly.* The doctor will see you now. Retrieved from http://www.thedoctorwillseeyounow.com/content/aging/art2080.html?getPage=2

Marks, J. W. (2014). *Constipation.* Medicinenet.com. Retrieved from http://www.medicinenet .com/constipation/article.htm

Case 15.5 ■ Hiatal Hernia

*M*r. Frank Lynch is an 83-year-old male who has experienced severe gastroesophageal reflux disease (GERD) for 6 months. Mr. Lynch comes to the community health clinic complaining of regurgitation, sore throat, cough, and a sour taste in his mouth. Mr. Lynch was seen for similar complaints 3 months ago. At that time, an upper GI series showed a hiatal hernia of 2 cm. After the initial x-ray, Mr. Lynch was instructed to sleep with the head of the bed elevated and use two pillows. He also was told to take over-the-counter (OTC) Prilosec (omeprazole) 20 mg daily.

Sam Alero, clinic admissions nurse, completes a health history and physical assessment. Mr. Lynch reports that in the past 3 months, he has been unable to exercise after eating. He says, "After meals, it feels like a burning chest pain right behind the breastbone, and up to my throat. My heartburn is worse after going to bed at night." Mr. Lynch reports that he eats three large meals per day, and has gained 20 pounds in the past 6 months. He has not slept on two pillows as instructed, due to neck pain. He smokes two packs per day.

Vital signs on Mr. Lynch include BP 138/88, heart rate 84, and respirations 20. He is 69 inches tall, and weighs 298 pounds. He has a dry, nonproductive cough. Mr. Lynch is wearing clothing that is too small for him; he has a pendulous abdomen that hangs over his belt.

1. ***What risk factors does Mr. Lynch have for the development of a hiatal hernia?***

2. ***What age-related changes can be associated with hiatal hernia?***

3. ***What history, laboratory results, or physical examination findings should be of the greatest concern to the admissions nurse?***

4. ***What dietary instructions should the nurse give to Mr. Lynch? Give five examples of foods that Mr. Lynch should limit or eliminate from his diet.***

5. ***What other instructions should the nurse give to Mr. Lynch? Give five examples of lifestyle changes that Mr. Lynch could make to reduce his GERD symptoms.***

Mr. Lynch returns to the clinic in 1 month. He tells Sam, "I am having a lot of trouble swallowing food." Mr. Lynch admits that he has not been able to stop smoking, but has "cut down" on the size of his meals and has decreased his coffee intake to 6 cups a day. He has put a foam wedge on his bed. Mr. Lynch asks, "Why do I have so much trouble swallowing?"

6. *What information can Sam give to Mr. Lynch?*

Mr. Lynch is scheduled for a gastroscopy. He asks Sam, "Why does the doctor want me to have this test?"

7. *What can Sam teach Mr. Lynch about the use of gastroscopy to evaluate dysphagia?*

Sam does some online research on esophageal stricture. He wants to find information that he thinks might be helpful to Mr. Lynch.

8. *Go to the following website, www.healthline.com/health/esophageal-stricture-benign#Overview1 (Giorgi, 2012), and find at least four facts that you think that Sam should share with Mr. Lynch.*

Mr. Lynch's esophagus was dilated by passing a dilator through an endoscope. It required three attempts to restore the lumen of the esophagus. Mucosa changes consistent with Barrett's esophagus were not found.

9. *After this procedure, what are the most important instructions that Sam can give Mr. Lynch regarding his current health practices?*

Suggested Resources

Gillson, S. (2014). *Top heartburn prevention tips.* About.com. Retrieved from http://heartburn .about.com/od/preventingheartburn/tp/heartburn_tips.htm

Giorgi, A. (2012). *Benign esophageal stricture.* Healthline. Retrieved from http://www.healthline .com/health/esophageal-stricture-benign#Overview1

Knott, L. (2014). *Hiatal hernia.* Patient.co.uk. Retrieved from http://www.patient.co.uk/health/ hiatus-hernia-leaflet

Lehrer, J. K. (2006). *Esophageal stricture—benign.* Retrieved from http://www.nlm.nih.gov/ medlineplus/ency/article/000207.htm

Quinn, K. L. (2014). Management of patients with oral and esophageal disorders. In J. L. Hinkle & K. H. Cheever (Eds.), *Brunner's and Suddarth's textbook of medical–surgical nursing* (13th ed., pp. 1251–1254). Philadelphia, PA: Lippincott.

Slowik, G. (2012). *GERD: How are the complications treated?* eHealth.com. Retrieved from http://ehealthmd.com/content/how-are-complications-treated#axzz3AkzzqfwX

Tomson, N. (2014). *Excellent advice for reducing the symptoms of acid reflux.* Acid Reflux Mentor. Retrieved from http://www.acidrefluxmentor.net/2014/03

Wedro, B. (2013). *Hiatal hernia overview.* MedicineNet.com. Retrieved from http://www .medicinenet.com/hiatal_hernia_overview/page2.htm

Case 15.6 ■ Hydration Management

*M*rs. Williams is an 88-year-old African American woman admitted to the acute care unit with dehydration following acute gastroenteritis. Her sister found her at home this morning, very weak, unable to walk without assistance, and confused. Mrs. Williams indicates that she's had nausea, vomiting, and diarrhea for several days and a feeling of "bloating" for a couple of months.

Before hospitalization, Mrs. Williams was living alone on the third floor of an apartment complex for older adults. She no longer drives. Her social history includes being widowed with one daughter who lives in another state and one sister who lives within walking distance from Mrs. Williams's apartment complex. Mrs. Williams is a retired office worker and her income consists of her monthly Social Security benefit check and a small pension. She is described by her sister as limited in activities such as shopping, traveling, and cooking because of fatigue and periods of confusion. She reports fatigue associated with activities of daily living (ADL).

Mrs. Williams has a medical history of hypertension treated with furosemide and an ACE inhibitor, as well as osteoarthritis (particularly of knees) treated with OTC ibuprofen. Her sister also reports that Mrs. Williams has lost "a good bit" of weight in the past 6 months. Mrs. Williams agrees that she has a decreased appetite but is unsure how many pounds she has lost. On admission to the nursing unit, she is oriented to person but not to place or date. Vital signs on admission are BP 100/56, HR 94, R 12, T 100.2°F orally. Weight is 130 pounds, height 5 feet 2 inches. Her complete blood count (CBC) is within normal limits with WBCs $8.1 \times (10)^3$, RBCs $4 \times (10)^6$, HGB 12 g/dL, HCT 42%, and platelets $400 \times (10)^3$.

> **1. What risk factors does this patient have for dehydration?**
>
> **2. Given Mrs. Williams's age and history, what assessments and laboratory tests should be done to further evaluate her fluid status at the time of admission?**
>
> **3. Mrs. Williams's sister asks whether the elevated temperature indicates that her sister needs antibiotics. What understanding should form the basis of the nurse's response?**

Mrs. Williams is at risk for both acid–base and fluid–electrolyte disorders. Whether Mrs. Williams exhibits hyponatremia or hypernatremia will depend on the relative severity of the vomiting and diarrhea she experienced, and her ability to drink and absorb water. It is essential that her electrolytes be evaluated thoroughly both at baseline, and as treatment progresses.

> **4. Explain why Mrs. Williams is at risk for each of the following disorders, and what the laboratory and clinical findings would**

likely be if the condition existed: hypokalemia, hypernatremia, hyponatremia, metabolic acidosis, metabolic alkalosis.

5. **What instructions should the RN give the certified nursing assistant (CNA) when delegating aspects of Mrs. Williams's care?**

Mrs. Williams's vomiting is controlled by antiemetics on admission to the unit, but she refuses oral intake other than occasional sips of water and chips of ice. She is started on an IV of 5% dextrose in 0.45% sodium chloride solution with 30 mEq K⁺/L at 150 mL per hour.

6. **What considerations should the nurse have in administering this fluid replacement?**

7. **The CNA asks whether a Foley catheter can be inserted to help keep Mrs. Williams dry. What are the advantages and disadvantages of use of a Foley catheter in this situation?**

8. **What assessments should be repeated once Mrs. Williams's fluid volume deficit is resolved?**

Following 3 days of IV fluid administration, antiemetics, and Imodium (loperamide), Mrs. Williams's vomiting, diarrhea, and fluid volume deficit have resolved. Her IV therapy is discontinued. Her confusion has decreased, but she still has trouble remembering date and place. She continues to experience anorexia and feeling that she's "full" although she refuses more than occasional sips of clear liquids. She continues to have weakness and apathy. Her abdomen is soft and diffusely tender, with active bowel sounds. Lab studies now reveal anemia, and her stool is guaiac positive for blood. Endoscopy with biopsy is performed, and gastric carcinoma is diagnosed. A CAT scan reveals metastasis to the liver and lungs. Physicians determine that Mrs. Williams's malignancies cannot be controlled, so cancer treatment will not be provided. Her daughter is notified, and all agree that Mrs. Williams's care will continue in an inpatient hospice setting.

9. **Using the National Cancer Institute's Fact Sheet (n.d.) at www .cancer.gov/cancertopics/factsheet/Support/end-of-life-care, what suggestions might you recommend to Mrs. Williams's daughter to provide emotional comfort to her mother?**

10. **There is conflicting research evidence regarding the efficacy of providing hydration at the end of life. How do you explain both points of view to Mrs. Williams's daughter?**

Some patients are more comfortable without artificial hydration, whereas others are more comfortable when artificial hydration is used. The driving forces in the decision to provide artificial hydration are often emotional, cultural, religious, and/or moral convictions on the part of patients, families, and caregivers. Mrs. Williams and her daughter request that hydration be attempted to see whether it could improve her cognitive status. The RN inserted a subcutaneous needle into her anterior thigh in order to administer fluids by hypodermoclysis. Mrs. Williams received 1 L of fluid within 24 hours, and improved her cognitive status. She died peacefully 3 days later.

11. **What are alternate routes of hydration when the oral route is no longer available? List the advantages and potential complications of routes for artificial hydration at end of life.**

Suggested Resources

Dalal, S., & Bruera, E. (2004). Dehydration in cancer patients: To treat or not to treat. *Journal of Supportive Oncology, 2,* 467–479.

Derrer, D. T. (2013). *Dehydration in adults.* WebMD. Retrieved from http://www.webmd .com/a-to-zguidess./dehydration-adults?page=4

Hospice and Palliative Care Nurses Association. (2011). *HPNA position statement. Artificial nutrition and hydration in advanced illness.* Retrieved from https://www.hpna.org/ displayPage.aspx?Title1=Position%20Statements

Mentes, J. C. (2012). Managing oral hydration. In E. Capezuti, D. Zwicker, M. Mezey, & T. Fulmer (Eds.), *Evidence-based geriatric nursing protocols for best practice* (4th ed., pp. 419–430). New York, NY: Springer Publishing Company.

Morrow, A. (2014). *Artificial nutition and hydration.* About.com. Retrieved from http://dying .about.com/od/lifesupport/a/artificialfeed.htm

Mulvey, M. (2014). Fluids and electrolytes: Balance and disturbance. In J. L. Hinkle & K. H. Cheever (Eds.), *Brunner and Suddarth's textbook of medical–surgical nursing* (13th ed., pp. 247–249). Philadelphia, PA: Lippincott Williams & Wilkins.

National Cancer Institute, U.S. National Institutes of Health. (n.d.). National Cancer Institute. *FactSheet: End-of-life care: Questions and answers.* Retrieved from http://www.cancer .gov/cancertopics/factsheet/Support/end-of-life-care

Shepherd, A. (2011). Measuring and managing fluid balance. *Nursing Times, 107*(28), 12–16. Retrieved from http://www.nursingtimes.net/Journals/1/Files/2011/8/1/Fluid%20balanceCorr .pdf.pdf

16

Cancer in the Older Adult

Case 16.1 ■ Chemotherapy and the Aged

*T*ally Ann Knight, a 68-year-old African American female, arrives at the outpatient cancer care center for her second round of chemotherapy for breast cancer. She had a left mastectomy for a Stage IIIA malignancy. Her medications include 5-fluorouracil (5-FU), Adriamycin (doxorubicin), and Cytoxan (cyclophosphamide). Zofran (ondansetron) is ordered for nausea.

1. *What special precautions should the nurse use when handling and administering chemotherapeutic agents?*

2. *Briefly describe the classifications and actions of these cancer treatment medications.*

3. *Find and cite a resource on your own, or watch the several-minute video available at www.videojug.com/interview/aging-and-disease-2#why-is-cancer-more-likely-among-the-elderly and identify reasons why cancer is more common with aging.*

4. *Ms. Knight hears the nurses refer to "nadir," a word she is unfamiliar with; how would you explain this to her?*

5. *What problems with chemotherapy is Ms. Knight more prone to because of her age, and how can the nurse prevent and treat these problems? Use the website www.cancer.net/patient/ Coping/Age-Specific+Information/Cancer+in+Older+Adults/ Cancer+Treatment or another source for your response.*

One of the major areas of health disparities for African American women is in recovery rates from cancer.

6. *Review the National Cancer Institute's Health Care Disparities fact sheet at www.cancer.gov/cancertopics/factsheet/cancer-health-disparities/ and reflect on this situation.*

> **7. Among the many assessment tools the nurses at the outpatient cancer care center use is the Kayser-Jones Brief Oral Health Status Examination (BOHSE) found at http://consultgerirn.org/ uploads/File/trythis/try_this_18.pdf Taub (2012). What is the importance of assessing Ms. Knight's oral cavity on a regular basis while on chemotherapy?**

Dorothy Hawk, RN, is the nurse assigned to Ms. Knight for today's visit. The client is alert and oriented to person, place, time, and event. Ms. Knight states that she doesn't feel well today. She has a sore throat and chills. Her vital signs are the following: BP 110/70, P 100, R 20, and T 102°F. Ms. Knight's height is 5 feet 7 inches, and she weighs 130 pounds. Labs ordered are a complete blood count, electrolytes, platelets, and a urinalysis.

> **8. What could be possible causes of Ms. Knight's symptoms?**

Ms. Knight is also complaining of pain from her mastectomy site, which is added to her "normal aches and pains" of having lived a "hard" 68 years. She was discharged home from the hospital 8 weeks ago with a prescription for Vicodin (hydrocodone 7.5 mg/acetaminophen 500 mg) and instructions to take one tablet every 6 hours as needed. She attempted to use them sparingly but ran out 10 days ago. She does not remember being asked to rate her pain on the first visit to the cancer care center.

Uncontrolled pain can be a tremendous problem for women with breast cancer, especially if the cancer metastasizes to the spine.

> **9. Find a resource pertaining to the ethical and legal issues of inadequate pain management in cancer. Could the patient's family be able to show that the lack of pain treatment was elder abuse?**

Following her third chemotherapy treatment, Ms. Knight made a major decision in her treatment plan based solely on her lifelong spiritual faith. She was overwhelmingly fatigued, had minimal appetite, and knew she was requiring a lot of extra time and attention from her daughter who worked full time and had three children at home. Therefore, she stopped all further chemotherapy treatments. Her alternate plan was to save as much of her Social Security income as possible for 10 months, which would allow her to afford a trip she very much wanted to take to a major city quite a distance from her home.

For decades, Ms. Knight had been a follower of a television evangelist and wanted to attend his program in person. She fully believed he would be able to heal her as he had done for so many others she witnessed through the years. Ms. Knight died in a hospice unit 9 months after her last treatment.

Suggested Resources

American Society of Clinical Oncology. (2012). *Cancer treatment*. Cancer.net. Retrieved from http://www.cancer.net/patient/Coping/Age-Specific+Information/Cancer+in+Older+Adults/Cancer+Treatment

National Cancer Institute. (2008). *Cancer health disparities*. U.S. National Institutes of Health. Retrieved from http://www.cancer.gov/cancertopics/factsheet/cancer-health-disparities/disparities

National Cancer Institute. (2011). *Cancer and the elderly*. Retrieved from http://www.cancer .gov/cancertopics/disparities/lifelines/2011/cancer-and-elderly-multicultural.pdf

National Cancer Institute. (2014). *Oral complications of cancer treatment: What the dental team can do*. National Institute of Dental and Craniofacial Research. Retrieved from http://www .nidcr.nih.gov/oralhealth/Topics/CancerTreatment/OralComplicationsCancerOral.htm

Taub, L. F. (2012). *The Kayser-Jones brief oral health status examination (BOHSE)*. Try this series: Best practices in nursing care to older adults. Hartford Institute for Geriatric Nursing. Retrieved from http://consultgerirn.org/uploads/File/trythis/try_this_18.pdf

Case 16.2 ■ Colorectal Cancer

October 20 is a date that has special meaning for Everett Manchester as it represents the day he was diagnosed with colorectal cancer 2 years ago. He had heard people talk about "life-changing events" in personal discussions, on television, or perhaps in the newspaper, and never gave it much thought, until something like this happened to him.

Mr. Manchester was 75 years old when he noticed blood on his toilet tissue three consecutive mornings. Although he knew this was abnormal, he did nothing about it for more than 2 weeks as he had a strong aversion to doctors and health care settings. This was likely due to many visits, procedures, and painful memories from his childhood as he was treated for polio, which resulted in paralysis of the left leg. He underwent a triple coronary artery bypass following myocardial infarction in his late 60s, has a history of acid reflux, and uses a diuretic, calcium channel blocker, and ACE inhibitor for hypertension. Following his bypass procedure, he reluctantly gave up alcohol, but made no dietary changes in his meat, potatoes, and dessert meals.

As far as other lifestyle behaviors, Mr. Manchester has never been a physically active person. He uses hand crutches for mobility and believes the extra effort required for walking, especially up and down the staircase in his home, uses a sufficient number of calories. He is 66 inches tall and weighs 195 pounds. He rates his life as a 2 (out of 1–10) in regards to stress. A long-term stable marriage, no financial concerns, several close friends, and attending church weekly are why he believes he rarely worries or gets upset about things.

1. ***What is the prevalence rate for colorectal cancer in the United States?***

2. ***Describe common risk factors for colorectal cancer and which ones pertain to Mr. Manchester.***

The physician monitoring hypertension and other health care needs for Mr. Manchester suggested long ago that he be screened for colorectal cancer, explaining this is a highly preventable disease if caught early.

3. What are the 2008 U.S. Preventive Services Task Force (USPSTF) recommendations for colorectal screening found at www.annals .org/content/149/9/627.full?

After contacting his medical internist, Mr. Manchester is referred to a colorectal specialist whom he speaks with over the phone initially. He is informed a colonoscopy is needed for visual inspection and the blood may be due to hemorrhoids, polyps, inflammation, or a tumor. In addition, it is requested he provide three consecutive specimens for fecal occult blood testing (FOBT). Preparation instructions for the scope will be mailed to his home with a prescription for the sodium sulfate and GoLytely (polyethylene glycol solution).

Mr. Manchester shares the news of his testing with a friend, Bill, over coffee. Bill tells him he can have a virtual colonoscopy "nowadays." Also, when he has a FOBT annually, there are medications and food restrictions to avoid a false-positive result. Although Bill is a good listener and shows concern, he really upsets Mr. Manchester when he makes the comment, "I sure hope you don't end up with a bag on the outside to collect your poop in; that would be awful."

4. Using Google or another source, find a short video showing a virtual colonoscopy. Compare and contrast this with the traditional procedure.

5. What medications and foods should be withheld 48 hours prior to giving hemoccult stool specimens?

6. What risks, especially for the elderly, are associated with a complete bowel cleansing and being NPO (nothing by mouth) prior to a colonoscopy?

Mr. Manchester's colonoscopy with biopsy resulted in a positive cancer diagnosis with a Stage II tumor (T2N1aM0) located in the descending colon. It was determined a colon resection (removal of the tumor and regional lymph nodes) with anastomosis could be provided with minimally invasive surgery (MIS) via laparoscopy.

7. Will a permanent colostomy be required with the colon resection?

8. What involvement with malignancy does Stage II represent? Interpret T2N1aM0 with the assistance of the following website: www.cancer.org/cancer/colonandrectumcancer/detailedguide/ colorectal-cancer-staged.

9. Preoperatively, what would you anticipate as expected nursing diagnoses (identify five)?

10. What are advantages of using MIS over a traditional approach (e.g., large abdominal incision)?

Mr. Manchester has no complications from the procedure other than generalized soreness and fatigue lasting for a week. An oncologist saw him the last day in the hospital and explained that chemotherapy was indicated related to his cancer staging; he wrote on a paper that the regime would entail FOLFOX4, standard combination drugs for colorectal cancer. Mr. and Mrs. Manchester did not have children, but are very close to a niece and nephew whom are aware of his situation. Several days prior to the oncologist visit, they have dinner together. His nephew is very vocal about refusing chemotherapy to "have a good quality of what life you have left." His niece totally disagrees and offers to accompany the couple to the oncology office to take notes, ask questions, and serve as a support.

The oncologist and a nurse practitioner review the chemotherapy drugs, treatment schedule, and adverse effects. A copy of the article, "Adjuvant Chemotherapy in the Elderly: Whom to Treat, What Regimen?" (Burdette-Radoux & Muss, 2006) is given to the group and discussed in lay terms. Mr. Manchester agrees to the treatment.

11. What chemotherapeutic drugs are included in FOLFOX4?

12. Access the journal article by Burdette-Radoux and Muss (2006) at http://theoncologist.alphamedpress.org/cgi/content/ full/11/3/234 and comment on the authors' conclusions in relation to assessment recommended for elderly individuals considering chemotherapy.

Suggested Resources

Burdette-Radoux, S., & Muss, H. B. (2006). Adjuvant chemotherapy in the elderly: Whom to treat, what regimen? *The Oncologist*. Retrieved from http://theoncologist.alphamedpress.org/ cgi/content/full/11/3/234

Centers for Disease Control and Prevention. (2014). *Colorectal cancer screening guidelines*. Retrieved from http://www.cdc.gov/cancer/colorectal/basic_info/screening/guidelines.htm

Lee, D. (2014). Virtual colonoscopy. *New England Journal of Medicine*. Retrieved from http:// www.medicinenet.com/virtual_colonoscopy/page3.htm

University of Chicago Medicine. (2013). *Minimally invasive colorectal surgery*. Retrieved from http://www.uchospitals.edu/specialties/minisurgery/colorectal

U.S. Preventive Services Task Force. (2014, October). *USPSTF A and B recommendations*. http:// www.uspreventiveservicestaskforce.org/Page/Name/uspstf-a-and-b-recommendations

Case 16.3 ■ HIV/AIDS

*R*ita and Pete live less than a mile apart in the same city, are the same age, and have a significant commonality; both are living with HIV. Their stories will be briefly shared as to the differences in origin of the illness and life thereafter.

Pete is 65 years old and has been HIV positive for 10 years. He lived in a heterosexual world the majority of his life. Married at age 22, Pete secured a position at his father's bank and generated a sizeable income in a short period of time. Two children were produced from the marriage, which lasted until his mid-50s. Pete was fully aware of his sexual preference for men since being a teenager, but never acted upon it until his wife died of ovarian cancer. He was raised in a strict Southern Baptist home, was a star athlete in high school, was well-known and respected in the community, and convinced himself that suicide was a better alternative than "coming out" as a gay male, but chose not to go that route.

Following his wife's death and knowing his adult children were secure, Pete spent weekends in a city several hours from his home and explored his homosexuality with many men.

He partnered with one individual who became quite ill a month later, with what Pete was told was pneumonia. In actuality, this man was admitted for *pneumocystis carinii*, an opportunistic infection of AIDS, and died at the hospital. Pete tested positive for HIV shortly thereafter.

Rita's life was quite a contrast, in particular with financial security. She had several unsuccessful marriages, which produced five children in total. Child support was a rarity, and she always struggled to provide her children with the basics. Rita was a nursing assistant for decades and on one shift incurred a needle stick injury. A medical resident put a syringe with a needle attached in a patient's trash bin following a bedside procedure. When emptying it, Rita was stuck to the point of bleeding heavily. Following protocol, the infection control nurse at the hospital checked both Rita and the patient for HIV using an enzyme-linked immunosorbent assay (ELISA). A week later, it was determined the patient was negative, Rita was not.

She had no choice but to disclose that, at age 64, she participated in unprotected sexual intercourse. On the night she buried her mother, she went to a local tavern for a drink to help "numb" her extreme sadness. A much younger man showed her a lot of attention, bought her multiple servings of alcohol, and she went home with him and had sexual relations. This was the only intimate encounter she'd participated in for a number of years, and no other risk factors existed that could result in HIV.

Use the website from the CDC, *HIV Among Older Americans* (2013) found at www .cdc.gov/hiv/risk/age/olderamericans/ to assist in answering the first three questions.

1. ***Comment on the growth rate of persons age 55 to 64 years living with AIDS in America.***

2. ***Discuss why HIV/AIDS is increasing in older people, including sexual risk factors.***

3. ***Why might the numbers of older persons with HIV/AIDS be much higher than actually reported?***

As stated, Pete has been living HIV positive for 10 years. He has been under medical surveillance with the same infectious disease specialist the entire time. His appearance is that of a healthy, well-groomed male looking perhaps in his late 50s. Pete eats three well-balanced meals a day, exercises five times a week, and has developed very effective stress management skills over the years. He doesn't smoke and keeps alcohol intake to three servings a week. His physician suggests he may continue on this pattern for many years, as long as he "follows his HAART."

4. ***What is HAART and how has it impacted life expectancy for individuals with HIV?***

Rita's lifestyle and daily habits are quite the opposite of Pete's. Her HIV diagnosis was devastating, and she immediately left her job due to embarrassment. Her health insurance covered only half the cost of antiviral medications, and therefore she chose not to use them, wanting to pay off debt before her death. She rarely leaves her apartment and drinks wine almost all her waking hours. Her oldest daughter, who visits regularly, is unaware of her mother's HIV status. She fears due to cognitive (specifically, memory) and physical (stumbling, occasionally falling) symptoms that Rita may have early Alzheimer's disease.

5. *What are the differences in AIDS-related dementia and Alzheimer's?*

Pete has also retired and is a voracious reader. He has attempted to stay informed about HIV and AIDS since the illnesses became known in the United States in the 1980s. He is aware in the early days of the global HIV epidemic treatment for people living with HIV focused on treating opportunistic infections, minimizing pain, and providing palliative care.

6. *What are the primary areas of focus currently with HIV? Use the article "HIV, Aging, and Co-morbidities" found at www.avert. org/hiv-ageing-and-comorbidities.htm for your answer.*

7. *What strategies does the Centers for Disease Control and its partners have for older adults in relation to HIV/AIDS through the High Impact Prevention program?*

Not a day goes by that Rita doesn't feel anger about being with the male she encountered at the tavern. She was never able to find him to inquire whether he knowingly gave her HIV. The infection control nurse at the hospital was so kind and empathetic toward her, especially on the topic of disclosure. Literature was provided to Rita about telling a potential partner one's status in relation to HIV/AIDS. The nurse also informed her she was legally obligated to report the information to the state health department.

8. *If an individual of any age asked you, as a nurse, where HIV testing was available in your community, could you tell him or her? A helpful resource is found at http://locator.aids.gov.*

9. *In your state of residence, are criminal charges filed if an HIV-positive person knowingly infects another human? A helpful resource may be found at http://aids.about.com/od/ dataandstatistics/fl/HIV-Criminal-Laws-by-State.htm.*

Suggested Resources

AVERT. (2014). *HIV, aging and co-morbidities.* Retrieved from http://www.avert.org/about-avert.htm

Centers for Disease Control and Prevention. (2013). *HIV among older Americans.* Retrieved from http://www.cdc.gov/hiv/risk/age/olderamericans

Cichocki, M. (2014). *HAART—Highly active antiretroviral therapy.* About.com: AIDS/HIV. Retrieved from http://aids.about.com/od/hivaidsletterh/g/haartdef.htm

Kennard, C. (2009). *How does HIV/AIDS dementia differ from Alzheimer's?* OurAlzheimer's.com. Retrieved from http://www.healthcentral.com/alzheimers/c/57548/62546/aids-alzheimer/2

Case 16.4 ■ Hospice Care

*J*ane Johnson is a 79-year-old female who was diagnosed 6 weeks ago with a recurrence of breast cancer, and she now has liver and bone metastases. Her past medical history includes hypertension, osteoarthritis, and type 2 diabetes, all of which are well controlled with medications. Jane is widowed and has three children, who all live within 1 hour of her suburban apartment. Her children and grandchildren are all active in her life and visit weekly. Jane is involved in the senior center activities in her community and has many friends in her neighborhood as well as the church she attends. Hospice care has been mentioned as an option to Jane by a friend whose husband died while receiving hospice benefits from a local not-for-profit organization. Jane has minimal experience with hospice care and does not fully understand the implications of choosing the hospice benefit, which is offered as an option on her health care plan. Jane has just recently told her family that she is considering the option of hospice care. Her only concern is that she lives alone and is afraid of pain. She states, "I am not afraid to die, it is just how I am going to die that scares me."

1. *What are the goals of hospice? The American Cancer Society website, www.cancer.org, has a well-prepared overview of hospice—search the term "hospice" on the website. In addition, review the National Hospice and Palliative Care Organization (NHPCO) and the Hospice and Palliative Nurses Association (HPNA) websites at www.nhpco.org and www.hpna.org.*

2. *How can Jane obtain a referral for hospice care that will include an assessment by a hospice admission nurse?*

3. *Describe the services provided by the hospice interdisciplinary team.*

Jane understands that to be considered for the hospice benefit, two doctors need to diagnose her as being terminally ill. Jane understands that the life expectancy to be admitted to the hospice program is 6 months, but she wants to live for another year to be able to see her granddaughter get married. She would like the benefits that hospice provides, but she is fearful that this is not the right time to begin hospice care.

4. *Describe the Medicare benefit periods to Jane, and services that are provided.*

5. *One of the major concerns of the hospice team is symptom control. Identify the most common symptoms found in patients at the end of life.*

6. *How can the hospice nurse address Jane's fear of pain and her statement, "It is just how I am going to die that scares me"?*

7. *Jane's family does not want her to accept the hospice benefit as a basis for her continued care. They feel that hospice will allow Jane "to give up and die sooner." As a nurse, how do you address this family's concern?*

8. *Who should make the decision to accept or decline hospice services and how can this type of decision be accomplished considering Jane and her children? (Take into account decision-making capacity.)*

Suggested Resource

American Cancer Society. (n.d.). *Hospice care*. Retrieved from http://www.cancer.org/Treatment/ FindingandPayingfor Treatment/ChoosingYourTreatmentTeam/HospiceCare/index

17

Cognitive Impairment in the Older Adult

Case 17.1 ■ Acute Confusion (Delirium)

Sara Garnet is a 78-year-old woman who is accompanied by her daughter, Megan, to a preoperative visit for a scheduled total hip replacement. Sara had been active, playing bridge and taking daily walks, until about 6 months ago when her hip began hurting so much as to limit her activity. She states she had experienced sporadic pain for years, but the hip started "giving out" on occasion, resulting in several falls. Sara is in otherwise good health, though her daughter reports that she has noticed that Sara has been having some difficulty with her short-term memory recently. She is able to compensate for this loss by keeping an appointment calendar next to her phone and using Post-it notes to help her remember messages and daily tasks. Sara has a history of depression, which is treated with Celexa (citalopram), and hypertension, which is treated with Lopressor (metoprolol).

Lily Arnse, RN, performs some presurgical cognitive screening tests, the Geriatric Depression Scale (GDS), Mini-Cog, and Trails B. Sara's score of 1 on the GDS indicates that her depression is well managed with her current medications. She struggles with three-item recall and the Clock Draw Test, as she is able to recall only two of three items and cannot correctly position the numbers on the clock. She is almost completely unable to perform the Trails B test.

1. *What is delirium?*

2. *How common is delirium in hospitalized, older adults?*

3. *Is Sara at high risk to develop postoperative delirium? What risk factors does she have?*

4. *How does surgery increase the risk for development of delirium?*

5. *Is delirium always reversible?*

6. *What negative sequelae can develop as a result of delirium?*

7. *An evidence-based guideline for recognizing, preventing, and treating delirium has been created through the Hartford Institute for Geriatric Nursing. Review this guideline, which is available at http://consultgerirn.org/topics/delirium/want_to_know_more (Tullmann, Fletcher, & Foreman 2012). How can Sara's risk for developing delirium during this hospitalization be reduced?*

8. *The Confusion Assessment Method is a valid and reliable tool for assessing delirium. Go to the Hartford Institute for Geriatric Nursing website, http://consultgerirn.org/uploads/File/trythis/try_this_13.pdf (Waszynski, 2012), to view this tool. Describe how to use the confusion assessment method (CAM) to make a diagnosis of delirium.*

9. *What medications are known to increase the risk of development of delirium?*

10. *Describe the cognitive screening tests that Lily performed. You can find the (a) GDS (Greenberg, 2012) at http://consultgerirn.org/uploads/File/trythis/try_this_4.pdf, the (b) Mini-Cog (Doerflinger, 2013) at http://consultgerirn.org/uploads/File/trythis/try_this_3.pdf, and (c) a description of the Trails B can be viewed at http://alzheimers.about.com/od/testsandprocedures/a/The-Trail-Making-Test-And-Its-Use-As-A-Screening-For-Dementia.htm (Heerema, 2014).*

Suggested Resources

American Association of Critical-Care Nurses. (2014). *Delirium assessment and management.* Retrieved from http://www.aacn.org/wd/practice/content/practicealerts/delirium-practice-alert.pcms?menu=practice

Doerflinger, D. M. C. (2013). *How to try this: The mini-cog.* The Hartford Institute for Geriatric Nursing. Retrieved from http://consultgerirn.org/uploads/File/trythis/try_this_3.pdf

Greenberg, S. A. (2012). *The Geriatric Depression Scale (GDS).* Hartford Institute for Geriatric Nursing. Retrieved from http://consultgerirn.org/uploads/File/trythis/try_this_4.pdf

Heerema, E. (2014). *The Trail Making Test and its use as a screening tool for dementia.* About.com Alzheimer's/Dementia. Retrieved from http://alzheimers.about.com/od/testsandprocedures/a/The-Trail-Making-Test-And-Its-Use-As-A-Screening-For-Dementia.htm

Tullmann, D. F., Fletcher, K., & Foreman, M. D. (2012). *Nursing standard of practice protocol: Delirium: prevention, early recognition, and treatment.* Hartford Institute for Geriatric Nursing. Retrieved from http://consultgerirn.org/topics/delirium/want_to_know_more

Waszynski, C. M. (2012). *The Confusion Assessment Method (CAM).* Hartford Institute for Geriatric Nursing. Retrieved from http://consultgerirn.org/uploads/File/trythis/try_this_13.pdf

Case 17.2 ■ Early Dementia

*C*laudine Everett, age 78, lives with her husband of 59 years in the home where they raised their four children. Her husband noticed (but kept to himself) that Claudine increasingly asked him questions about things she previously had no trouble remembering and that she was misplacing things with greater frequency. Sometime later, the couple's children, who live in different cities and only see her every few weeks, began to notice these same things, and Claudine even began to say, "You know I have a memory problem," when she couldn't remember something.

At a family meal one Thanksgiving season, Claudine was very slow in getting the meal prepared even with the usual help she received from her daughters. Everyone in the family noted that Claudine was having an unusual amount of difficulty organizing the meal and getting it ready to serve. She required recipes to follow for side dishes she had made from memory for decades, and did not set the table with the traditional cloth napkins, candles, and cornucopia centerpiece her daughters had become accustomed to seeing since they were very young children.

1. *According to the Alzheimer's Association website found at www.alz.org/alzheimers_disease_stages_of_alzheimers.asp, what stage of cognitive decline is Claudine experiencing at this point?*

Soon after this Thanksgiving meal, her family started talking among themselves about Claudine's apparently declining cognition. At this point, Claudine's husband revealed that he had actually been noticing this decline for a year or more. The family suspected that Claudine might have early Alzheimer's disease and decided to search out information online to determine the best course of action.

2. *Discuss the definition of dementia using the Hartford Institute for Geriatric Nursing Evidence-Based Practice website at http://consultgerirn.org/topics/dementia/want_to_know_more (Fletcher, 2012). What is the prevalence?*

3. *After conducting an Internet search, identify three reputable websites where Claudine's family can obtain information about Alzheimer's disease.*

Go to the Alzheimer's Association website, www.alz.org/index.asp to answer Questions 4 through 7.

The family finds a wealth of information online and gathers to discuss the warning signs for Alzheimer's.

> 4. *What warning signs (behaviors) for Alzheimer's disease does the family find on the Alzheimer's Association website at www.alz .org/10signs?*

The family determines that Claudine might be suffering from early Alzheimer's disease and believes that they need to have her examined by a qualified health professional in order to secure a diagnosis and to begin treatment as soon as possible.

> 5. *According to the Alzheimer's Association (2014c) at www.alz. org/alzheimers_disease_steps_to_diagnosis.asp, what kind of practitioner should Claudine visit?*

> 6. *What kinds of recommended treatments might Claudine's family anticipate to slow the progression of Claudine's disease? Find some of these at www.alz.org/alzheimers_disease_standard_ prescriptions.asp (Alzheimer's Association, 2014b).*

Claudine's grandson is getting married in a town several states away from their home. The family has decided it is not wise to take Claudine to the wedding, as she has made comments about opening the car door and jumping out during rides with family members. However, Claudine's daughters and her husband want to attend the wedding, in order to support the new couple. In addition, the daughters think it would be good for Mr. Everett to have a brief time away from Claudine since he has been caring for her around the clock for many months.

> 7. *What could you tell the family about potential respite services for them? Find information on these at www.alz.org/living_with_ alzheimers_respite_care.asp (Alzheimer's Association, 2014a).*

A month or two after returning from the wedding, Mr. Everett still declines offers to move Claudine out of their home; however, he is showing increasing signs of stress and reports that he does not "even have time to get a haircut."

> 8. *What are some reasons for which the nurse might recommend an adult day care center as a potential option for Mr. Everett to pursue? Find some of these in the Adult Day Center's pdf document linked from www.alz.org/living_with_alzheimers_respite_care.asp.*

The family asks you whether it is acceptable to leave Claudine at home alone for short periods of time on days when they do not have access to the adult day care center.

> 9. *What are three questions you would advise the family to consider as they grapple with this issue? You can find some of these at the website of the National Institute on Aging: www.nia. nih.gov/Alzheimers/Publications/homesafety.htm#safe.*

You enter Claudine's home one day and become aware that there are some things the family could do in the home to promote Claudine's safety. Particularly, you note some hazards as soon as you step inside the front door.

10. *What are two actions Claudine's family could take to promote safety in the home's entryway?*

The Everetts' oldest daughter, Mary, has announced to her father that she is ending her marriage of more than three decades. Mr. Everett is saddened by this news as he has always had a warm, friendly relationship with his son-in-law and worries for Mary's future as a single woman living alone. Mary insists her father not share this information with Claudine, stating, "Just make excuses why he doesn't attend family functions; Mom will never know the difference."

11. *What are your thoughts on how to best handle this situation in relation to Claudine knowing the truth?*

Suggested Resources

Alzheimer's Association. (2014a). *Respite care.* Retrieved from http://www.alz.org/living_with_ alzheimers_respite_care.asp

Alzheimer's Association. (2014b). *Standard treatments.* Retrieved from http://www.alz.org/ alzheimers_disease_standard_prescriptions.asp

Alzheimer's Association. (2014c). *Steps to diagnosis.* Retrieved from http://www.alz.org/ alzheimers_disease_steps_to_diagnosis.asp

Fletcher, K. (2012). *Nursing standard of practice protocol: Recognition and management of dementia.* Hartford Institute for Geriatric Nursing. Retrieved from http://consultgerirn.org/ topics/dementia/want_to_know_more

National Institute on Aging. (2014). *Home safety for people with Alzheimer's disease.* (NIH Publication No. 02-5179). Retrieved from http://www.nia.nih.gov/alzheimers/publication/ home-safety-people-alzheimers-disease/introduction

Reisberg, B. (2014). *Stages of Alzheimer's.* Alzheimer's Association. Retrieved from http://www .alz.org/alzheimers_disease_stages_of_alzheimers.asp

Case 17.3 ■ Dementia (Late Stage)

*N*ote: This is the same patient who was in the early stages of dementia described in a previous case study.

Claudine Everett, aged 85, lives in a skilled nursing care unit in a continuing care retirement community. She moved to this community about 5 years ago with her husband of 66 years after declining cognitive health resulted in her care being too difficult for the husband. Mr. and Mrs. Everett have three daughters who live near the retirement facility. For the past 5 years, with the help of the daughters, Mrs. Everett resided in an independent living apartment with her husband. She continued to decline cognitively, but her husband refused to move her to a higher level of care, insisting he could handle her. A few months ago she fell in her apartment, sustaining an ankle fracture that required surgery. Due to the level of care she needed after the fall, she was moved to the skilled nursing unit.

Within a few days of the fall and subsequent surgery, she suffered a bout with delirium, but this resolved after several days. However, since the move to the skilled care unit, her overall cognitive state has continued to decline. She often thinks her daughters are her siblings (many of whom have long since died), but usually recognizes her husband. Initially when moving to the skilled unit, her temperament was sometimes sour, a difference noted by the family. She threw her meal tray at times when frustrated, and repeatedly fell when getting out of her bed without assistance. She also begged to go with family members when they were leaving after a visit.

Questions 1 through 4 can be answered by going to the Alzheimer's Association (2014) website at www.alz.org. Click on "Professionals and Researchers." All of the handouts mentioned in the questions can be obtained under "Educational Materials."

1. *Obtain the pamphlet "Stages of Alzheimer's Disease." Based on this description, which stage of Alzheimer's disease does Claudine manifest?*

2. *Obtain the pamphlet "Behaviors" and list two ways the family can respond when Claudine exhibits confusion and calls family members by the wrong name.*

3. *The family also wants to know how to respond to her "begging" to go with them when they leave. Find a recommendation from the pamphlet "Behaviors" for the family to use in response to these repeated requests. What other ideas might work?*

Mr. Everett and his daughters participate in regular patient care conferences on the skilled unit. The nurse manager and the entire staff keep the family informed of Claudine's daily functioning. The family expresses gratitude for this level of communication, in addition to the physical and emotional support provided. In particular, they note the emphasis of maintaining an atmosphere conducive to individuals with advanced dementia.

4. *Discuss examples of providing a therapeutic and safe environment for an institutionalized individual with Alzheimer's disease.*

In the past month as she continues to decline, Claudine sometimes appears to be sleeping and is not readily arousable. Her family reports great distress seeing her in this debilitated state. The family insists that she be dressed each day and gotten out of bed. She must be fed now, and is sometimes incontinent of urine.

5. *Obtain the pamphlet "Communication" from the Alzheimer's Association website and identify two ways to best communicate with Claudine at this stage of her illness.*

Questions 6 through 9 can be answered by clicking on the section "Living With Alzheimer's" of the Alzheimer's Association website and then by clicking on "Late Stages of Care."

6. ***What recommendations are given for urinary incontinence?***

7. ***List three recommendations for helping Claudine eat and drink safely.***

8. ***Discuss three actions for keeping Claudine's skin healthy and free of skin breakdown.***

9. ***The family asks, "Is Claudine in pain?" What are some signs of pain in a person with Alzheimer's disease?***

10. ***Because Claudine is declining rapidly, the family wonders whether she would be eligible for hospice care while in the nursing home. Is hospice care available in a long-term care facility?***

11. ***What would be the purpose of involving hospice in her care since Claudine is already receiving long-term care?***

Suggested Resources

Alzheimer's Association. (2014a). *Behaviors. How to respond when dementia causes unpredictable behaviors.* Retrieved from http://www.alz.org/national/documents/brochure_behaviors.pdf

Alzheimer's Association. (2014b). *Stages of Alzheimer's.* Retrieved from http://www.alz.org/alzheimers_disease_stages_of_alzheimers.asp#stage7

American Cancer Society. (2014). *Where is hospice care given?* Retrieved from http://www.cancer.org/treatment/findingandpayingfortreatment/choosingyourtreatmentteam/hospicecare/hospice-care-settings

Fletcher, K. (2014). *Nursing standard of practice protocol: Recognition and management of dementia.* Hartford Institute for Geriatric Nursing. Retrieved from http://consultgerirn.org/topics/dementia/want_to_know_more

Case 17.4 ■ Wandering/Need for Movement

*M*ary Cottrell is a 73-year-old female who lives at home with her husband of 48 years, Wayne, in a small suburban town. She has one son from a previous marriage who lives approximately 15 minutes from her home and assists with the care of his mother when needed. Mary was diagnosed 3 years ago with probable Alzheimer's disease, the most common form of dementia, and has shown a steady decline in memory abilities as well as a fluctuation of mood. Although she is experiencing a marked decline in instrumental activities of daily living (IADL; Lawton & Brody,

1969) and one activities of daily living (ADL) item (Katz, Down, Cash, & Grotz, 1970), her physical strength remains unchanged, and she has a strong will to maintain her independence. She currently takes the following medications: Aricept (donepezil) 10 mg orally daily and vitamin E 400 IU orally daily.

At Mary's scheduled visit with her family physician, Wayne reports to Carol, the nurse manager whom she has increasingly mentioned, that she wants to "go home" even though she remains at the home she has lived in for the past 38 years. He reports that she has wandered away from their home four times at night over the past month,with the most recent resulting in the police finding her walking along the main highway in town. She told the police officers she was trying to "go home" but got lost, so they drove her around the neighborhood until she saw her house. She was able to identify her home at that moment in time and was satisfied that she was there. Wayne asks Carol for ideas on how to keep Mary safe and secure within their home, especially at night when he is asleep and doesn't know when she wanders. Carol offers several ideas, including having deadbolt locks on the doors that can only be accessed with a key or placing a sliding lock on the upper part of the doors where she cannot reach it. Carol also suggests that Wayne call the Alzheimer's Association or visit the website at www.alz.org to obtain more information on the behavior of wandering and a new GPS tracking service that is currently offered (www.alz.org/comfortzone/about_comfort_zone.asp) for individuals with dementia. Wayne is open to these suggestions, which will offer him peace of mind at night. However, he is hesitant of the locks due to the safety concerns of an emergency situation such as evacuation during a fire. He also does not want Mary to feel that she is locked or caged in her own home, but decides that it is necessary during the nighttime hours only when he is unable to watch after her.

At the following physician visit, Wayne reports to Carol that Mary continues to wake a few nights a week now, but does not wander outside due to the sliding locks he installed on the top of the two exterior doors of their home. She walks around the home with her purse under her arm and states she wants to "go home," and he has to convince her she is home and needs to go back to bed. He has also contacted the Alzheimer's Association to set up the new GPS tracking service for Mary in case she does wander away from home.

1. *What other ideas might the nurse suggest in order to keep Mary from wandering away at night?*

2. *Discuss how behavior modification may be helpful in this situation.*

3. *Locking a person in his or her home can present some ethical dilemmas. Discuss these issues while weighing them against the need for safety.*

4. *What national alert system resource might the nurse suggest if Mary ever wanders away from home and can't be immediately located?*

5. *Discuss how modifying the decor of the home environment may help the person with dementia stop wandering and "going home"?*

6. *If a person with dementia does wander out of the home, day or night, then what preventative measures can one take to maximize a safe return?*

7. *Where can Carol instruct Wayne to look for additional help and information about Mary's declining mental status and wandering behavior?*

8. *Why do individuals with dementia seem to wander often during the night?*

Suggested Resources

Alzheimer's Association. (2014). *Wandering and getting lost*. Retrieved from http://www.alz.org/care/alzheimers-dementia-wandering.asp

deWerd, M. M., Boelen, D., Rikkert, M. G. O., & Kessels, R. P. C. (2013). Errorless learning of everyday tasks in people with dementia. *Clinical Interventions in Aging, 8*, 1177–1190. Retrieved from http://www.ncbi.nlm.nih.gov/pmc/articles/PMC3775624

Katz, S., Down, T., Cash, H., & Grotz, R. (1970). Progress in the development of the index of ADL. *Gerontologist, 10*(1), 20–30.

Lawton, M., & Brody, E. (1969). Assessment of older people: Self-maintaining and instrumental activities of daily living. *Gerontologist, 9*, 179–186.

Mayo Clinic Staff. (2012). *Alzheimer's: Understand and control wandering*. Retrieved from http://www.mayoclinic.org/healthy-living/caregivers/in-depth/alzheimers/art-20046222

Wynn, L. (2014). *How does spaced retrieval therapy work?* Gray Matter Therapy. Retrieved from http://graymattertherapy.com/spaced_retrieval_therapy

Case 17.5 ■ Agitation and Aggression

Darryl Ison is a 73-year-old male living in an extended care facility on the Alzheimer's unit. He came here 2 weeks ago from several states away at his only child's insistence. Mr. Ison was living at home previously, his residence for five decades, and safety issues became a concern. His daughter, Melissa, provided the following history about her father.

Mr. Ison was an electrician and retired from his company at age 66. His wife died when he was 70 and had provided him with a wonderful life. He was pampered and catered to in every respect. Melissa describes her father as an intelligent and generous man, but not always easy to get along with during her years growing up. He was prone to be critical and sulk for hours if something didn't go his way. After her mother's death, several live-in housekeepers were hired; the longest stayed 3 months. All of the workers quit due to Mr. Ison's temper and argumentative nature.

Melissa coordinated meals to be prepared by a local chef and a week's worth delivered at a time, all laundry to be sent out, and cleaning of the home to occur twice a month. This method sufficed for 2 years.

On a weekend visit with her father, Melissa noted a number of issues that concerned her. A stack of overdue bills were found, his appearance was disheveled, he had not refilled prescription medication, and his short-term memory was noticeably impaired. He became angry and emotionally charged when he could not find an item such as his wallet, always accusing the cleaning service of stealing.

Melissa carefully negotiated three major changes with her father over the next several months. First, she convinced him to quit driving as it was a constant anger-provoking source (other drivers), and he forgot how to get home from well-known places on several occasions. A private chauffeur service was used, although having to arrange transportation in advance kept Mr. Ison constantly complaining.

She arranged for a home health service to divide out his medicines in a pill box designated by the days of the week every Monday. This strategy was only partially beneficial; Mr. Ison did not take the bedtime doses several times a week.

Finally, she had her father agree to answer the phone and speak with her three times a day so that she would know he was "okay"; this method never was successful as Mr. Ison either could not find the phone, or was asleep, or expressed anger toward Melissa for living so far away to even require this system of communication.

The final consequence of Mr. Ison's anger before moving away resulted in a criminal charge (which was eventually dropped). He handed a bank teller a check to cash and, in an effort to be friendly, the employee said, "How are things going today, Darryl?" Mr. Ison initially demanded to know how the teller knew his name; when told it was on the check, he became enraged that he was referred to by his first name, which was disrespectful behavior. He began swinging at the teller and cursing loudly. When a security guard approached him, Mr. Ison kicked him; thus, the police were called and took him away in handcuffs.

Melissa found a long-term care facility near her home and, within a week, had her father admitted. He had a physical, functional, and behavioral assessment and scored very high on the GDS. He was classified as having mild to moderate dementia. The decision was made to start off with a private room until his agitation and aggression was under better control. Melissa came to visit for an hour after dinner (7 p.m.–8 p.m.) on weekdays and stayed longer on the weekends.

1. ***In reviewing the client's past 7 years, what life changes likely contributed to his diagnosis of depression?***

2. ***What examples in the case reflect the onset of dementia?***

3. ***Adult children being caretakers of an elderly parent is common; was there anything you believe Melissa should have done differently over the previous several years?***

4. ***Explain how agitation is contrasted with aggression.***

Melissa finds her father's mood and functional ability to be much better when she visits him on Saturday mornings and early Sunday afternoons. One evening when she was leaving after a visit, she heard a nursing assistant remark, "He's starting to sundown" and asked the charge nurse what this term meant.

5. *Describe what Sundowner's syndrome entails and at least three contributing factors that may be associated.*

Mr. Ison's agitation continues at the long-term care facility. He complains loudly and curses over his food preparation, having to get dressed and bathe, and when he cannot find things such as his eyeglasses or the few family photos he brought to the facility. There have been no incidents of aggression insofar as attempting to physically assault, throwing items, or pounding his fists, such as occurred preadmission. Melissa chose a restraint-free facility for her father and talked at length before moving him there about treatment options for his agitation and periods of aggression. She preferred medications, in particular those with sedation properties, be used only as a last measure. A handout developed for family was provided that explained the facility's treatment approach, based on the Progressively Lowered Stress Threshold (PLST) Model (Hall & Buckwalter, 1987). Use www.rosalynncarter.org/caregiver_intervention_database/dimentia/individualized_plan_of_care_based_on_progressively_lowered_stress_threshold_model/ for Questions 6 through 8.

6. *What is an important assumption inherent in Hall and Buckwalter's (1987) PLST Model?*

7. *The PLST Model identifies six sources of stress for persons with dementia; what are they?*

The guiding principles of the PLST Model were developed to allow caregivers of persons with dementia to provide timely and appropriate interventions for agitated and aggressive behaviors.

8. *These principles include the following. Select all that apply.*

    a. *Maximize safe function by supporting losses in a prosthetic manner*

    b. *Provide unconditional positive regard*

    c. *Avoid foods, drinks, and medications that are known stimulants*

    d. *Teach caregivers to observe and "listen" to the patient*

    e. *Modify environments to support losses and enhance safety*

    f. *Provide ongoing support and assistance for informal and formal caregivers*

9. *An older male client with dementia has become physically aggressive triggered by a urinary tract infection. How would you position yourself in an enclosed room in an attempt for de-escalation?*

Geriatric "fiblets" (aka "white lies") are mentioned throughout the literature as a therapeutic approach to dealing with a dementia client experiencing agitation or aggression. For example, an individual who needs to move to a facility due to extreme wandering behavior is told, "Your apartment building is being renovated so you have to stay somewhere else for awhile."

10. What are your thoughts for using fiblets in dealing with a client who is displaying agitation or aggression?

Suggested Resources

Buckwalter, K. C. (2009). *Individualized plan of care based on Progressively Lowered Stress Threshold (PLST) model (Buckwalter)*. Rosalynn Carter Institute of Caregiving. Retrieved from http://www.rosalynncarter.org/caregiver_intervention_database/dimentia/individualized_plan_of_care_based_on_progressively_lowered_stress_threshold_model

Hall, G. R., & Buckwalter, K. C. (1987). Progressively lowered stress threshold: A conceptual model for care of adults with Alzheimer's disease. *Archives of Psychiatric Nursing, 1*(6), 399–406.

National Institute on Aging. (n.d.). *Coping with agitation and aggression*. Retrieved from http://www.nia.nih.gov/sites/default/files/Alzheimers_Caregiving_Tips_Coping_with_Agitation_and_Aggression.pdf

Novack, M. (2012). *The ethics of geriatric fiblets*. Moving Solutions. Retrieved from http://www.movingsolutions.com/2012/09/05/the-ethics-of-geriatric-fiblets

Warchol, K. (n.d.). *The "Progressively Lowered Stress Threshold" model—Understanding and minimizing challenging behaviors*. Crisis Prevention, CPI. Retrieved from http://www.crisisprevention.com/Resources/Article-Library/Dementia-Care-Specialists-Articles/Behavior-Management/The-Progressively-Lowered-Stress-Threshold-Model

18

Cultural Diversity

Case 18.1 ■ Culturally Specific Care—Part I

*T*he Part I case study for culturally specific care explores various facts, definitions, and concepts necessary for the student nurse (and eventual RN) to acquiesce the most holistic and caring skills possible when interacting with individuals from a variety of cultures. The Part II case addresses a situation whereby these skills can be applied.

A group of four nursing students share an apartment located in dormitory housing at a large, state university. The roommates often study together, with each person rotating as the group leader. Today's topic is culture-based nursing care; a combination multiple-choice/short-essay exam for their Intro to the Profession class is scheduled in 2 days.

In addition to the assigned chapter reading and PowerPoint notes the students received, the nursing instructor suggested another source for the class to be familiar with in relation to culture and the elderly client. It is from the Hartford Institute for Geriatric Nursing located at http://consultgerirn.org/topics/ethnogeriatrics_and_cultural_competence_for_nursing_practice/want_to_know_more, authored by Melen McBride.

Mary initiates the study time by asking whether everyone can remember the difference between the terms *culture* and *ethnicity*. She repeats the example given in class that culture represents the nonphysical inheritance, while ethnicity represents physical aspects of who we are as well as unique social characteristics, symbols, and behavior patterns, which may not be fully understood or shared by others. There are numerous definitions available for "culture," but two tenets hold steady: Culture is constantly changing, and it represents a complex whole comprised of many parts, all related to one another.

1. Identify a minimum of five components that are generally included in the definition of culture.

Next, Casey approaches another new term presented in class, *ethnocentric*. She reminds the group of the examples the instructor presented that helped her better understand this concept. Casey predicts there will be a multiple-choice question where they will have to choose one of the four statements that best represents the term.

2. After reviewing the definition, share an ethnocentric remark you have heard recently, or develop one as an example.

The nursing instructor shared a graph in class depicting current and future trends in diversity rates in America. She encouraged discussion about how the changing demographics may impact the students' careers: in particular, the need for cultural sensitivity, cultural appropriateness, and the goal to be culturally competent.

3. Using the website http://kff.org/disparities-policy/slide/ distribution-of-u-s-population-by-raceethnicity-2010-and-2050, transfer the statistics to the following table.

Table 18.1 Distribution of U.S. population by Race/Ethnicity, 2010 and 2050

	2010	2050
% White, non-Hispanic		
% Hispanic		
% Black, non-Hispanic		
% Asian		
% Other (Native Hawaiian, Pacific Islander, American Indian or Alaskan Native, individuals of two or more races		

Source: Kaiser Family Foundation (2013).

4. What impact do you believe the changes projected for 2050 may have on the profession of nursing?

The study group talked about an in-class exercise each of them completed. Mary found filling out the Heritage Assessment Tool (Cultural Care Guide, 2014) very valuable. Morgan agreed, stating, "It was a great way to increase our self-awareness which was a major focus of the class." The instructor collected the assessment tools with the intention of combining all responses and sharing the aggregate results confidentially. Morgan adds, "Like she said, we think of ourselves as homogenous; all nursing students, close in age, a 90% female class, but our heritages will definitely show the unique traits we possess."

5. Take several minutes to fill out the Heritage Assessment Tool at http://wps.prenhall.com/chet_spector_cultural_7/94/24265/6211875 .cw/index.html. As the instructions indicate, add the positive responses and briefly discuss your personal identification with traditional heritage versus a North American, modern culture.

Techniques for establishing trust prior to using an assessment tool of any kind was addressed in the students' reading. In particular, specific strategies in working with older patients of diverse cultures such as a calm approach, showing humility versus an air of authority, and taking sufficient time were all recommended.

> 6. *What additional strategies would be appropriate in preparing to assess culture in an older person? Select all that apply.*
>
> a. *Addressing the individual by the first name.*
>
> b. *Avoid any type of informal conversation (aka "chit-chat")*
>
> c. *Avoid the "invisible patient syndrome"*
>
> d. *Ask for help in understanding the client's cultural components as needed.*

Another major section of the upcoming students' test involves working with the older client to maximize verbal and nonverbal communication in regard to providing culturally sensitive care. They each recall examples discussed in class and visit the website the instructor recommended to gain additional information.

> 7. *For each of the following categories, list one strategy the nurse should implement for a specific identified cultural group: physical distance, eye contact, emotional expressiveness, and body movements.*

The group's last topic for review is cultural competence, defined in their assigned reading: "To be culturally competent the nurse needs to understand his or her own world views and those of the patient, while avoiding stereotyping and misapplication of scientific knowledge. Cultural competence is obtaining cultural information and then applying that knowledge. This cultural awareness allows you to see the entire picture and improves the quality of care and health outcomes" (Transcultural Nursing, 2012).

Terry, another roommate, states she feels certain a short-essay question will be present on the exam asking why cultural competency is so important. Notes from class emphasized health care systems where cultural competency is valued have improved health outcomes and quality of care and can contribute to the elimination of racial and ethnic health disparities. The foursome finishes their studying by discussing a video shown in class on the topic.

> 8. *Watch the video at www.youtube.com/watch?v=MTh3pe8N3DQ and comment on any new information you acquired or your reaction to the content.*

Suggested Resources

Cultural Care Guide. (2014). Pearson Education. Retrieved from http://wps.prenhall.com/chet_spector_cultural_7/94/24265/6211875.cw

Kaiser Family Foundation. (2013). *Distribution of U.S. population by race/ethnicity, 2010 and 2050*. Retrieved from http://kff.org/disparities-policy/slide/distribution-of-u-s-population-by-raceethnicity-2010-and-2050

McBride, M. (n.d.). *Ethnogeriatrics and cultural competence for nursing practice.* Hartford Institute for Geriatric Nursing. Retrieved from http://consultgerirn .org/topics/ethnogeriatrics_and_cultural_competence_for_nursing_practice/ want_to_know_moreractice/want_to_know_more

Spector, R. E. (2009). Heritage assessment tool. In R. Spector (Ed.), *Cultural care: Guide to heritage assessment and health traditions* (5th ed.). Upper Saddle River, NJ: Pearson Education/ PH College.

Transcultural Nursing. (2012). *Cultural competency.* Retrieved from http://www.culturediversity .org/cultcomp.htm

Case 18.2 ■ Culturally Specific Care—Part II

*T*he following story features Hosea Rivera, a 70-year-old Hispanic male, as he has an initial health care visit with a focus on the ethnogeriatric components used to assist him in acquiring the medical attention he seeks. Two websites can be used as references to answer the questions, or other sources may be sought (and appropriately cited). These include the following: *Health and Health Care of Hispanic/Latino American Elders,* www.stanford.edu/group/ethnoger/ index.html (Talmantes, Lindeman, & Mouton, 2001), along with *Ethnogeriatrics and Cultural Competence for Nursing Practice* (McBride, n.d.) located on the Hartford Institute for Geriatric Nursing website: http://consultgerirn.org/topics/ ethnogeriatrics_and_cultural_competence_for_nursing_practice/want_to_know_more.

1. ***Ethnogeriatrics may be a term students and nurses are unfamiliar with. Provide a definition.***

2. ***Mr. Rivera was noted as being Hispanic. What further definition is used to note the countries included for this ethnicity category?***

Mr. Rivera has come to a mental health clinic previously used with positive results by another Hispanic relative several years ago. He is well groomed, appropriately dressed for the weather, appears to be younger than his stated age, and is height and weight proportionate. His adolescent grandson was to accompany him; however, he had difficulty awakening at 9 a.m., so Mr. Rivera came to the appointment alone.

The geropsych nurse practitioner seeing the client today is Brody Hyatt. He begins by greeting Mr. Rivera, shaking his hand, and escorting him to a private room. From experience, Brody knows it is quite important to determine Mr. Rivera's level of acculturation prior to taking a history. A standard practice is to obtain vital signs on all new clients. Mr. Rivera participates in this process with no apparent hesitation. When asked about the presence and rating of pain, there is a moment of silence. Brody follows with the questions in Spanish, and Mr. Rivera nods "yes." When asked where, the client holds his hand over the left chest and his facial expression is one of sadness. Finally, Brody asks in Spanish for a pain rating and is told "10."

3. Describe what a "level of acculturation" entails. Why is it important to know?

4. What is recommended as informal indicators of acculturation that can be used quickly by a health care provider for assessment?

Brody learns Mr. Rivera has been in the United States for less than 10 years. In his apartment reside his mother, sister, daughter-in-law, and two grandchildren. The grandsons and their mother are fluent in English; the others speak Spanish exclusively to one another. Brody knows he needs assistance in communication in order to provide quality care.

5. Will an interpreter or a translator be contacted to assist with the health intake interview?

Cultural competency in geriatrics is a very important skill Brody strives to achieve in his everyday practice with Hispanic clients. For an individual serving as a direct provider, this involves (a) awareness of one's personal biases and their impact on professional behavior; (b) knowledge of (1) population-specific health-related cultural values, beliefs, and behaviors; (2) disease incidence, prevalence, or mortality rates; and (3) population-specific treatment outcomes; and (c) skills in working with culturally diverse populations (McBride, n.d.).

6. Which of the following is included in suggestions for successful communication with an elderly Hispanic or Latino client? Select all that apply.

a. Gesturing with the hands is encouraged

b. Addressing the individual by his or her last name

c. Knowing some persons nod "yes," but do not comprehend the message

d. Realizing questioning of authority may be considered unacceptable

Although he makes an effort to continuously learn the Spanish language, Brody still requires help. Adults of all ages are discouraged from bringing a child in to serve as an interpreter, yet this continues to happen with regularity. He has attended many seminars and used self-study programs to be as informed as possible. Being very knowledgeable of cultural themes and incorporating them into his interactions with clients is one example of his efforts.

7. Complete the following table using the information found at http://web.stanford.edu/group/ethnoger/index.html.

Table 18.2 Description of Hispanic or Latino Cultural Themes

Cultural Theme	Description
Familismo	
Personalismo	
Jerarquismo	
Presentismo	
Espiritismo	

Source: Talmantes, Lindeman, and Mouton (2001).

With assistance from the clinic's interpreter, Brody learns that Mr. Rivera's pain rating is heartache associated, not cardiac in origin. His only son, who also lived with the nuclear family, died in a tragic accident last month. Mr. Rivera explains they were best friends and depended on one another for emotional support. In addition, the loss of income (and no life insurance) has worried the women in the family.

Mr. Rivera's mother is 87 years old and is bedbound from a variety of chronic illnesses. His sister attends to her toileting and bathing needs, and he assists with feeding, turning, medication administration, and trying to keep her comfortable in general. He shares that since his son's death, he has not been sleeping at night and fatigue has made him irritable toward family members. In addition, he is a non-insulin-dependent diabetic and self-monitors glucose levels, which have been erratic the past month.

Brody administers the Spanish version of the Geriatric Depression Scale and finds Mr. Rivera scoring a "9," indicative of depression. He inquires about suicide ideation, and it is denied firmly. As far as past coping mechanisms, Mr. Rivera states talking, joking, and just spending time with his son was always used successfully in times of stress or grief. Brody asks whether the client can come in weekly for perhaps 2 months, and he agrees. The clinic has a group therapy session for male Hispanics, which Mr. Rivera turns down. On his own accord, he decides to begin attending an early morning Catholic mass at a parish in the neighborhood, stating going each Sunday gives him a little comfort, so perhaps more often would be beneficial.

Mr. Rivera asks about medication, and Brody reviews the antidepressant options with him. He includes adverse affects for the drug Zoloft (sertraline), which the clinic uses regularly, for the reduced rate at which they can purchase it. When Brody mentions erectile dysfunction (impotence) as a possibility, Mr. Rivera says "No, no, no."

Mr. Rivera returned for only one other visit to the mental health clinic. The family did not have a phone, which ruled out contacting him via this route. He chose to forgo "American medicine" and began seeing a *curandero* who recommended he continue attending mass daily, along with using herbs for his depression.

8. What role does a curandero serve in the Hispanic culture? Provide at least two herbs commonly used for depression as a complementary health measure.

Suggested Resources

McBride, M. (n.d.). *Ethnogeriatrics and cultural competence for nursing practice.* Hartford Institute for Geriatric Nursing. Retrieved from http://consultgerirn.org/topics/ethnogeriatrics_and_cultural_competence_for_nursing_practice/want_to_know_more

Motel, S., & Patten, E. (2012). *The 10 largest Hispanic origin groups: Characteristics, rankings, top counties.* Pew Research. Retrieved from http://www.pewhispanic.org/2012/06/27/the-10-largest-hispanic-origin-groups-characteristics-rankings-top-counties

Talmantes, M., Lindeman, R., & Mouton, C. (2001). *Health and health care of Hispanic/Latino American elders* (2nd ed.). Stanford Geriatric Center. Supported by the Bureau of Health Professions Health Resources and Services Administration U.S. Department of Health and Human Services. Retrieved from http://www.stanford.edu/group/ethnoger/index.html

Case 18.3 ■ The Homeless Aging

Two 66-year-old men are sitting next to one another at a cafeteria-style table eating lunch provided by a service known as "Loaves and Fishes." This is a faith-based program that feeds the homeless and hungry every weekday. The men have discovered some similarities by sharing information about their pasts. Lee and Kirk grew up only several miles apart, although each attended a different high school. Upon graduation, Lee went to work for his father's painting company while Kirk attended the state university. From that point, their lives were quite different . . . until recently.

Lee was introduced to marijuana by his older brother; within a year he used it daily, in addition to heavy alcohol intake and "downers" on the weekends. He was able to function relatively well until he fell off a ladder while painting one day; the emergency room ran a drug test and reported high levels of several substances. His father fired him and demanded he leave his parents' home. For three decades, Lee went from one temporary manual labor job to the next, as well as lived with one woman after another. He fathered four children and paid child support sporadically. In his early 50s, Lee was introduced to one of the few substances he hadn't tried: crystal methamphetamine. He resorted to theft in order to support this need; as a result, he was imprisoned for 10 years. Lee has been homeless for 2 years.

Kirk graduated with a degree in finance and was hired by a nationally known investment company. He married at age 23 and was a father shortly thereafter, followed by two other children. His wife was a beautiful woman from a wealthy upbringing, and he constantly strived to please her. This entailed living far beyond their means: expensive home, furnishings, cars, private schools, an abundance of trendy clothes, jewelry, and so forth. Kirk had stock holdings in the company for which he worked but no savings and loads of debt that over more than three decades grew to an amount that he could no longer handle. His wife was never employed and adamantly refused to ask her family for assistance. Kirk considered suicide on several occasions as a way out of his highly stressed situation. Instead, he resorted to theft, diverting clients' investment funds to a falsified account for his own needs. He was caught for embezzlement during the same period the nation's banking industry fell apart; all of his stock holdings were worthless. His wife and children disowned him. Like Lee, he served 10 years in prison, to be released as a homeless elder.

1. ***The Housing and Urban Development (HUD) department has suggested changes to how homelessness is defined. Using the website, www.endhomelessness.org/library/entry/changes-in-the-hud-definition-of-homeless, describe the current definition.***

Use the article "Aging and Housing Instability: Homelessness Among Older and Elderly Adults," found at www.nhchc.org/wp-content/uploads/2011/09/infocus_ september2013.pdf, for assistance with the next three questions.

2. ***The number of elderly homeless is on the rise and is projected to increase tremendously by 2050. What is the reason for this?***

3. ***Discuss how health care utilization is affected by homelessness.***

The article notes, "The consequences of weathering on health status emerge with age. Unstably housed adults over 50 experience higher rates of geriatric syndromes at younger ages than the general population of older adults, such as falls and memory loss."

4. ***Describe what these geriatric syndromes entail and the potential outcome of experiencing them.***

5. ***Advance care planning is challenging for an older homeless individual; what aspect in particular is addressed in the article?***

6. ***Kirk and Lee became homeless from very different directions. What are other causes do you believe may contribute to this plight?***

7. ***What resources are available in the area where you live for homeless individuals? If there are none, what would you suggest to someone in need of assistance?***

8. ***Watch the video,* A Day in the Life of the Homeless, *produced by Eric Miller (2009), found at www.youtube.com/ watch?v=27Gf5HAg6_0. Which individual featured had the most impact on you and why?***

Suggested Resources

Miller, E. (2013). *A day in the life of the homeless* [Video file]. Retrieved from https://www.youtube .com/watch?v=27Gf5HAg6_0

National Alliance to End Homelessness. (2012). *Changes in the HUD definition of "homeless."* Retrieved from http://www.endhomelessness.org/library/entry/changes-in-the-hud-definition-of-homeless

National HCH Council. (2013). Aging and housing instability: Homelessness among older and elderly adults. *A Quarterly Research Review of the National HCH Council, 2*(1). Retrieved from http://www.nhchc.org/wp-content/uploads/2011/09/infocus_september2013.pdf

Case 18.4 ■ The Baby Boomer Culture

*T*his case study will focus on a group of people, rather than an individual client. The group (aka cohort) are those persons born between the years of 1946 and 1964, referred to as the baby boomers. It has been predicted by the U.S. Census Bureau that 71.4 million people will be age 65 or older in 2029. This means that the elderly ages 65 and older will make up about 20% of the U.S. population by 2029, up from almost 14% in 2012 (Pollard & Scommengna, 2014). "So what?" you might ask. The growth in population of older adults in the next couple of decades represents both the largest number in history, as well as representing the recipients in need of health care services for nurses graduating during that same time period.

A generational cohort represents groups of people who were born in the same date range and share similar cultural experiences. "Generational profiles, while not infallible, help us to understand how the life experiences of a generation capture the attention and emotions of millions of individuals at a formative stage in their lives and ultimately affect personal core values. Although there is no absolute beginning or end to generational groups, they typically span 15 to 20 years" (Duchscher & Cowin, 2004). The historical, political, and social events experienced by generational cohorts are important to know and appreciate by nurses who provide health care services to these groups.

The study of generational diversity and published analyses are predominantly driven by the field of sociology. In reviewing the literature, articles in nursing journals comparing and contrasting generational cohorts are most abundant shortly after the millennium. The focus at that time was a multigenerational workforce and the consequences for nursing leadership (Duchscher & Cowin, 2004; Hart, 2006; Sherman, 2006; Ulrich, 2001; Weston, 2001; Wieck, Prydun, & Walsh, 2002).

Each of the generational cohorts has the commonality of events that have an impact on all members of the generation in one way or another during their formative years. However, it is important, as has been stressed from "day one" in any nursing program, to always view the person as an individual. Demographic profiling is essentially an exercise in making generalizations about groups of people. Please keep in mind, as with all such generalizations, many individuals within these groups will not conform to the profile.

What types of things comprise a generation to receive a specific label? Sociologists study defining characteristics that are largely attributed to the social spheres at that point in time. The groupings of generational cohorts identified since 1900 are:

- G.I. Generation 1901–1924
- Silent Generation: 1925–1945
- Baby Boomers: 1946–1964
- Generation X: 1965–1980
- Millennial Generation: 1981–2000

1. *Prior to focusing on the baby boomer generation, find the defining characteristics of your generation (or any other) using the Internet and cite the source.*

2. *According to the author, what was the single defining historical event during the baby boom generation?*

3. *What two cultural events united the early (1946–1955) leading-edge boomers with those born from 1956–1964, known as the shadow boomers?*

4. *What are several examples of how this generation shaped the political arena like no other group previously?*

5. *What are the growth industries for companies wanting to market to the boomers? How do you see yourself as a part of this future market?*

6. *Briefly summarize the information pertaining to baby boomers and second careers.*

7. *What impact is predicted for Social Security and Medicare funds by the aging of the baby boomers?*

8. *Describe what is meant by an "ethical will."*

9. *What trends regarding end-of-life choices are baby boomers creating?*

Suggested Resources

Duchscher, J. E., & Cowin, L. (2004). Multigenerational nurses in the workplace. *Journal of Nursing Administration, 34*(11), 493–501.

Hart, S. M. (2006). Generation diversity: Impact on recruitment and retention of nurses. *Journal of Nursing Administration, 36*(1), 10–12.

Neilsen, D. (2014). *Baby boomers: All you ever needed to know.* HowStuffWorks.com. Retrieved from http://health.howstuffworks.com/wellness/aging/baby-boomers/baby-boomers.htm

Pollard. K., & Scommengna, P. (2014). *Just how many baby boomers are there?* Population Reference Bureau. Retrieved from http://www.prb.org/Publications/Articles/2002/JustHowManyBabyBoomersAreThere.aspx

Sherman, R., (2006, May 31). Leading a multigenerational nursing workforce: Issues, challenges and strategies. *OJIN: The Online Journal of Issues in Nursing, 11*(2), Manuscript 2.

Ulrich, B. T. (2001). Successfully managing a multigenerational workforce. *Seminars for Nurse Managers, 9*(3), 147–153.

Weston, M. (2001). Coaching generations in the workplace. *Nursing Administration Quarterly, 25*(2), 11–21.

Wieck, K. L., Prydun, M., & Walsh, T. (2002). What the emerging workforce wants in its leaders. *Journal of Nursing Scholarship, 34*(3), 283–288.

19

Pain Management in the Older Adult

Case 19.1 ■ Undertreatment of Pain

John Jones, age 84, has been in a long-term care facility for 4 years after the death of his wife who was his primary caregiver. Mr. Jones has a history of hypertension, type 2 diabetes (controlled by diet) with the long-term or chronic complication of peripheral neuropathy, osteoarthritis (OA), and gastroesophageal reflux disease. His medications include aspirin (acetylsalicylic acid) 81 mg every morning, Lasix (furosemide) 20 mg twice a day, Tylenol (acetaminophen) 650 mg every 4 hours as needed for pain, and Prilosec (omeprazole) 20 mg twice a day.

Mr. Jones becomes agitated when he is assisted out of bed in the morning and winces with pain. He often complains of his hands, knees, and lower legs hurting. The pain he describes in his hands and knees can be considered pain from arthritis. He takes Tylenol for arthritis pain when offered but states there is little relief. He rates the pain in his hands and knees as a "6" (on a scale of "0" being no pain and "10" being the worst pain possible), and it decreases to a "4" after the Tylenol is given. He rates the pain in his lower legs as a "10," and this pain decreases to a "7" after taking Tylenol. When reviewing his medication records, you notice that he takes the Tylenol twice a day, usually in the morning with breakfast and at bedtime. The nurse caring for Mr. Jones notes that he will take medication when asked whether he is in pain, but otherwise he does not complain of pain. Mr. Jones states, "I can deal with the pain in my hands and knees, but my legs hurt all the time." As a nurse, you are aware that pain is a significant problem in the older adult population as at least 50% of community-dwelling older adults, and as many as 85% of nursing home residents, suffer from pain and that pain is often undertreated in this population (Horgas, Yoon, & Grall, 2012).

1. Identify four myths or misconceptions about pain and the management of pain in the older adult population that may have an effect on the undertreatment of Mr. Jones's pain and discuss why these myths may occur.

It is clear that the pain Mr. Jones is experiencing is not being managed in a way that will provide him comfort. Pain is often undertreated in the older adult population related to factors found in health care providers as well as patients themselves.

2. *Discuss the factors that add to the problem of undertreatment of pain in the older adult population.*

3. *What are some of the major problems for the older adult who suffers from untreated pain?*

4. *Mr. Jones has been offered morphine as well as other adjuvant medications for the pain in his legs, but he refuses as he states, "I don't want to get addicted to that stuff." How would you describe the use of morphine for pain and the potential for addiction?*

As a nurse, you understand that the Joint Commission on Accreditation of Health Care Organizations requires nursing assessment of pain as a requirement to be in compliance with regulatory guidelines for pain management.

5. *Describe how you would assess Mr. Jones's pain and a tool that can be used to assess pain in the older adult.*

6. *Describe the World Health Organization's Three-Step Analgesic Ladder for pain management, considering the pain that Mr. Jones is experiencing. He is having a moderate level of pain, "6," on a scale of 1–10 related to the arthritis in his hands and knees. He is also experiencing a severe level of pain in his lower extremities related to diabetic neuropathy (he rates his pain as a "10" [on a scale of 1–10]).*

In addition to pharmacological pain relief measures, Mr. Jones could benefit from nonpharmacologic measures to decrease both his arthritis pain as well as the neuropathic pain in his lower extremities.

7. *Discuss several nonpharmacological techniques for pain management.*

Suggested Resources

Horgas, A. L., Yoon, S. L., &, Grall, M. (2012). *Nursing standard of practice protocol: Pain management in older adults.* Hartford Institute for Geriatric Nursing. Retrieved from http://consultgerirn.org/topics/pain/want_to_know_more

Thielke, S., Sale, J., & Reid, C. M. (2012). AGING: Are these 4 pain myths complicating care? *The Journal of Family Practice, 61*(11), 666–670. Retrieved from http://www.chronicpainperspectives.com/articles/feature-article/article/aging-are-these-4-pain-myths-complicating-care/0bf757e1f76f31745e78b94866999973.html

World Health Organization. (n.d.). *WHO's cancer pain ladder for adults.* Retrieved from http://www.who.int/cancer/palliative/painladder/en/

Case 19.2 ■ Side Effects of Opioids

*H*elen Neuschwander, age 77, is in an inpatient hospice facility with the diagnosis of end-stage lung disease. Her husband of 56 years is with her on a daily basis, and her children are also able to visit almost daily. She is awake and alert, able to eat small amounts, but is beginning to withdraw from her family. She is talking less and sleeping for short periods of time throughout the day. Morphine (1 mg every 4 hours) around the clock is being used to decrease the sensation of shortness of breath and manage pain she is experiencing. When the first two doses of morphine are given, Helen complains of nausea that subsides after she eats several crackers.

1. *As a nurse, what would you teach Helen about the side effect of nausea, which may occur when an opioid narcotic is given?*

2. *What is the most common side effect of opioid analgesics? What nursing interventions can act to prevent this unwanted side effect?*

Mrs. Neuschwander's family is concerned that the morphine being used to treat her shortness of breath and pain is causing her to sleep more. As the nurse caring for Helen, you have seen a decline in her overall condition and a decreased level of pain; in addition, she is breathing comfortably with a rate of 16 breaths per minute.

3. *How will you discuss the side effect of sleepiness with her family?*

For more than 4 weeks, the family notices that when Helen's pain increases, the dosages of morphine are also increasing. They are fearful of the higher doses and that Helen may suffer an "overdose." You have assessed Helen and find that her blood pressure is 110/70, heart rate 86, and respirations are 16 (regular and nonlabored).

4. *Describe the term "tolerance" that is found with narcotic medications and how you would discuss this term with Helen's concerned family.*

Mrs. Neuschwander begins to have a decreased urine output despite no change in oral intake. You assess her abdomen and find that her bladder is distended and firm. She states that she "feels like I have to go" but cannot urinate.

5. *What side effect of the opioid, morphine, may be occurring? Why is this occurring; and what nursing interventions will you implement?*

One month later, it is apparent that her overall physical condition is declining and that she is "actively dying," which means that death is going to occur. The family has been provided support and teaching about Helen's decline in function and impending death. Two months after beginning morphine for pain and shortness of breath, Mrs. Neuschwander becomes somnolent and begins to have jerking motions in her upper and lower extremities.

> 6. *What is the medical terminology for this type of jerking motion, why may it be occurring, and what can be done about this side effect of opioid use?*
>
> 7. *The final side effect of opioid analgesics that must be addressed is the potential for respiratory depression. How do you define and assess for respiratory depression? What medication is used to reverse respiratory depression? Who is at highest risk to develop respiratory depression?*

Suggested Resources

American Cancer Society. (2014). *Pain control.* Retrieved from http://www.cancer .org/Treatment/TreatmentsandSideEffects/PhysicalSideEffects/Pain/PainDiary/ pain-control-opioid-pain-medicines

Wells, N., Pasero, C., & McCaffery, M. (2008). Improving the quality of care through pain assessment and management. In R. G. Huges (Ed.), *Patient safety and quality: An evidence-based handbook for nurses.* Retrieved from http://www.ncbi.nlm.nih.gov/books/NBK2658/

Case 19.3 ■ Adjuvants for Pain Control

*F*rank James is a 78-year-old male who is living at the home of his youngest daughter after surgery for a right below-the-knee amputation related to a long-term complication of peripheral vascular disease. Frank has a history of depression that continues to affect his mental health despite the use of Celexa (citalopram hydrobromide) 10 mg orally once a day for 3 years. Frank was diagnosed 2 years ago with type 2 diabetes (which is well controlled with oral medications) and coronary artery disease. Frank also has a long-standing history of low back pain from compression fractures as a result of osteoporosis. In addition to these medical diagnoses, Frank has periods of severe muscle discomfort in his back and lower extremities when he suffers from a decreased mobility related to uncontrolled pain. As Frank has a multitude of chronic pain syndromes, a palliative care nurse practitioner who is experienced in gerontological nursing has been consulted to see Mr. James for pain control. The nurse practitioner will assess Mr. James's pain and suggest treatment measures that will include the use of adjuvant medications. As a practicing home care nurse, you need knowledge of pain control measures that utilize adjuvant medications to treat pain.

> ### 1. How would you describe an adjuvant medication that is used for pain control to Mr. James and his daughter?

Four causes or types of pain that the palliative care nurse practitioner has identified that Mr. Jones is experiencing are neuropathic pain, bone pain, phantom limb pain, and muscle spasticity that is causing an increase in pain.

> ### 2. Describe these four types of pain as they relate to Mr. Jones and how they are often managed with adjuvant medications.

> ### 3. Identify three common classifications of adjuvant medications that are commonly used for pain control. Within these classifications, identify the generic and trade names of common drugs used for pain management.

> ### 4. Identify benefits of using adjuvants for pain control.

> ### 5. Identify general precautions that need to be considered when utilizing adjuvants for pain control in the older adult population.

> ### 6. Identify potential side effects of nonsteroidal anti-inflammatory drugs (NSAIDs) as used for pain management in the older adult population.

> ### 7. Identify potential side effects of antidepressants as used as an adjuvant for pain management in the older adult population.

> ### 8. Identify potential side effects of corticosteroids as used as an adjuvant for pain management in the older adult population.

> ### 9. Identify potential side effects of anticonvulsants as used as an adjuvant for pain management in the older adult population.

> ### 10. Identify potential side effects of muscle relaxants as used as an adjuvant for pain management in the older adult population.

Suggested Resources

Boomershine, C. S. (2013). *Adjuvant nonopioid medications for managing chronic pain.* Pain Medicine News. Retrieved from http://www.painmedicinenews.com/download/Adjuvant_PMNSE13_WM.pdf

Candiotto, K., Gitlin, M. C., & Ciliberti, M. M. (2011). *Opioid adjunvans for multimodal pain management.* McMahon Publishing. Retrieved from http://www.painmedicinenews.com/download/NonOpioid_PMNSE11_WM.pdf

Case 19.4 ▪ Noninvasive Interventions for Pain

Marie Taylor is a 72-year-old woman who was diagnosed with OA in 1994. She is 66.5 inches tall, and weighs 226 pounds. She has come to the community health clinic to be seen for increasing pain in both knees. Miranda Fuller, clinic admission nurse, takes a health history.

Ms. Taylor says she is a retired nursing assistant, has never been married, and lives with her sister. She states that pain interferes with recreational activities and work. Weight management has been difficult; she cannot walk long distances and has difficulty with stairs, particularly descending. She states that her knees are stiff for about 30 minutes when she gets out of bed in the morning, and for a few minutes after getting up from a chair. Although sitting and resting reduce her pain, she becomes stiff if she stays in one position for too long. Ms. Taylor reports that she takes Tylenol Extra Strength (acetaminophen) 500 mg every 4 hours for pain. She states, "My pain wakes me up in the night, so I take it twice at night." Miranda notes that Ms. Taylor has great difficulty rising from a chair, and audible crepitation is heard when Ms. Taylor bends her knees.

1. *What history or physical examination findings should be of the greatest concern to the admissions nurse?*

2. *What risk factors did Ms. Taylor have for developing OA?*

Ms. Taylor shares, "My sister rubs my knees twice a day to make the pain better. It does not help, but she says it always works for her."

3. *What other interventions might relieve Ms. Taylor's knee pain? Go to the following website, http://consultgerirn.org/topics/pain/want_to_know_more#item_8, and identify some nonpharmacologic interventions that Miranda might suggest that Ms. Taylor use to relieve her chronic knee pain (Horgas, Yoon, & Grall, 2012).*

Ms. Taylor tells Miranda, "I wear magnets on my knees to help the pain. I also take glucosamine every day, because I read in a magazine that it really helps cure arthritis."

4. *What does research show about the effectiveness of Ms. Taylor's self-care practices? Go to the following website, http://nccam.nih .gov/research/results/gait, and identify information about the use of magnets and glucosamine plus chondroitin for the relief of pain from OA (National Institutes for Health: National Center for Complementary and Alternative Medicine, 2012).*

Ms. Taylor tells Miranda that she feels "useless," because she cannot work and has difficulty with activities of daily living (ADL). She states, "All I do is sit around, which makes things worse. I used to belong to a quilt club, and the senior center."

5. What lifestyle changes can Miranda suggest to Ms. Taylor? Write out a complete teaching plan for Miranda to give to Ms. Taylor.

Ms. Taylor reports that her symptoms are worse on cold days, and she frequently feels as if both of her knees will "give out."

6. Identify the ways that referrals to physical therapy or occupational therapy might be of assistance to Ms. Taylor.

7. What other referrals might Miranda make to assist Ms. Taylor?

Ms. Taylor tells Miranda that she lives in a two-story house, with one full bathroom on the first floor, and all bedrooms and another bathroom on the second floor. She says, "My sister has to help me take a bath, because we are both afraid that I might fall. She would never be able to get me off the floor."

8. What modifications to Ms. Taylor's home environment might be helpful?

Ms. Taylor returns to the clinic in 1 month. She has lost 5 pounds and says that she does quadriceps exercises while sitting in the chair. She has reduced her use of Tylenol (acetaminophen) to no more than eight 500 mg capsules per day. Ms. Taylor asks whether there is anything else that she can do to relieve her knee pain. She says, "There has to be something else I can do."

9. Go to the following website, www.webmd.com/osteoarthritis/ guide/national-institute-arthritis-musculoskeletal-skin- diseases?page=13, and identify information about scientific studies of complementary and alternative treatment for the management of chronic pain. What can Miranda tell Ms. Taylor about these studies?

10. Some lifestyle and self-care practices may worsen chronic pain. What should Miranda teach Ms. Taylor to avoid?

Suggested Resources

Horgas, A. L., Yoon, S. L., & Grall, M. (2012). *Nursing standard of practice protocol: Pain management in older adults*. Hartford Institute for Geriatric Nursing. Retrieved from http://consultgerirn.org/topics/pain/want_to_know_more#item_8

National Center for Complementary and Alternative Medicine. (2012). *Glucosamine/chondroitin arthritis intervention trial* (GAIT). Retrieved from http://nccam.nih.gov/research/results/gait

National Center for Complementary and Alternative Medicine. (2013). *Chronic pain and complementary health approaches: What you need to know*. Retrieved from http://nccam.nih.gov/health/pain/chronic.htm#hed2

National Institute of Arthritis and Musculoskeletal and Skin Diseases. (2013). *Handout on health: Osteoarthritis*. Retrieved from http://www.niams.nih.gov/Health_Info/Osteoarthritis

20

Sleep Disturbances in the Older Adult

Case 20.1 ■ Restless Legs Syndrome

JoAnn Gibson is a 79-year-old widow who resides with her youngest daughter's family. She agreed to give up her home and live with her daughter, Kim, when her son-in-law became unemployed 2 years ago. The grandchildren in the family are ages 17, 15, and 12. JoAnn is very content with the living arrangements and often thinks of the contrast of this nuclear family compared to how she raised her own.

Kim returned to teaching high school math and tutors students several evenings a week and Saturday mornings. Her husband, a former bank manager, lost a lucrative position due to the nation's economic crisis. He keeps very busy providing much of the house and yard work, helping his elderly parents who live nearby, and attending the children's school events. All of the grandchildren are involved in sports and clubs, and maintain above average grades.

JoAnn's primary duties in the household include doing all of the family's laundry and assisting with meal preparation. In addition, she provides transportation for the youngest child's activities as the older two share an automobile. She has her own bedroom on the second floor where the children also sleep. Kim and her husband use a former dining room on the main floor as a master bedroom.

Socially, JoAnn attends a support group for widows or widowers and sees former neighbors once a month. She has noticed other widows not being as friendly toward her since moving into her daughter's home; after a period of time, she mentioned this to the group's leader. Her remark was, "They are obviously jealous of you."

1. What may be the underlying reason for this behavior toward JoAnn?

JoAnn has been experiencing problematic sleep in recent months. She has a long-term habit of retiring at 10 p.m. and awakening at 6 a.m. Although she falls asleep easily, she awakens shortly thereafter due to an unpleasant feeling in her legs. She finds herself needing to constantly move her legs due to a combination of a tugging sensation and a creepy-crawling up and down each extremity. Some nights, she has generalized itching. Moving her legs constantly for 20 minutes or so provides relief; however, only temporarily. JoAnn dozes back to sleep, then awakens within an hour to start the process over again.

Eventually, JoAnn will get up and apply moisturizing lotion, take an Advil (ibuprofen) 200 mg tablet, and walk around her small room. Often she thinks about going downstairs to have something to eat, watch TV, or even fold laundry; however, this may wake Kim and her son-in-law, so she refrains from doing so. She has never experienced any of her symptoms during the daytime hours. On nights when the sensation is worse, JoAnn typically falls asleep deeply around 4 a.m. and struggles to awaken at 6 a.m. to begin fixing breakfast for the grandchildren and start her daily duties.

Believing her daughter and son-in-law have enough worries and responsibilities, JoAnn does not share what she has been experiencing. One afternoon after a rough night, she decides to take a brief nap prior to picking up her grandson from basketball practice. She slept deeply for several hours and awoke in a panic when she looked at the clock. Her daughter picked up the child after another parent loaned him a cell phone to call for a ride. JoAnn felt terribly guilty and told her daughter about the problem with her legs. Kim investigated the symptoms on the Internet and said, "Mom, it appears you have restless legs syndrome."

Use the Restless Legs Syndrome Fact Sheet (National Institute of Neurological Disorders and Stroke, 2014) found at the website http://www.ninds.nih.gov/disorders/restless_legs/detail_restless_legs.htm for Questions 2 through 4.

2. Left untreated, what psychosocial issues and problems with activities of daily living can occur?

JoAnn makes an appointment with a health care provider. When she phoned to be seen, the receptionist inquired about the need for a visit. JoAnn stated that she thought she had a muscular problem in her lower extremities keeping her awake at night.

3. Restless legs syndrome (RLS) is associated with what body system?

JoAnn is initially seen by an RN at the internal medicine practice. She shares that her daughter searched the Internet and found four criteria describing RLS, and she experiences all of them. The nurse asks what nonpharmaceutical practices have been used to give her relief from the unpleasant sensations in her legs and itching.

4. What are the four criteria used in diagnosing RLS?

The article found at http://emedicine.medscape.com/article/1188327-overview (Bozorg, 2014) can be helpful for answering the remaining questions.

5. What is the name of the device recently given approval by the Food and Drug Administration to help with the symptoms of RLS, and how does it work?

JoAnn takes prescribed medication for osteoporosis, hypertension, hyperlipidemia, and acid reflux. Her body mass index (BMI) is 22; surgical history includes an abdominal hysterectomy, laparoscopic cholecystectomy, and a bunionectomy. She takes pride in her physical appearance and believes she looks younger than her actual age. She has never smoked, uses alcohol minimally, and avoids sun exposure. Until the age of 55 when moderate hypertension was diagnosed, JoAnn consumed 10 to 12 cups of coffee per day. She reluctantly reduced the amount by half in an effort to lower her blood pressure.

JoAnn has multiple questions related to RLS and asks whether this is an "old person's condition." The nurse explains that up to 12 million Americans are affected, with a higher incidence in those of middle to older age (Diebold, Fanning-Harding, & Hanson, 2010). The client inquires whether she will have an MRI as she is quite claustrophobic. The nurse reassures JoAnn that she will have lab tests initially to rule out underlying causes of RLS such as diabetes, hypothyroidism, and chronic renal failure. Further contributing problems include iron deficiency anemia and folate/B12 deficiency, which will be tested for as well.

6. What diagnostic tests will be ordered for JoAnn?

Several days later, JoAnn receives a phone call from the internist at the medical office. He asks her for additional information about her history of acid reflux, stating, "You have few of the common risk factors for this problem. Can you tell me when you began taking medicine and for what symptoms?" JoAnn explains that 5 years ago after her husband died, she experienced bad heartburn almost constantly. She wasn't eating much of anything due to grief and lost 10 pounds over several months. "I pretty much lived on coffee until I accepted my husband's death." A prescription for Prilosec (omeprazole) 40 mg was ordered, and she has used it daily since that time.

The physician goes on to relay to JoAnn that her lab tests showed a mild drop in B12. This deficiency can be caused by insufficient stomach acid, which is necessary to separate B12 from ingested protein. It is the most common cause of B12 deficiency in the elderly and individuals on drugs that suppress gastric acid production. The physician states, "Between your caffeine intake and using a proton-pump inhibitor, I feel pretty certain it's affecting your B12 levels. In return, low B12 has been indicated as contributing to restless legs syndrome."

JoAnn agrees to stop taking her medication for acid reflux and have no caffeine intake. Vitamin B12 is ordered as a 2,000 mcg tablet on a daily basis. She also seeks ways to increase the vitamin in her daily nutrition.

7. Create a lunch or dinner menu that is high in vitamin B12.

8. A Task Force of the International Restless Legs Syndrome Study Group (IRLSSG) has developed evidence-based guidelines for long-term pharmacologic treatment of RLS. These medications are not needed at this time for JoAnn. What are the recommendations?

At a 6-month follow-up visit, JoAnn tells the RN at the medical office, "My restless legs have really settled down. I have no heartburn and feel well rested. But, I sure do miss my coffee! I found a local support group on the Internet. I hope to be able to encourage others by attending and make some new friends at the same time."

9. What complementary health measures might be suggested for an individual with RLS?

Suggested Resources

Bozorg, A. M. (2014). *Restless legs syndrome treatment & management.* MedScape. Retrieved from http://emedicine.medscape.com/article/1188327-overview

Chase, B. (2014). *B12 and reestless leg syndrome.* Progressive Health. Retrieved from http://www.progressivehealth.com/rls-b12.htm

Diebold, C., Fanning-Harding, F., & Hanson, P. (2010). Management of common problems. In K. Mauk (Ed.), *Gerontological nursing competencies for care* (2nd ed., p. 496). Sudbury, MA: Jones and Bartlett Learning.

National Institute of Neurological Disorders and Stroke. (2014). *Restless legs syndrome fact sheet.* Retrieved from http://www.ninds.nih.gov/disorders/restless_legs/detail_restless_legs.htm

Case 20.2 ■ Insomnia

*F*ollowing several months of academic work and team effort, today is the "big day" for a group of undergraduate nursing students to highlight their senior teaching project. The team consists of five students: Lindsay, Jessica, Stacey, Kyle, and Branden. They have prepared a 3-hour program, handouts, an intricate PowerPoint, and a pre- or posttest for an audience of 100 senior citizens. The session is being filmed by the university's media services with the specific intent of using the teaching information repeatedly in the future.

The focus of the presentation is insomnia. The group took several days to select this topic, employing a variety of methods. Using their gerontology textbook, they immediately ruled out the majority of disorders affecting the elderly, which left a pool of eight broad choices. With those topics, they surveyed the local senior center where the program will be offered and another 50 individuals comprised of their grandparents, neighbors, and church members ranging in age from 65 to 92 years old. This informal needs assessment showed an overwhelming interest in the topic of sleep disorders, specifically insomnia.

Next, the group made a list of all the associated tasks necessary to implement the teaching project and distributed them per volunteer basis. In addition, a timetable showing expected completion of drafts, sending out announcements of the program, xeroxing materials, and so forth, was generated. The title, "Overcoming Insomnia Through Healthy Solutions" was agreed upon as the students desired to take a primary care approach for the project.

Lindsay started off the program and her focus was predominantly a review of the physiology and age-related changes pertaining to sleep. She began by emphasizing how common insomnia is by stating, "Sixty-four percent of people report experiencing a sleep problem at least a few nights a week, and of those, 41% report problems every night, or almost every night" (2009 Sleep in America Poll). The 2010 Sleep in

America Poll focused on four ethnic groups in relation to sleep problems. Lindsay shared the following statistics with the seniors from the survey: "Asians were the most likely ethnic group to say they get a good night's sleep at least a few nights a week (84% vs. 72% Hispanics, 68% Whites, and 66% Blacks)."

Next, she reviewed the physiology of REM and presented a PowerPoint slide with the stages of non-REM (NREM) sleep, such as found in this table.

Stages of NREM Sleep

	Characteristics
Stage I	
Stage II	
Stage III	
Stage IV	

1. Fill in this table with information describing the characteristics of each stage.

Lindsay pointed out to the group that Stage IV NREM sleep is the one most affected by increasing age and also provided an overview of circadian rhythm. She emphasized that often older people tend to become sleepier in the early evening and wake earlier in the morning compared to younger adults. This pattern is known as advanced sleep phase syndrome. The sleep rhythm is altered so that 7 or 8 hours of sleep are still acquired, but the individuals will wake up much earlier because they have gone to sleep quite early. Jessica's part of the teaching seminar focused on assessing and diagnosing sleep disorders. She described what is involved with having an overnight sleep study; one gentleman in the audience stated he underwent this test 5 years ago to rule out obstructive sleep apnea. An example of a sleep log, or diary, was shown on the screen with information pertaining to the importance of tracking events. Jessica then proceeded to explain that an individual would keep a record of about a dozen events for 2 weeks.

Examples include the time the person tried to fall asleep, the time the person thinks sleep onset occurred, and the number, time, and length of any nighttime awakenings. One lady in attendance stated, "I'd be writing all night and never get any sleep if I had to do that."

The audience broke out in laughter and Jessica changed the focus to a different type of assessment tool: The Pittsburgh Sleep Quality Index (PSQI), which she found on the Hartford Institute for Geriatric Nursing website in the *Try This* series. She brought a copy of the instrument for everyone attending and encouraged them to fill out the form and take it to their health care provider as a means for giving a personal history about their insomnia. Jessica also told the group someone else could read the questions to them and record the answers if necessary.

2. Using the website http://consultgerirn.org/uploads/File/trythis/ try_this_6_1.pdf (Smyth, 2012), view the PSQI. What elements of sleep quality are measured by this assessment? What makes this a user-friendly tool for both the client and the nurse?

The next nursing student to present was Stacey. She generated a lot of participation in the room with her section of the program. Stacey began by asking the question, "What are common reasons you believe may contribute to insomnia with older people?"

3. *Identify a minimum of five events commonly associated with insomnia among geriatric clients.*

4. *Next, Stacey reviewed common myths about older persons and sleep. What might be included? (use a table found at www .gmhfonline.org/gmhf/consumer/factsheets/hlthage_sleep.html).*

The next area addressed at the program was health promotion as it pertains to sleep. Kyle created large colorful poster boards based on an article for 32 sleep solutions he found at http://greatist.com/health/cant-sleep-advice-and-tips (Newcomer, 2014).

5. *What sleep hygiene instructions were available in this brochure that was new information for you?*

The audience appeared to be quite divided on the suggestion in the sleep solutions article to designate a "Worry Time" as a means to promote better sleep. A group of women near the front of the room expressed interest and actual enthusiasm for trying this method; a group in the back of the room had quite the opposite opinion.

6. *What are your thoughts on incorporating a routine "Worry Time" in one's life? Is this a recommendation you might share with an older individual?*

Kyle assisted Branden in searching the literature for material relating to the last section of the insomnia program. These students wanted to share only evidence-based information in relation to treatment or recommended therapies for older persons with sleep problems. The group made a unanimous decision to not recommend or discuss in detail pharmacological methods requiring a prescriptive source. They believed the pharmokinetics could affect people quite differently based on co-morbid conditions or other medications they took, and wanted to solely keep a primary care focus for the project.

Kyle found an article by Lie (2013) titled "Sleep Disorders: Can Complementary and Alternative Medicine (CAM) Help?" Use the information to answer the following question.

7. *Evidence-based practice supports which of the following complementary therapies that have been effective based on objective sleep measures? Select all that apply.*

   a. Magnetic therapy

   b. Tai chi

   c. Valerian

  d. Aromatherapy

  e. Music therapy

  f. Auricular acupuncture therapy

One lady in the audience shared she had a very difficult time falling asleep for years. She began taking a warm bath with lavender oil in the water prior to bedtime and also had lavender potpourri beside her bed. Her claim was the lavender helped her to relax and fall asleep within a half hour.

  8. What additional complementary therapies can you find in the literature for problems with insomnia that may not be evidence-based but are commonly used?

Kyle closed the program with further evidence-based guidelines. He explained the standard nonpharmacological approach to insomnia should focus on the following: (a) stimulus control, (b) sleep restriction, (c) sleep hygiene, (d) sleep environment improvement, (d) relaxation training, (e) remaining passively awake and (f) biofeedback.

  9. Provide a brief description of each of these modalities found on the Mayo Clinic site: www.mayoclinic.org/diseases-conditions/insomnia/in-depth/insomnia-treatment/art-20046677.

The entire audience applauded the students when the program was over. Many seniors came forward with heartfelt gratitude and personal stories afterward, and it was another 45 minutes before the students left the facility. They decided to have dinner together at a nearby restaurant to celebrate and go over the program evaluations as a group. Lindsay raised her water glass to make the following toast to her classmates, "Here's to our 'big day,' effective team work, and . . . to a good night's sleep!"

Suggested Resources

Diebold, C., Fanning-Harding, F., & Hanson, P. (2010). Management of common problems. In K. Mauk (Ed.), *Gerontological nursing competencies for care* (2nd ed., p. 496). Sudbury, MA: Jones and Bartlett Learning.

Lie, D. A. (2013). *Sleep disorders: Can CAM help?* Medscape. Retrieved from http://www.medscape.com/viewarticle/803722_5

Mayo Clinic staff. (2014). *Insomnia treatment: Cognitive behavioral therapy instead of sleeping pills.* Retrieved from http://www.mayoclinic.org/diseases-conditions/insomnia/in-depth/insomnia-treatment/art-20046677

Newcomer, L. (2014). *32 solutions for when you can't sleep.* Retrieved from http://greatist.com/health/cant-sleep-advice-and-tips

Smyth, C. A. (2012). How to try this: Evaluating sleep quality in older adults. *American Journal of Nursing, 5*(108). Retrieved from http://consultgerirn.org/uploads/File/trythis/try_this_6_1.pdf

Case 20.3 ■ Hypersomnia

Mack Dunlevy left his primary health care provider's office with an unfamiliar word, "hypersomnia," written on a prescription pad. He sought help due to an ongoing problem of being very tired and sleepy during the daytime. He is 67 years old and retired from a manufacturing position 5 years ago. He has been a very active man most of his adult life, but over the past 6 months he finds himself predominantly sedentary.

1. What other terms are used to define excessive sleepiness?

Mack was divorced in his 50s and has dated Diane for more than 7 years. Diane retired from the local university a year ago. Their relationship has experienced a lot of conflict recently as Diane planned on the couple traveling, providing volunteer work, playing with grandchildren, and generally being together the majority of the time once she no longer worked. She gave Mack an ultimatum to seek medical help about his excessive sleepiness or the relationship would end. Diane also gave him the nickname "Narc" as she has repeatedly told him he is suffering from narcolepsy.

2. Compare and contrast hypersomnia with narcolepsy.

Based on the history taken by a nurse practitioner at the office, Mack's health status was considered above average for his age group. He had two surgeries many years ago, which included an inguinal hernia repair and appendectomy. His height is 68 inches with his weight at 200 pounds. He has never smoked, used tobacco products, or tried recreational drugs. When asked about alcohol use, Mack told the nurse practitioner he had "one or two" servings of bourbon prior to bedtime. In actuality, since his relationship with Diane has been strained, he consumes double or more of that amount. Mack believes alcohol helps him sleep better at night, which allows him to stay awake during the day. This has not been the case, however.

Current prescribed medications include Flomax (tamsulosin) 0.4 mg orally daily, Nexium (esomeprazole) 40 mg oral daily, and Lasix (furosemide) 20 mg orally every other day. Medication used on a prn basis includes Motrin (ibuprofen) 400 mg orally for occasional muscle soreness and Benadryl (diphenhydramine) 25 mg orally for seasonal allergy-based rhinitis.

3. Watch the 1+ minute video at www.healthysleep.med.harvard .edu/video/sleep07_duffy_problems/wm-hi and take note of the underlying medical conditions causing sleep problems in older adults. What, if any, are applicable to Mack?

4. Describe how the as-needed medications listed could result in daytime sleepiness.

5. What are age-related physiological changes affecting the circadian rhythm of older adults?

The nurse practitioner who evaluated Mack at the office asked him questions pertaining to hypersomnia using the Epworth Sleepiness Scale (ESS) authored by Smyth (2012). Mack's score was a "12."

6. Go to http://consultgerirn.org/uploads/File/trythis/try_this_6_2.pdf in order to interpret what this finding means.

Many other questions were asked at the office in an effort to find a cause for Mack's excessive daytime sleepiness. He was wearing a cotton button-up shirt, and the nurse practitioner inquired about the neck size of this piece of clothing. Mack was quite surprised at such a question but good-naturedly replied, "Why in the world does that matter?" The nurse practitioner explained perhaps obstructive sleep apnea may be a contributing factor for his hypersomnia.

7. What bearing would neck size have with this condition?

8. What other risk factors for obstructive sleep apnea does Mack possess based on the information provided?

Another topic explored was the presence of snoring. Mack stated he was unaware if deep, pronounced snoring woke him up repeatedly during the night. He stated his dating partner, Diane, complained about this problem. "We sleep all night together a couple times a year when visiting my family out of state. Diane carries on and on about my snoring so I bought her ear plugs. But she is such a light sleeper; I doubt my snoring is any different than most men."

A sleep study is arranged for Mack at a local hospital for the following week. The nurse practitioner reviewed safety issues as a priority concern for this client.

9. What activities related to excessive daytime sleepiness should Mack use caution with, or avoid altogether?

Obstructive sleep apnea was confirmed following diagnostic testing. Mack began using a continuous positive airway pressure (CPAP) machine immediately.

10. Visit the Hartford Institute for Geriatric Nursing evidence-based guidelines at http://consultgerirn.org/topics/sleep/want_to_ know_more (Chasens & Umlauf, 2012). What action is suggested for optimizing the use of CPAP?

Mack experienced a dramatic improvement in his daytime sleepiness following treatment. He began golfing, playing cards, and watching sports with his male buddies once again. He and Diane enjoyed daytime trips, volunteering at their church, and attending local events. Mack was so busy experiencing life again, he lost 15 pounds and rarely thought about taking a nap in his favorite recliner.

Suggested Resources

Chasens, E. R., & Umlauf, M. G. (2012). *Nursing standard practice protocol: Excessive sleepiness.* Hartford Institute for Geriatric Nursing. Retrieved from http://consultgerirn.org/topics/sleep/want_to_know_more

Duffy, J. (2007). *Sleep problems in older adults* [Video file]. Healthy Sleep. Retrieved from http://healthysleep.med.harvard.edu/video/sleep07_duffy_problems/wm-hi

Johns, M. W. (1991). A new method for measuring daytime sleepiness: The Epworth sleepiness scale. *Sleep, 14,* 540–545.

Lifetips. (2014). *The difference between hypersomnia and narcolepsy.* Retrieved from http://sleepdisorders.lifetips.com/faq/120851/0/what-is-the-difference-between-hypersomnia-and-narcolepsy/index.html

Mayo Clinic staff. (2012). *Sleep apnea.* Retrieved from http://www.mayoclinic.com/health/sleep-apnea/DS00148/DSECTION=risk-factors

Smyth, C. (2012). *The Epworth sleepiness scale (ESS).* Hartford Institute for Geriatric Nursing. Retrieved from http://consultgerirn.org/uploads/File/trythis/try_this_6_2.pdf

21

Aging Issues Affecting the Family

Case 21.1 ■ Caregiver Burden

Annually, there are 65.7 million unpaid or informal caregivers (29% of the American population). Most of these caregivers are middle-aged women, with 48 years being their average age. They are usually caring for a family member: an aging parent or spouse (Family Caregiver Alliance, 2012a). Motivations for caregiving, such as love or obligation, are often based on culture and ethnicity and influence the caregivers' willingness to provide needed care (Pierce & Lutz, 2009). Caregiving may bring family members together, but it also may be a stressful time.

The term "caregiver stress or burden" refers to the person's emotional response to changes and demands that occur as they give help and support to the person in need of care. The burden of caring for another can result in anxiety, depression, difficulty with coping, and problems with physical health. Signs of this burden can include sleeping problems, weight loss or gain, fatigue, irritability, withdrawal, or vague physical symptoms, stomach upset, or headache (Reinhard, Given, Petlick, & Bemis, 2008).

Tom Ketron is the caregiver for his wife Asa, who is a 68-year-old Nigerian woman. Tom is African American and is 5 years younger than his wife. Neither of them graduated from high school; both worked at various factory jobs for the same manufacturing company. Several years ago, the plant unexpectedly closed and they were released without any benefits or pensions. They live in a tiny two-story home in a small rural town in one of the southern states. Asa shares that they own the home and have Social Security and Medicare for income and insurance. Asa has some current medical bills that they are trying to pay week by week; monthly, Asa sends money to her family members in Nigeria; and they have a small amount of money in a bank for a "rainy day." Asa and Tom have many brothers and sisters; however, they live in western states or in other countries. They have no children. They report that they live day-to-day by relying on a strong faith and having a small circle of church friends.

Asa has heart disease (congestive heart failure and coronary artery disease) that has caused increasing fatigue, shortness of breath, and angina-type pain over the past 3 years. Her health has declined and she has lost weight. Frequently, Asa describes "colds and coughs" that have increased her shortness of breath to the point of using continuous portable oxygen in the home. She is unable to climb stairs due to her exhaustion. The living room was converted to her bedroom; she uses a wheelchair for mobility. Tom placed a portable commode nearby her wheelchair and bed, but he has difficulty transferring her from bed to chair to toilet. He is worried about her safety in that she could fall and injure herself. If she fell, he is concerned that he could not assist her.

Tom tells that he has "suffered numerous small strokes" this past year; he is also overweight and has a herniated disc. He did see a physician for his health concerns but he refuses to take "Western medicines." Tom started to follow a regimen of herbal medicines for stroke prevention, including ginkgo biloba (believed to help prevent blood clots from developing and increase the blood flow to the brain); garlic (thought to help reduce blood pressure and lower cholesterol levels, and act as an anticoagulant); and willow bark (called herbal aspirin and a reported anticoagulant). He has refused surgical treatment for his back pain, stating that he is not willing to leave his wife for any large amount of time. His friend, who recently died from a massive heart attack, told him before he died that he read about devil's claw and willow bark as effective back pain remedies. Tom already takes willow bark and he is thinking about adding devil's claw to his herbal daily schedule to help manage his back pain.

Tom shares that he feels alone in caring for his wife as his friends are "passing." He states that if family members lived closer, they would "pitch-in and help." However, he is feeling hopeless and helpless without the family members and friends' support. He also shares that he is short-tempered and is tired all the time. He is upset as he begins to think that he can no longer care for his wife at home, because of her increasing weakness and his health issues. However, he promised her that he would never place her in a nursing home, stating that "family takes care of family."

In the next month, Asa's health continues to decline and she is hospitalized again for difficulty breathing and chest pain. The physician talks with Tom about a do not resuscitate (DNR) agreement. Asa and Tom together decide that they agree to the DNR order, as she does not want the "machines to keep her alive." Tom realizes that he cannot continue to care for Asa in their home. He is angry about placing Asa in a nursing home at discharge from the hospital, but he can see no alternatives. He believes that it is truly "raining" and that he needs to use the money in the bank for Asa's care, but how? Tom contacts the nurse case manager for guidance.

1. *Name at least one reason why informal African American caregivers prefer to provide home care to family members.*

2. *Which is NOT a sign of caregiver burden?*

   a. *Weight loss*

   b. *Headache*

   c. *Fatigue*

   d. *Hunger*

   e. *Irritability*

3. *On the Hartford Institute for Geriatric Nursing website, Onega (2013) presents a tool for measuring caregiver strain. Describe why this is considered the "best tool." Use the link http:// consultgerirn.org/uploads/File/trythis/try_this_14.pdf.*

4. *As Tom continues to care for his wife, identify a few potential costs.*

5. *Suggest some ways that Tom might continue to care for his wife at home.*

6. *What are some first strategies that Tom should do as a caregiver to take care of himself?*

7. *Discuss positive ways of coping that caregivers may use.*

8. *Search the Internet and choose at least one educational website for emotional coping strategies to lessen caregivers' burden.*

9. *Name an alternative to home care that caregivers may consider.*

Suggested Resources

AgingCare. (2009). *Cost of caring for aging parents could be next financial crisis.* Retrieved from http://www.agingcare.com/News/133372/Cost-of-Caring-for-Aging-Parents-Could-be-Next-Financial-Crisis.htm

Clark, D. (2014). *Counseling options and opportunities for caregivers.* Retrieved from http://www.agingcare.com/Featured-Stories/126208/Caregiver-Support.htm

Family Caregiver Alliance. (2012a). *Selected caregiver statistics.* Retrieved from https://caregiver.org/selected-caregiver-statistics

Family Caregiver Alliance. (2012b). *Taking care of YOU: Self-care for family caregivers.* Retrieved from http://www.caregiver.org/caregiver/jsp/content_node.jsp?nodeid=847

Given, C., Given, B., Stommel, M., Collins, C., King, S., & Franklin, S. (1992). The Caregiver Reaction Assessment (CRA) for caregivers to persons with chronic physical and mental impairments. *Research in Nursing & Health, 15*(4), 271–283.

Helpguide.org. (2014). *Caregiving support and help.* Retrieved from http://www.helpguide.org/elder/caring_for_caregivers.htm

Montgomery, R. J. V., Borgatta, E. F., & Borgatta, M. L. (2000). Societal and family change in the burden of care. In W. T. Liu & H. Kendig (Eds.), *Who should care for the elderly? An east-west value divide.* Singapore: The National University of Singapore Press.

Onega, L. L. (2013). *The Modified Caregiver Strain Index (MCSI).* Hartford Institute for Geriatric Nursing. Retrieved from http://consultgerirn.org/uploads/File/trythis/try_this_14.pdf

Pierce, L., & Lutz, B. (2009). Family caregiving. In P. Larsen (Ed.), *Chronic illness impact and intervention* (7th ed., pp. 191–229). Boston, MA: Jones and Bartlett.

Reinhard, S. C., Given, B., Petlick, N. H., & Bemis, A. (2008). Supporting family caregivers in providing care. In R. G. Hughes (Ed.), *Patient safety and quality: An evidence-based handbook for nurses.* Agency for Healthcare Research and Quality. Retrieved from http://www.ahrq.gov/professionals/clinicians-providers/resources/nursing/resources/nurseshdbk/ReinhardS_FCCA.pdf

Zarit, S., Reever, K. E., & Bach-Peterson, J. (1980). Relatives of the impaired elderly: Correlates of feelings of burden. *Gerontologist, 20*(6), 649–655.

Case 21.2 ■ Ineffective Family Coping

*E*llen Lang is an 88-year-old single woman who lives in a continuous care community. She originally moved into an independent-living condo, but a year ago transferred into the assisted living center. Ellen has always been fiercely independent, often vocally judgmental, and has always had a verbal "mean streak." She is quite healthy, completely independent in all activities of daily living (ADL), and takes no medications. She had bilateral mastectomies for breast cancer, but has had no evidence of further malignancy for many years.

Six years ago, Ellen moved to Grand Junction, Colorado, to be near her youngest daughter, Ruth, her son-in-law, Bill, and their three children. She bought a condo about a mile from Ruth and Bill's house and was a big help to Ruth and Bill and their children, ages 7, 10, and 12. Ellen watched the children after school, drove them to activities, and did some shopping for the family. She would also have the family over for dinner at least once a week and participated in many family activities and holiday events. She also cared for the family's miniature schnauzer, Jackie, taking him to veterinarian and grooming appointments, and caring for him in her condo when the family was out of town. Ellen loved Jackie, whom she has named her "grand-dog," and the dog loved visiting Ellen. In addition to helping her daughter's family, Ellen's primary social activity was attending her local Catholic church. She participated in two church activities every week in addition to Sunday mass.

Ellen's move to assisted living was precipitated by a progressive decline in her abilities. Her memory declined rapidly over the past 2 years. She began drinking more alcohol at home and fell twice while impaired, once breaking a rib. Her neighbors reported that she frequently appeared confused and had locked herself out of her condo several times. Ellen was seen by her primary physician and had a complete neurological work-up, which revealed only age-related changes in her brain. She took prescribed Aricept (donepezil) for a while, but then stopped because it did not seem to help and caused her to have nightmares. As her memory problems increased, she could no longer live on her own, prompting Ruth and her siblings to convince Ellen to move into the assisted living center. Ruth also convinced Ellen to give up driving.

> 1. *As a nurse working with Ellen in assisted living, what general assessments would be important to complete to help direct your nursing care?*
>
> 2. *Review the American Association of Colleges of Nursing (AACN) website on caring for older adults located at www.aacn.nche. edu/geriatric-nursing/aacn_gerocompetencies.pdf (pp. 11–12) and identify four competencies that you can use to guide her care and promote family involvement.*

Ellen's move to assisted living and subsequent changes in her behavior affected all of the family members. Ellen's behavior became more intolerable. Several times she was critical of Bill and Ruth's children, especially the boys. She complained about their driving and belittled them about school and girls. The boys, now 16 and 18, refused to drive their grandmother to their home for family functions. When Bill and Ruth brought Ellen over for dinner, the boys often found reasons to dine elsewhere. Ellen's granddaughter, Melissa, was now 13 years old. Melissa and Ellen previously had a close relationship, because Melissa was only 7 when Ellen initially moved to Grand Junction. Of all the children, Melissa was the most disturbed by her grandmother's decline and resented that Ellen frequently contacted her when she was confused. Ellen sometimes called Melissa 10 times a day; as a result, Melissa refused to take her calls.

3. *Go to the website www.youtube.com/watch?v=Tgv4VhC4Bl4 and, after viewing the video, identify ideas to help a young person such as Melissa understand and cope with her grandmother's dementia.*

4. *At "How Can We Spend Time Together," provided on the website www.afateens.org/coping.html, what can the nurse recommend for Melissa to share with her grandmother so that both will find meaningful?*

After moving into assisted living, Ellen no longer participated in Catholic church activities and she rarely saw her beloved grand-dog, Jackie. She resented these losses, and often isolated herself, spending most days alone in her room. She called Bill and Ruth almost daily and asked them to "bring me a bottle of wine," which Bill and Ruth refused to do as they did not want her to injure herself, embarrass the family, or be asked to leave the assisted living facility. Ellen also resented no longer being included in many family activities.

> Older adults often need to find a way to cope with serious illnesses and end of life issues while re-evaluating life and spirituality. Research has shown that patients rely on their religion to help them cope with their illnesses and want their clinicians to ask about their spiritual concerns. Spirituality, however defined by the patient, is often a component of reminiscing that may reinforce meaning and value to a person's life. (Borneman, 2011, p. 1)

5. *Nurses use assessment prior to interventions. Find the assessment tool known as the FICA Spiritual History Tool (Puchalski, 2006) located at http://consultgerirn.org/uploads/File/trythis/try_this_ sp5.pdf. What are the four categories assessed?*

6. *Following assessment, what interventions do Kaplan and Berkman (2013) recommend in their article, "Religion and Spirituality in the Elderly," at www.merckmanuals.com/ professional/geriatrics/social_issues_in_the_elderly/religion_ and_spirituality_in_the_elderly.html?*

7. *How might staff at the assisted living facility intervene so that Ellen is not so isolated?*

Bill and Ruth fought regularly about Ellen as they struggled with managing three teenage children and Ellen's declining mental status. They felt guilty about no longer including Ellen in family activities and resentful of her criticisms and need for increased care, all of which placed more strain on their family. Bill and Ruth also frequently disagreed on how to best handle Ellen and the children, and each felt the other was undermining his or her efforts.

8. *You decide that working on forgiveness would be beneficial for all family members. Access information on this concept at www .mayoclinic.com/health/forgiveness/ MH00131. Discuss some of the benefits of forgiveness.*

Suggested Resources

Alzheimer's Association. (2011). Teens look at Alzheimer's disease: What can I expect and how can I deal with it? [Video file]. Retrieved from https://www.youtube.com/watch?v=Tgv4VhC4Bl4

Alzheimer's Foundation of America. (2013). *Coping.* Retrieved from http://www.afateens.org/ coping.html

American Association of Colleges of Nursing. (2010). *Recommended baccalaureate competencies and curricular guidelines for the nursing care of older adults: A supplement to the essentials of baccalaureate education for professional nursing practice.* Retrieved from http:// www.aacn.nche.edu/geriatric-nursing/aacn_gerocompetencies.pdf

Borneman, T. (2011). *Assessment of spirituality in older adults: FICA spiritual history tool.* Hartford Institute for Geriatric Nursing. Retrieved from http://consultgerirn.org/uploads/ File/trythis/try_this_sp5.pdf

Kaplan, D. B., & Berkman, B. J. (2013). *Religion and spirituality in the elderly.* Merck Manual. Retrieved from http://www.merckmanuals.com/professional/geriatrics/social_issues_in_ the_elderly/religion_and_spirituality_in_the_elderly.html

Mayo Clinic. (2011). *Forgiveness: Letting go of grudges and bitterness.* Retrieved from http:// www.mayoclinic.org/healthy-living/adult-health/in-depth/forgiveness/art-20047692?pg=2

Puchalski, C. (2006). Spiritual assessment in clinical practice. *Psychiatric Annals, 36*(3), 150–155.

Case 21.3 ■ Emergency Preparedness for the Elderly and Their Families

*M*att Lawrence is a senior nursing student who will graduate in less than 6 weeks. He has completed a community health teaching project, which had a tremendous amount of personal meaning to him. His nursing instructor assisted him in obtaining a

$3,000 grant for the project and wrote in her reference letter, "I've never had a student more passionate about providing a public health service in 20 years of teaching."

In the late summer of 2012, when Matt was in high school, he attended a huge family reunion on the Jersey shore. His paternal grandfather, Bill, lived in the area and close to 40 people traveled to celebrate his grandfather's 65th birthday. It was a fun-filled week but the last time anyone would ever see the man alive.

Bill lived on the coast on the first floor of a high-rise senior housing facility. He functioned independently in spite of having a long-term history of chronic lung disease and a below-the-knee amputation. Matt's family lived in the Great Lakes area and followed the news closely regarding the impending devastation of Hurricane Sandy.

Several days prior to the storm's arrival, Matt's father talked to Bill about planning for evacuation. He assured Matt's dad that he had been through a number of similar situations and would be fine. He also threw in, "I made it home from the Vietnam War in one piece, so this will be a piece of cake." Bill could not be reached on his cell phone the 24 hours prior to the storm, which flooded his building. The family had no other people to contact in the area to check on his safety. They were notified by the Red Cross a few days later that Bill's body was found in his apartment with his German Shepherd dog lying across him.

When preparing for his project, Matt used the following quote as evidence of the need or significance of his work.

> Elderly residents were hit especially hard, with close to half of the people who died age 65 or older. In New York City, the majority of deaths occurred in Queens and on Staten Island, and most people perished at the height of the storm, drowned by the surge. (Josh Keller, reporter the *New York Times*, November 17, 2012)

1. Using the following article, sponsored by the Centers for Disease Control, *www.cdc.gov/aging/pdf/disaster_planning_tips.pdf*, identify factors associated with the aging process, which may increase an older person's vulnerability to a disaster.

Matt's family was convinced that his grandfather did not evacuate his apartment because he was a pet owner. His beloved dog was older and had special needs, in addition to being fearful of storms. This is a common situation with many elderly people living alone.

2. What action did Congress take following Hurricane Katrina in regards to pets and disasters?

Matt secured, reviewed, and printed off a multitude of "Disaster Preparedness Checklists" for his project. Most contained the same information, which listed items necessary for a 3-day time span. His plan was also to include items specifically geared toward the elderly.

3. Think of supplies you would have ready for 3 days at home in the event of a disaster. Compare your list with what the American Red Cross or another source suggests. What did you omit? What might an older person need in addition to the standard items?

Rather than handing out lists and general guidelines related to emergency planning, Matt wanted something he believed would not get lost, accidentally tossed out, or damaged as easily as paper. Through his search online, he found an item known as the Emergency Readiness Wheel for seniors that he thought was ideal. He ordered a multitude of these resources, which could be kept on a refrigerator with the magnet attached at the top; the cost was covered by the grant monies he secured. One side of the wheel contains information relating to preparedness, whereas the other side focuses on response.

> ***4. The EAD & Associates wheel can be found at http://eadassociates .com/wheels.html. Spin the wheel and document major categories of information on each side. Do you believe this would be a useful resource for senior citizens?***

Matt's uncle found a small fireproof safe at his grandfather's residence after the hurricane. Inside were a variety of papers kept in a plastic zip-lock bag that remained undamaged from the flooding waters.

> ***5. What documents are suggested to be kept together in the event of a disaster? An excellent resource is located at www.gmhfonline .org/gmhf/consumer/disaster_prprdns.html, provided by the Geriatric Mental Health Foundation.***

Matt's plan for reaching out to senior citizens was to present multiple teaching sessions around the tri-state area in which he lived. In particular, he invited "snowbirds" (seniors who spend the cold months in a southern state such as Florida), which included hundreds of individuals and couples in the area. This strategy would focus on disasters such as floods, blizzards, and tornadoes, which were more common in the Great Lakes area, as well as provide information about evacuation and preparation for hurricanes.

> ***6. Watch the video, 5 Disaster Prep Tips for Older Americans found at www.aarp.org/aarp-foundation/our-work/housing/info-2012/ emergency-disaster-preparedness-plans-for-seniors.html. What were the suggestions?***

A brochure Matt used as a guideline for PowerPoint slides shown at the teaching sessions was well received, primarily by family members of elderly persons attending. He found the organization Eldercare Locator provided lots of helpful information. Review the brochure titled "How Will I Know Mom and Dad Are Okay?" at www .adph.org/ALPHTN/assets/113011bStay.pd

> ***7. What acronym (and its interpretation) from the brochure is used to promote safety in crisis situations?***

Along with the rest of the nation, Matt was saddened to hear about the number of elderly persons who lived in residential care facilities and died during Hurricane Sandy. Not far from his town, a nursing home was recently heavily damaged by a fire, which left many residents injured. He decided to end his program with information that both the elderly and their family members could use when choosing, or currently residing in, a facility. His resource, the National Consumer Voice for Quality Long-Term Care (NCCNHR), emphasizes residents and their families should inquire about the facility's emergency preparedness and evacuation plans.

8. *Review the organization's website at www.theconsumervoice .org/sites/default/files/advocate/Emergency-Preparedness.pdf theconsumervoice.org/uploads/files/family-member/Emergency-Preparedness.pdf. Do you think most residents and/or their caregivers ask the suggested questions? If not, why?*

Suggested Resources

AARP Foundation. (2014). 5 Disaster prep tips for older Americans [Video file]. Retrieved from http://www.aarp.org/aarp-foundation/our-work/housing/info-2012/emergency-disaster-preparedness-plans-for-seniors.html

Administration on Aging, U.S. Department of Health and Human Services. (n.d.). *How will I know mom and dad are okay?* Eldercare Locater. Retrieved from http://www.eldercare .gov/Eldercare.NET/Public/Resources/Brochures/docs/INTOUCH_brochure.pdf

Geriatric Mental Health Foundation. (2009). *Older adults and disaster: Preparedness and response.* Retrieved from http://www.gmhfonline.org/gmhf/consumer/disaster_prprdns.html

Keller, J. (2012, November 17). Mapping hurricane Sandy's deadly toll. *New York Times.* http://www.nytimes/interactive/2012/11/17/region/hurricane-sandy-map.html?_r=0

Case 21.4 ■ Leaving the Homestead: Challenges and Solutions

*I*t is Thanksgiving eve, and Lillian Perry is preparing several pies in her kitchen while also preparing how to best share an important decision she has made with her family tomorrow. After living 74 years, Lillian has decided to give up the home she has occupied since 1950. Following her husband's death a few years ago, her interest in housekeeping, yard work, and living alone has declined. In addition, her house is in the best shape it can be for its age. New interior paint throughout, a kitchen update, bathroom tile, and fixtures replaced; all will add to the sale price, which she will need for her new residence.

A senior independent living complex opened over a year ago outside of Lillian's town. Lillian has toured the facility and believes it will be an ideal place to live as she ages. Each unit has a large bedroom and an open-living concept for the public areas. She figures 15 to 20 people can easily visit at a time (in the same area), which is a selling point she will share with her family. Currently, in her Cape Cod style home, the layout does not allow everyone to be together in one place. In addition, there is a party room, an indoor pool, exercise facilities, a large patio area, and space for a barbeque outside. Lillian will buy her unit outright and also pay a monthly $150 fee (home owner's association). Half of the 100 units are designated for independent living and the other half for assisted living; Lillian hopes it will be a long time before she requires those services.

> ### 1. Compare and contrast the two approaches to housing for the elderly: independent versus assisted living. Cite your source.

> ### 2. What are the qualifications for individuals to be eligible for independent living?

Lillian and her husband worked together for close to three decades. Fred owned a hardware store downtown, and she was there from 8 a.m. to 2 p.m. during the school year, serving customers, stocking items, and also taking care of the accounting. When a large retail "mega" store opened, it was the demise of their business. Lillian provided family income in the summers while the children were growing up by making a variety of jellies and jams from the fruit trees and garden the couple tended, and sold the products to the local tourist welcome center. After their business closed, she worked every morning until noon as a church secretary for her parish. At age 72, when Fred died, Lillian retired. She provides care for a great-grandchild 2 days a week now, which she is willing to continue.

Each generation in America has been "labeled" by researchers as to the trends, social influences, and historical events occurring during the period of birth through adulthood. People of Lillian's age group have been coined "The Silent Generation."

> ### 3. Using the article "The Silent Generation Explores Retirement Community Options" on the following website, www. seniorcitizensguide.com/articles/chicago/silent-generation-retirement-community.htm, explain how this label came about. What characteristics do Lillian's background present that are "typical" for her generation?

Lillian's immediate family consists of three children: Jack is married and has twin daughters, Betsy is divorced and has a son, and Karen is married with four children. All of these family members and the seven grandchildren live within 50 miles of Lillian and see one another at least monthly. Sunday dinner get-togethers were a tradition while Fred was alive. Holidays were celebrated at Lillian's routinely, and it is common for at least two or more individuals to stop in briefly most days of the week. Lillian fears this may change with her proposed move.

She shares her intentions the next day and is quite unprepared for the response. Questions are fired at her by several family members at once; her youngest daughter begins crying, Jack tenses up and leaves the room, and it is more than she can cope with reasonably. She had handwritten a list of items she was taking to the independent care unit and tells the group, "Everything else is yours for the taking; as soon as the house is sold, we'll establish a certain weekend to clear out all the contents."

The next day, Lillian receives a phone call from her daughter-in-law. Jack's wife requests an extensive list of items she wants from Lillian's home. This includes many family heirlooms such as china and crystal, 100-year-old quilts, vases, antique bedroom sets, and another dozen or more objects. She asks Lillian to commit to her that the oldest child, and only son, has the first choice in material goods. Lillian tells her she will "think it over" and hangs up the phone, shaking.

Christmas arrives, and it is celebrated at Lillian's home since it is the last opportunity. Lillian finds herself choking up when putting out decorations in their designated spots around her home, looking over a multitude of handmade ornaments from her children and grandchildren, and wondering if future celebrations could ever match the comfort gained from familiarity with traditions.

She also is having difficulty sleeping, which was related to worry. Over and over, Lillian thinks about the requests her daughter-in-law made in regards to taking family heirlooms and other items. She tries to think of a system of equitable means for everyone to have what they want, yet there is always reason for concern. She has no friends or extended family members to ask for suggestions; their belongings were either divided upon death, or they still lived in a home surrounded by personal possessions. A few people in their 70s or 80s she knew had moved so often in their lives, most of their personal belongings had been kept minimal.

> **4. Use the following resource from the U.S. Census Bureau, www.apartmenttherapy.com/moving-stats-us-census-bureau-153381, to comment on the average number of moves an adult makes in his or her lifetime. Do you believe Lillian's situation of residing in a home 50+ years will be a rarity in the 21st century?**

The winter months are especially difficult as Lillian is inside the majority of the time, and her worrying increases. Everywhere she looks and everything she touches brings back decades of memories. Her oldest granddaughter loved looking and talking about her Avon collection of perfume bottles when she was a preschooler; should Lillian offer them to her? Another grandchild adored a set of cookie cutters in animal shapes; would he want them now?

Lillian was a list-maker most of her life in order to keep organized and productive. She attempts to fill a notebook with items from each room of the house, thinking it might be helpful when her home goes on the market in a few months. She also is a woman of faith and uses prayer several times a day when feeling overwhelmed. In addition to these struggles, be it due to weather or perhaps their own sadness, her kids and grandchildren are not stopping in nearly as often.

> **5. Describe a situation in your family, or someone else's, where material property had to be divided. What system was used? Did it go smoothly or cause conflict? (If no experience is available, describe how you would suggest it be done in Lillian's family.)**

Lillian's youngest daughter hears about a method for allocating personal property from a friend, which the family eventually uses when the house is sold. Everyone workes together cohesively through this process, although Jack's wife pouts and whines at times when certain family heirlooms are given to Lillian's daughters.

> **6. Visit the website www.edivvyup.com/edivvyup_overview .php. Describe this service and your opinion of the potential usefulness.**

After attending mass one morning, Lillian stops by the health ministry office to have her blood pressure checked. She is familiar with the parish nurse, Anne, as she assisted the family with coordinating Fred's care during the last months of his life. Anne immediately comments on the weight loss she observes, as well as stating, "You look so pale and stressed." Lillian responds in a manner very unlike herself; she starts to cry.

Anne sits with Lillian for over an hour that morning and predominantly listens. One positive sentence such as, "I know moving will be a so good for me," is followed by a worrisome one, "What if I miss my backyard?" She states her house was to go on the market in early April, just 6 weeks away, and fears she may change her mind.

Anne validates Lillian's emotional conflict and praises her for making a life change that many elderly persons consider, yet never have the courage to implement. She believes Lillian would be an ideal candidate for a Reminiscence Group, which meets in a nearby town twice a month. Lillian shares that she would not feel comfortable in this type of setting as she is a "private" person and would feel too vulnerable in front of strangers to share her worries.

The parish nurse makes a referral to a social worker trained in Reminiscence Therapy, and Lillian attends one-on-one sessions for five visits. Along with the change in seasons, Lillian feels a sense of renewal as spring arrives. Her three children and all the grandchildren host a special party for her the weekend before she moves, humorously referring to the event as a "closed house."

> **7. Briefly describe what Reminiscence Therapy entails.**

> **8. Identify a minimum of five positive outcomes of reminiscing and cite the source.**

Suggested Resources

Apartment Therapy. (2011). *Moving stats*. U.S. Census Bureau. Retrieved from http://www .apartmenttherapy.com/moving-stats-us-census-bureau-153381

Crossing, S. (n.d.). *The silent generation explores retirement community options*. Senior Citizen's Guide to Chicago. Retrieved from http://www.seniorcitizensguide.com/articles/chicago/ silent-generation-retirement-community.htm

Rose, A., de Benedictis, T., & Russell, D. (2010). *Independent living for seniors. A guide to retirement communities and homes*. Helpguide.org. Retrieved from http://www.ftfhousing.com/ images/FCKUploads/file/IndependentLiving_for_Seniors_%20A_Guide_to_Retirement_ Communities_and_Homes.pdf

Case 21.5 ■ Long-Distance Caregiving

*M*arion Hatcher is a 60-year-old woman facing a major dilemma in her life. She has a spouse who has lived in a long-term care facility since he incurred a head injury several years ago from a fall off a ladder, as well as a 20-year-old son with Down syndrome requiring around-the-clock supervision. Marion resides 700 miles from her father, who lives alone and is in his mid-80s. She was contacted by his primary care physician this morning stating he is showing signs of mild to moderate dementia, has lost 5% of his body weight since his last visit, and perhaps should not be living alone.

The first thought Marion had as she hung up the phone was a frequent one in her life. Where would she get the money to go visit her father? Another multitude of worries shortly followed related to the care of her son if she left home for awhile, the potential effect missing her daily visits would have on her husband, and wondering just how seriously debilitated her father had become.

Marion learned long ago an effective short-term coping mechanism to use in times such as this when yet another crisis came into her life. She spent the rest of the morning doing a variety of housekeeping chores to keep her distracted. At 2 p.m. when she was changing her clothes before she and her son were to visit her husband, Marion could barely button her blouse due to the trembling of her hands.

At the facility, Marion sees the director of nursing, Mrs. Wilson, shortly after arriving. This is a woman about her age and someone much admired by all the staff, residents, and family members. The director is out and about in the facility all day long, ensuring policies are followed and nursing care is delivered in a safe, effective manner. Despite her strict ways and business focus, she has a warm and friendly personality. Mrs. Wilson comments on Marion looking particularly stressed, which immediately brings her to tears. She shares the morning news about her father and states, "I just don't know what to do. This is more than I can handle." Mrs. Wilson initially responds with a term Marion is unfamiliar with and asks for clarification.

1. Marion is referred to as being a member of the "sandwich generation"; what does this mean?

Mrs. Wilson takes Marion into her office while her son goes with the activities director to work on puzzles. She takes notes on what Marion relays and picks up the phone to call the facility receptionist and social worker to join them. Both employees have experienced similar situations in the past year with a parent out of town needing medical assistance and a change in living arrangements. They gladly agree to share examples of how they dealt with challenges they experienced to give Marion some beginning advice and support.

The social worker recommends the use of a professionally prepared individual, knowledgeable in geriatrics, to make an initial assessment of Marion's father before she travels to see him. He believes since her dad lives in a major city, he can find someone who will accept Medicare reimbursement for this consultation, and leaves to do a computer search.

2. Describe the role of a professional geriatric care manager.

3. Using the website www.caremanager.org/displaycommon .cfm?an=1&subarticlenbr=306, can you find someone near your own home fulfilling this role?

The receptionist gives Marion a copy of a book she secured known as *So Far Away: Twenty Questions for Long-Distance Caregivers* (Schuster, 2014), which she received from the parish nurse at her church. She encourages Marion to go through it this evening in order to start making some definite plans for her father in the next few days. The book contents can be found at www.nia.nih.gov/HealthInformation/Publications/ LongDistanceCaregiving. The following three questions relate to information within the guide.

4. How common is long-distance caregiving in our country? What change in demographics has occurred in regard to who serves as caregivers?

5. The second question addressed in the book will be the target of information obtained by the geriatric care manager during a home visit. What assessments will be necessary?

6. What suggestions does the book have for adult children whose parents ask to promise never to put them in a nursing home facility?

The Alzheimer's Association is another source for information pertaining to long-distance caregiving. Use the following resource, www.alz.org/care/alzheimers-dementia-long-distance-caregiving.asp, for answering the next two questions.

7. What suggestions are available for long-distance caregivers in relation to "making the most of a visit" for those living away?

It is determined Marion's father had a chronic urinary tract infection, which was the underlying cause for his behavioral changes as well as weight loss. Following antibiotic treatment, he returned to his previous level of functioning. Marion knows she must think ahead and discusses several options with her father for when the time comes; he does require daily assistance. He tells her that he would consider moving and living with her as long as he has his own bedroom.

8. What considerations are suggested to explore prior to moving a loved one into your home? Of these, which topic is a high priority in Marion's situation?

Marion's father eventually moves to her home. After several months, he realizes how much he misses the small group of friends he had coffee with each morning and meals with at the local diner. He goes to the long-term care facility with Marion and her son often when she visits her spouse. Over time, he makes the decision to move into an assisted living apartment connected to the facility to be around others his age, and adjusts quite well.

Suggested Resources

Alzheimer's Association. (2014). *Long-distance caregiving*. Retrieved from http://www.alz.org/living_with_alzheimers_long_distance_caregiving.asp#4

National Association of Professional Geriatric Care Managers. (n.d.). *Find a care manager near you*. Retrieved from http://www.caremanager.org/displaycommon.cfm?an=1&subarticlenbr=306

Schuster, J. L. (2014). *So far away: Twenty questions for long-distance caregivers*. National Institute on Aging. Retrieved from http://www.nia.nih.gov/HealthInformation/Publications/Long DistanceCaregiving

Case 21.6 ■ Relationships and Aging

*I*t is generally accepted that having close relationships throughout life is a positive, if not necessary, component of healthy living. Someone to share stories with, enlist an opinion or physically help with a task, remember us on special occasions, and so on, are several examples. Our relationships likely change as we age; for elderly persons, they may gradually decrease in numbers as family, friends, work colleagues, and neighbors' lives end or communication halts. Divorce, relocation, and failing health can impact long-term relationships in a short period of time. As a consequence, one might believe growing old is the loneliest time period of life.

In the United States, the loneliest people are adolescents and young adults. Loneliness actually declines with age—at least until people are well into the later stages of old age, when it may begin to increase. Although this association between youth and loneliness goes against our stereotype of the elderly lonely, it is not really so surprising when we think about it. Young people face the enormously difficult task of defining their own identity as individuals. *Without a solid sense of self, it is all too easy to feel unappreciated and unloved by others.* Moreover, young people are constantly having to develop new relationships as they go through schools and into employment settings—and each new social situation creates the possibility of feeling lonely. *Finally, it may be that younger people have greater expectations about their relationships than do older people, who have learned to live with less than perfect understanding and compatibility* (University of Missouri-Kansas City, Center on Aging Studies Without Walls, 2014). Relationships. Retrieved from http://cas.umkc.edu/casww/

> ***1. Please reflect on this statement in relation to your own adolescence period. Do you believe social media (e.g., Facebook) can help counteract loneliness in young people's lives or perhaps enhance it due to the "virtuality" of friendships?***

  2. What is your definition of loneliness? If needed, find one on the Internet and cite the source.

  3. A common myth in our society is that most older people live alone. Use the information found at www.aoa.gov/Aging_Statistics/Profile/2013/6.aspx to counter this misconception.

Use the website http://cas.umkc.edu/casww/sa/Relationships.htm for the remainder of the questions related to relationships and aging.

  4. Studies of relational benefits have focused on three types for social support. What are they?

  5. Siblings (especially sisters) provide what type of benefits to emotional health?

  6. What themes form the basis for adult friendships?

  7. Cite the statistics associated with being a grandparent and great-grandparent in the United States.

  8. The reading includes the statement: "Intergenerational relationships tend to be reciprocal." What does this mean to you personally? If not applicable, create an example.

In the late 19th century, Florence Nightingale wrote: "A small pet animal is often an excellent companion for the sick, for long chronic cases especially. A pet bird in a cage is sometimes the only pleasure of an invalid confined for years to the same room" (Nightingale, 1969, p. 103).

  9. What healthy outcomes can be brought about from an older person's relationship with a pet?

Suggested Resources

Cherry, K. (2014). *Loneliness: Causes, effects and treatments for loneliness*. About Education. Retrieved from http://psychology.about.com/od/psychotherapy/a/loneliness.htm

Nightingale, F. (1969). *Notes on nursing: What it is, and what it is not*. New York, NY: Dover.

University of Missouri-Kansas City, Center on Aging Studies Without Walls. (2014). *Relationships*. Retrieved from http://cas.umkc.edu/casww

Case 21.7 ■ Geriatric Specialists for the Family

*T*he junior nursing class at a midwest university has a big project ahead, and a reputation to uphold for planning and implementing a "Celebrate Aging Week." For almost a decade, the last week of October has been scheduled for the event, which has a different focus each day. Monday is utilized for a service-learning activity. The entire class participates in a Repair Affair; helping senior citizens with small improvements to their homes, yard work, painting, and so on. On Tuesday, a free immunization clinic is offered in conjunction with the local health department. Recipients may choose to receive one free vaccine for any of the following: influenza, herpes zoster, diphtheria/tetanus, or pneumococcal if they are 65 years and older. Wednesday is set aside for a health fair; a variety of local agencies focusing on elder care are invited and a number of screenings are offered as well. On Thursday, it is Senior Arts and Entertainment Day. About a dozen older adults perform songs, dance routines, or music. In addition, handmade items are sold with the proceeds going to charity.

Friday is set aside for education. Each year the junior class chooses a new topic. The entire school of nursing attends as well as interested persons in the community. Recent topics have included dementia, housing options, polypharmacy, and nutritional needs of the elderly.

This year, the group decided to have a panel presentation of speakers. With the field of geriatric health care growing, it was determined that learning about a variety of specialist roles would be advantageous.

Your Assignment

Each speaker will give an overview of his or her role in working with older clients/family members, along with what training or education is needed. In addition, one of the nurse educators at the school will provide information on becoming certified in geriatric nursing.

Use the Internet to describe what each of these speakers would likely share:

1. Geriatric clinical nurse specialist

2. Geriatric nurse practitioner

3. Geriatrician

4. Geropsychiatrist

5. Geriatric care manager

6. Gerontology certification: who administers, what is required, and how to renew

Index